Pediatric Psychopharmacology

The Use of Behavior Modifying Drugs in Children

Edited by

JOHN S. WERRY, M.D.

Professor of Psychiatry
University of Auckland
(New Zealand)

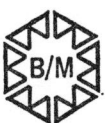

BRUNNER/MAZEL, Publishers • New York

To My Parents
Edith K. (Scott) Werry & Chace C. Werry

Library of Congress Cataloging in Publication Data

Main entry under title:
Pediatric psychopharmacology.

  Bibliography: p.
  Includes index.
  1. Psychopharmacology.   2. Child psychiatry.
I. Werry, John S.   [DNLM: 1. Psychopharmacology—In infancy and childhood.   QV77 P371]
RJ504.7.P4   615'.78   77-26626
ISBN 0-87630-162-6

Copyright © 1978 by John S. Werry

Published by
BRUNNER/MAZEL, INC.
19 Union Square West
New York, New York 10003

All rights reserved. No part of this book may be reproduced by any process whatsoever, without the written permission of the copyright owner.

MANUFACTURED IN THE UNITED STATES OF AMERICA

PREFACE

Pediatric psychopharmacology or the use of behavior modifying drugs in children is very different from psychopharmacology in adults—the indications for and actions of drugs are quite different. It merits special consideration. The purpose of this book is to bring together, in one volume, the usable, formal knowledge in this rapidly expanding field which hitherto has been found only scattered through various texts and articles in pediatrics, child psychiatry, child psychology, special education, and so on, or buried, as an afterthought, in books devoted primarily to adults. Because the distinctiveness of pediatric psychopathology and psychopharmacology is most marked *before the onset of puberty*, for the purposes of this book children have been defined as aged 12 years or less, though much of what is said is still applicable in the first few years of adolescence, though it is at this developmental stage that most adult disorders, such as schizophrenia and true depression, first appear in any frequency.

This text is unashamedly medical since, whatever may be the accoutrements from other disciplines, the core of pediatric psychopharmacology is, and must be, medical. However, considerable effort has been made to make most of the contents (except perhaps the chemistry and pharmacology of the drugs) comprehensible by all those who work professionally with children or are in training for such professions. The emphasis of the book is also unashamedly scientific and consists primarily of a series of critical reviews of the state of knowledge in the particular topic covered. However, there is a wealth of clinical information and anyone interested in how to go about actually prescribing a particular drug will find what he or she seeks, particularly at the end of the chapters relating to particular drugs.

Special thanks must go to Eileen, Joan and Karen who cheerfully (or almost so) deciphered strange calligraphic shapes, typed, retyped, cross checked references and struggled with the ordinary business of a medical school department as well. The editor would like to express his appreciation, too, to the Medical Research Council of New Zealand which underwrote some of the expenses incurred and which has permitted him to maintain his research interest in pediatric psychopharmacology since his return from North America in 1970; also, to CIBA-GEIGY, who have helped him to keep contact with colleagues overseas. Finally, he would like to express his gratitude to all the children and their parents who have been his patients and who helped temper his need for precision and certainty with commonsense and humanity, and to the students at the School of Medicine, University of Auckland, who keep asking questions.

JOHN S. WERRY
Auckland, New Zealand

January, 1978

CONTRIBUTORS

MICHAEL G. AMAN, M.A.
    University of Auckland

ROBIN H. BRIANT, M.D.
    University of Auckland and Auckland Hospital

DENNIS P. CANTWELL, M.D.
    University of California at Los Angeles

GABRIELLE A. CARLSON, M.D.
    University of California at Los Angeles

RACHEL GITTELMAN-KLEIN, Ph.D.
    Queens College, City University of New York and Long Island Jewish-Hillside Medical Center

EDWIN J. MIKKELSON, M.D.
    U.S. National Institute of Mental Health

JUDITH L. RAPOPORT, M.D.
    U.S. National Institute of Mental Health

ROBERT L. SPITZER, M.D.
    New York State Psychiatric Institute

ROBERT L. SPRAGUE, Ph.D.
    University of Illinois at Urbana-Champaign

GREGORY STORES, M.D.
    University of Oxford and U.K. National Center for Children with Epilepsy, Park Hospital

JOHN S. WERRY, M.D.
    University of Auckland and Auckland Hospital

BERTRAND G. WINSBERG, M.D.
Long Island Research Institute and State University of New York at Stony Brook

LUIS E. YEPES, M.D.
Long Island Research Institute and State University of New York at Stony Brook

CONTENTS

Preface iii

Contributors v

Introduction ix

I. BASIC PRINCIPLES

1. An Introduction to Clinical Pharmacology 3
   Robin H. Briant

2. Measures in Pediatric Psychopharmacology 29
   John S. Werry

3. Drugs, Learning and the Psychotherapies 79
   Michael G. Aman

4. Principles of Clinical Trials and Social, Ethical and Legal Issues of Drug Use in Children 109
   Robert L. Sprague

5. Diagnostic Classifications and Psychopharmacological Indications 136
   Rachel Gittelman-Klein, Robert L. Spitzer and
   Dennis P. Cantwell

II. INDIVIDUAL DRUGS

6. Stimulants 171
   Dennis P. Cantwell and Gabrielle A. Carlson

7. Antidepressants 208
   Judith L. Rapoport and Edwin J. Mikkelsen

8. Antipsychotics (Major Tranquilizers, Neuroleptics) 234
   Bertrand G. Winsberg and Luis E. Yepes

9. Antiepileptics (Anticonvulsants) 274
   Gregory Stores

10. Antimanic, Antianxiety, Hallucinogenic and Miscellaneous Drugs 316
    Judith L. Rapoport, Edwin J. Mikkelsen and John S. Werry

References 357

Index 401

INTRODUCTION

Historical

Pediatric psychopharmacology may be said to have begun in 1937 when, working at the Emma Pendelton Bradley Home, a residential treatment center for exceptional children in Providence, R.I., Bradley published his findings on the use of the stimulant amphetamine (Benzedrine) in children with a variety of diagnoses. To have thought to use such a drug in children in the first place may cause some surprise now, but this was the beginning of the Benzedrine era which kept Allied and German armies alike alert in World War II, but also ultimately led to drug abuse problems in postwar Japan and Sweden.

So meticulous were Bradley's observations that his findings are as valid today as they were then and set a model for clinical pediatric psychopharmacology. Unfortunately, Bradley's papers appeared at a time when the extreme psychoanalytic era in child psychiatry was also beginning. Little more seems to have been done apart from the solitary efforts of Bender at Bellevue Hospital in New York, whose interest, however, was primarily with psychotic children who were, and still are, relatively unresponsive to any kind of treatment, physical or psychological. Bender's work was carried on after her retirement around 1960 by Fish and, in turn now, by Campbell.

With the advent of the first so-called tranquiliser, reserpine, a naturally occurring plant-derived drug (or Galenical as such are called), the psychopharmacological era in psychiatry began in earnest in 1950. Chlorpromazine, the first of the phenothiazine antipsychotics, a by-product of the search for better drugs in anesthiology, and the so-called minor tranquilisers such as meprobamate (Equanil, Miltown), which are said by some cynics to have been one of the major influences upon Washington in the Eisenhower years, quickly followed; then the antidepressants, lithium and the benzodiazepines (Valium and Librium)—all within the space of a few years. However, there has been no important new developments in psychopharmacology and all drugs appearing since then resemble one of those which first appeared in that hectic decade.

Preoccupied with intensive, individual psychotherapy, child psychiatry was slow to evince any interest in all these new psychotropic drugs. Such early work as was done was mostly with institutionalised mentally retarded children, was uncontrolled, of generally poor quality and aimed mostly at behavioral control within the institution.

In 1959, Knobel first reported on the use of methylphenidate (Ritalin) in hyperkinetic children, beginning what some, particularly the British, regard as a peculiar obsession in current American child psychiatry. About the same time, Eisenberg began his classic studies at Johns Hopkins and in a move which portended future developments in pediatric psychopharmacology, was soon joined by a clinical psychologist, Conners, who is now probably the best known and most prolific contributor to the field.

In 1962, in the last year of our residency in child psychiatry at the Montreal Children's Hospital, with the active encouragement of the head of the department of child psychiatry (Dr. Taylor Statten) and of the pediatrician-in-chief (Dr. Alan Ross), Dr. Gabrielle Weiss and the author began a series of psychopharmacological studies. Because of our concern about the possible effects of psychotropic drugs upon mental alertness, Virginia Douglas, Ph.D., of McGill University was invited to join us. Also, because of the need for a well-defined, relatively easily measurable target for the drugs we intended to use, it was decided to concentrate on hyperactive children, operationally defined as children whose motor activity was the source of complaint at home and at school. The editor's association with the Montreal group ended in 1968, but their pioneering work in pediatric psychopharmacology and the study of hyperactivity has continued. From 1964 on, he began a fruitful association with Robert L. Sprague, Ph.D., at the University of Illinois at Urbana, an association which has continued despite a distance of 10,000 kilometers, since 1970.

Since the early 1960s, the number of investigators interested in pediatric psychopharmacology has grown steadily, particularly in the last five years. Fortunately, too, the quality of investigation has improved greatly, though there are still too many amateurs in the field who seem to know little of measurement of behavior and cognition, of experimental designs, and of statistical methods used in the behavioral sciences. One thing is clear—clinical child psychologists have achieved preeminence in the field of pediatric psychopharmacology to date and the best research comes from teams where they operate with physicians as colleagues of equal status following the example originally set by Eisenberg and Conners. This preeminence is not likely to continue since pediatric psychopharmacology needs to enter a true pharmacological era if it is to advance beyond fumbling empiricism. To do this, pharmacologists, neuroscientists, pediatricians and biologically-oriented child psychiatrists need to join hands. While the psychological side of pediatric psychopharmacology must remain, the biological side must be upgraded to a comparable level and a serious attempt made to relate modern knowledge of structure and function of the brain to the behavioral and cognitive effects of psychotropic drugs.

Social Aspects

No introduction to a volume like this could fail to note the *anti-medication movement* of the 1970s. This is discussed in detail in Chapter 4 by Dr. Robert Sprague who, as Chairman of the Pediatric Psychopharmacology Subcommittee of the U.S. Food and Drug Administration, has been in the thick of it. Only a few remarks will be made here. As a foreigner, the editor can perhaps be forgiven for noting that Americans are romantics. The essence of romanticism is a belief in the superiority of emotions and sensibility over the intellect and in the uniqueness and worth of the individual and his private experience or, to put it in current parlance, in doing your own thing. The discovery in the sixties by a whole generation of Americans of injustice, poverty, racism, sexism, imperialism, exploitation, and ecological irresponsibility has led to many positive attitudes and developments but it has also resulted in a new form of totalitarianism based on anti-intellectualism and a contempt for patiently established truth, especially by the scientific method.

While much of deviant behavior in children is, indeed, the result of social oppression and disadvantage, some is intra-organismic and some intrafamilial. In the end, however, considerations of etiology are of much less importance than the possibility of ameliorating, albeit only slightly, the individual child's psychological distress and social disease. If this can be done painlessly, economically, safely and without dulling the human mind and spirit through the use of medication, should one eschew such treatment and simply wait for the *Revolution to Free All Peoples?*

The essence of a good doctor is his or her ability to elicit and listen to all the requisite evidence and to treat the patient as a whole person. Many doctors do and will continue to fall short of this desideratum, but, if individual clinical judgment is to be subject to supervisory committees, or doctors are to be constantly vilified, taken to court and generally distrusted, the best in clinical judgment will go. No doctor expects unquestioning obedience and respect, but medical practice depends, in the end, on a spirit of mutual trust between doctor and patient.

Also, much of the anti-medication movement not only views doctors as mere tools of the System, but regards the scientific method with suspicion. This epistemological tool—which is all that the scientific method is—certainly has its faults but it is unsurpassed in preventing the accumulation of knowledge based solely on superstition or self deception. Behavior and emotions, like any other natural phenomenon, can be measured and the uniqueness of human beings is limited and, to anyone who has lived as long as the author, less striking than their many similarities.

When psychotropic or behavior modifying drugs are properly indicated and properly given to children, they can produce admittedly small, but often significant benefits. To dismiss them *a priori* makes about as much sense as removing penicillin or vitamin B_{12} from the market because they are frequently misused.

Names of Psychotropic Drugs

Psychopharmacology is concerned with psychotropic, psychiatric or psycholeptic drugs, all of which synonyms emphasise that, though their action is mediated physically, the therapeutic target is psychological or behavioral.

A drug has a *chemical* name which describes its structure and which is usually unpronounceable and extremely long, a *generic* name, often a pronounceable contraction of the chemical name, and a *proprietary* or *trade* name under which it is marketed and which, not surprisingly, is euphonious, often reflects the purported purpose and is subject to a substantial amount of advertising. While different brands of the same drug may vary in quality, there is no evidence that this is so to any great extent with psychotropic drugs produced in the major Western countries. On the other hand, while quality does not vary much, prices may do so considerably. Trade names may vary from one country to another. For all these reasons, in keeping with the practice of medical journals, generic names (in lower case letters) will be used throughout this book. When a drug is first mentioned, its trade names will be given in parentheses and identified by an initial upper case letter. If a generic name or trade name needs to be cross identified, the index should be consulted where both are listed together.

INTRODUCTION   xiii

CLASSIFICATION OF PSYCHOTROPIC DRUGS

There is no universally accepted or satisfactory way of classifying psychotropic drugs. Medicine, in general, is moving towards classification based on *therapeutic indication* with subgroups defined on a *chemical* base nested within major therapeutic groups, and this is happening in psychiatry too. This type of classification has some obvious disadvantages. The most important is that the drug may have more than one therapeutic use and, in pediatric psychopharmacology, the therapeutic indications are usually very different from those in adults. Antipsychotics are used primarily in non-psychotic conditions and symptomatically rather than specifically; antidepressants are used in enuresis and hyperactivity; antimanics may be useful against episodic aggression and stimulants are used as antiactivity drugs. However, any alternative classification is equally disadvantageous—tranquiliser; for example, is a term which no longer has any precise meaning pharmacologically and has acquired certain pejorative social connotations. While an argument could be made for developing a new terminology in pediatric psychopharmacology such as anti-inattentionals for stimulants or antiactivitys for antipsychotics, pediatric psychopharmacology is too small a field to be able to impose its particular classification on psychopharmacology in general. It cannot afford to go its own way in a sort of infantile autism.

So, albeit reluctantly, the *adult-derived therapeutic-based* classification of psychotropic drugs has been used throughout this volume, but no therapeutic action should be presumed despite the apparent meaning of a term like antipsychotic. Within each group, particular drugs are further subclassified by a chemical group or occasionally a functional one if there is more than one member of that particular subgroup and then finally further categorised by its generic name. The major groupings and some examples are set out in Table 1.

Though antiepileptic drugs are not strictly psychotropic drugs, they are sometimes proposed and quite commonly used as such. Because of this and the intimate association of epilepsy with certain psychopathological states of childhood and with mental retardation, they have been included in this volume (Chapter 9).

ABOUT THIS BOOK

This book is designed as an authoritative, critical text comprehensible to any professional working or training to work with exceptional children aged 12 or less. It is divided into two main sections. The first is devoted to *basic principles of pediatric psychopharmacology*—general pharmacology

TABLE 1
Terminology and Classification of Psychoactive Drugs Used in Children

Therapeutic Classification	Chemical or Functional Classification	Generic Name	Trade Name
Stimulants	Sympathomimetic Amines (and similar)	amphetamine dextroamphetamine methamphetamine methylphenidate pemoline	Benzedrine Dexedrine Desoxyn Ritalin Cylert
	Xanthines	caffeine	
	Acetylcholine Analogs	deanol	Deaner
Antipsychotics (Major Tranquilizers)	Phenothiazines	chlorpromazine thioridazine trifluoperazine	Thorazine, Largactil Mellaril Stelazine
	Butyrophenones	haloperidol	Haldol, Serenace
	Thioxanthenes	thiothixene chlorprothixene	Navane Taractan
Antidepressants	Tricyclics	imipramine amitriptyline desipramine	Tofranil Elavil Pertofran, Norpramin
Antianxietys (Anxiolytics) & Sedatives	Barbiturates	phenobarbital	
	Benzodiazepines	diazepam chlordiazepoxide oxazepam nitrazepam	Valium Librium Serax, Serapax Mogadon
	Propanediols	meprobamate	Miltown, Equanil
	Antihistamines	diphenhydramine hydroxyzine	Benadryl Vistaril, Atarax
Antimanics	Lithium	lithium	Priadel Lithicarb

(Chapter 1); measurement and measures (Chapter 2); drugs and cognitive processes, drugs and learning (Chapter 3); drugs and other psychological treatments (Chapter 3); social, legal and ethical issues (Chapter 4); the principles of clinical trials (Chapter 4); diagnostic classifications and indications for psychopharmacology (Chapter 5). The second section looks at *individual drugs* grouped therapeutically (for adults, that is) into stimulants (Chapter 6); antidepressants (Chapter 7); antipsychotics (Chapter 8); antiepileptics (Chapter 9); antimanic, antianxiety and miscellaneous drugs such as sedatives, hallucinogens, vitamins and so on (Chapter 10).

Each of the chapters in Section II follows the same general format: types and chemical structures of the groups of drugs, pharmacology, clinical effects, treatment-emergent or side effects, drug interactions, clinical indications, non-indications and contraindications, clinical administration, social and ethical issues (where relevant).

In general, the editor has edited each chapter substantially to give it uniformity, accuracy and comprehensiveness. Throughout, the emphasis has been on fact rather than on opinion. However, the subsection on *clinical administration* in each of the chapters in Section II has been left very much as written by the particular authors. These sections are matters of opinion and, read as a composite, give some perspective on differing modes of practice within the field of pediatric psychopharmacology. Occasionally the editor has disagreed with a matter of opinion or policy and, if he considers both opinions or policies tenable or inevitable, he has added a footnote, but in general his opinions are seeded throughout the text.

Lest offense be taken, it should be said that the term *child psychiatric* is used here only as a convenient, less clumsy, more familiar synonym for child psychopathological or emotionally disturbed. It in no way implies any restriction to medical disorders or practice.

One last point: The book is organised around *drugs, not around diagnostic conditions or symptoms*. However, if the starting point is the latter, the necessary information about drugs is readily available in Chapter 5 (Table 5) and/or by consulting the index which has been compiled with this particular use in mind.

I.
BASIC PRINCIPLES

1

AN INTRODUCTION TO CLINICAL PHARMACOLOGY

ROBIN H. BRIANT, M.D.

INTRODUCTION

The understanding of pharmacologic principles has lagged far behind the introduction and use of powerful drugs; thus, many decisions about drug use, such as size and frequency of dose, have been empirically based. However, increasing knowledge about what happens to drugs in the body is gradually allowing a more rational approach to drug use in all fields of therapy.

This chapter introduces the reader to the important clinical pharmacologic determinants of drug use in terms comprehensible to readers with only elementary knowledge of chemistry and biology. Since most available information refers only to healthy young adults, and data on the clinical pharmacology of children are quite insufficient, much has had to be extrapolated from experience with adults.

More extended discussions can be found in standard pharmacological texts such as Goodman and Gilman (1975).

PHARMACOKINETICS

Pharmacokinetics describe the *movement* of drugs into, around, and out of the body.

For a drug to achieve systemic effect it must be absorbed into the body, and it must enter the organ or tissue where it exerts its effect. For the effect to be terminated, the drug must be rendered inactive, or be excreted from the body. Thus *absorption, distribution, metabolism* and *elimination* are the *kinetic* determinants of drug effects. Elemental to these processes is the ability of drug molecules to cross cell membranes.

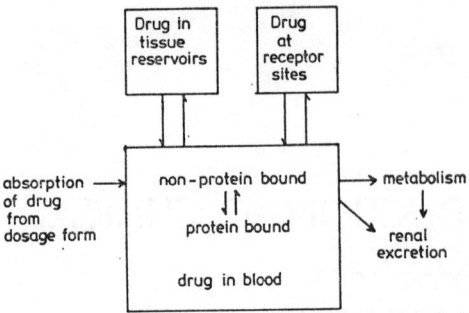

FIG. 1: Representation of drug movements into, around and out of the body.

Passage of Drug Across Cell Membrane

Cell membranes comprise a biomolecular lipid sheet, bound on each side by protein and probably interspersed with minute water-filled channels or pores. The overall thickness of the membrane is about 100Å (10^{-8}m.).

Transfer of molecules across membranes may be active or passive, but, since it is the more usual, only *passive* transfer need be considered. The membrane plays no active part in such transfer, which proceeds as a result of, and in proportion to, difference in drug concentration on each side. Small water soluble molecules (M.W. 100-200) may pass through the water-filled pores, but larger molecules must dissolve in the lipoid membrane to achieve this transfer.

The degree of lipid (fat) solubility is an inherent property of any compound, and is expressed by the *lipid:water partition coefficient* (the extent to which the substance will concentrate in the oil portion of an oil/water mixture); the greater the partitioning, the more readily will the drug dissolve in cell membrane, and the faster will transfer occur, all other factors being favourable.

Most drugs are weak acids or weak bases and so when in solution will be in either ionised (charged) or unionised forms depending upon environmental pH.

Each drug has another intrinsic property, its dissociation constant (pKa), which describes the pH at which the compound is 50% ionised. The degree of ionisation has important effects on transfer across membranes, for, in general, unionised molecules are lipid soluble but ionised molecules are not.

An example of the importance of pKa and pH on drug movements is shown in Figure 2.

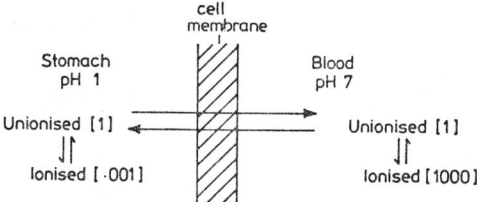

FIG. 2: Schematic account of pH-dependent passage of drug across a membrane. An acidic compound, *acetylsalicyclic acid with pKa 3.5* is predominantly unionised at gastric pH about 1, and predominantly ionised at blood pH about 7. Only the unionised form of the drug equilibrates across the membrane. The ratio of total drug concentration [ ] is approximately 1000:1 in favor of absorption from stomach to blood stream.

Absorption

To have an effect on the whole organism, a drug must be absorbed into the systemic circulation.

INTRAVENOUS ROUTE

The most efficient means of achieving this is by intravenous injection, introducing the whole dose directly into the bloodstream. Not only is this route efficient but it is rapid, the drug possibly reaching the brain very swiftly which may be vital as with diazepam (Valium) in epilepsy (see Chapter 9). The practical limitations of this method are obvious, especially in children; also dangerous toxicity can occur when high concentrations of potent agents reach vital organs.

ORAL ROUTE

The majority of drug administrations are *oral*, thus allowing self-administration by the patient or his parents, but having the limitation that incomplete absorption may occur. The rate and extent of absorption depend upon the drug and its formulation, and upon factors inherent in the patient.

The drug must be able to withstand intestinal digestion and must be provided in a formulation which disintegrates in the gastrointestinal tract. The drug particles must dissolve in intestinal fluid before they can be absorbed. Numerous influences may prevent or slow the process; changes in stomach acidity, the presence of food or other drugs, inadequate blood supply or rapid passage through the intestine as in gastroenteritis may all interfere with the process.

It is difficult in any situation to predict just how any particular change in the upper gastrointestinal tract will affect absorption. Therefore, for optimal absorption, all potential interferences should be avoided as much as possible and, except in some special cases, medication should be taken at least one hour before or two hours after food.

INTRAMUSCULAR OR SUBCUTANEOUS ROUTE

Intramuscular or subcutaneous injection of a drug does not necessarily avoid absorption problems, for the solution, although suitable for injection, may not provide the appropriate pH for optimum lipid-solubility of the compound. Such physiological factors as the blood supply to the site provide additional variables.

In some instances the poor solubility of a compound is used to advantage; depot preparations of antipsychotic phenothiazines (see Chapter 8), for example, are made with very low solubility salts (e.g., decanoate) and the active principle is only slowly absorbed from the injection site; thus the action of the one administration can span many days.

BIOAVAILABILITY

Some drug formulations are superior to others in ability to give up their contained drug in such a way that it is completely absorbed in active form. This capacity is termed *bioavailability* and is another important determinant of drug absorption and effect. Where two formulations of the same drug are shown to have different bioavailability, as is occasionally the situation, there is a strong case for departing from the principle espoused in the introduction to this book and prescribing by trade name, rather than generic name, to ensure consistent drug effect.

Distribution

COMPARTMENTS

Drug molecules, once absorbed into the circulation, are distributed to various body *compartments,* the degree and sites of distribution depending largely upon characteristics of the drug itself. Compartments are best thought of in *physiological*, not *anatomical* terms, for in pharmacokinetics they represent areas to which the drug distributes in concentrations, or at rates, different from other areas. They do not have anatomical boundaries and are not necessarily one type of tissue.

However, some physical aspects of drug distribution can be defined in rather general terms. For instance some drugs, particularly acidic ones, are largely confined to the vascular system or compartment and, if lipid soluble, may bind to plasma albumin, as they do not dissolve adequately in plasma water. Many drugs pass easily through the capillary membrane and from the vascular system to distribute throughout the extracellular water which separates capillaries from tissues and many tissues from each other, there achieving the concentrations equal to free (non-protein bound) drug in plasma. Other drugs may leave the vascular system to concentrate in parenchymal (non-structural) tissue (e.g., basic compounds like the tricyclic antidepressants), or to concentrate in fat depots (e.g., the extremely lipophilic barbiturate drug, thiopentone).

Drug distribution is an important determinant of both *efficacy* and *toxicity*. For example, to be effective an antibiotic must reach the site of infection, and in epilepsy an antiepileptic drug (see Chapter 9) must enter the brain; alternatively a fetus might be affected by drugs taken by a pregnant woman if the drug crosses the placenta. In fact, few drugs are excluded from reaching the fetal circulation, for the placenta presents little barrier to the movement of lipid-soluble compounds (Mirkin, 1973).

BRAIN AND OTHER TISSUES

Entry of drugs to the *brain* is less readily achieved, for brain capillaries are invested with a layer of close-knit glial (supporting) cells which provide an additional series of lipid layers for the drug to cross, constituting the so-called *blood-brain barrier*. As might be expected, highly lipid-soluble compounds such as diazepam (see Chapters 9, 10) find this no barrier at all and rapidly enter the brain. At the other end of the scale dopamine is totally excluded from the brain and, as in the treatment of Parkinsonism (see Chapter 8), must be given as its lipid-soluble precursor levo-dopa for access to the central nervous system. Between these two extremes are many compounds which gradually enter cerebrospinal fluid and brain and equilibrate to the concentration of *free* drug in plasma.

Distribution throughout *other organs* or tissues can also be a source of variability of drug effect. For example, much of the cardiac drug, digoxin, in the body is found in skeletal muscle, so a reduction in muscle mass may lead to a rise in plasma concentration. Likewise, changes in body water either in development or disease can affect the distribution of certain compounds. Such changes are implied in the studies of Liddell et al. (1975) which demonstrate a reduced volume of distribution of the analgesic phenazone (Antipyrine) in elderly women.

BINDING OF DRUGS

Plasma protein binding of drugs has been studied more than tissue binding, so more is known of this phenomenon and its influence on drug effects. Drugs are bound reversibly to protein and the ratio of bound to unbound drug is in dynamic equilibrium. The degree of protein binding may be described by the fraction of the total drug concentration represented by protein-bound molecules; hence, at body temperature and in therapeutic concentrations, the anticoagulant warfarin is 99% protein bound, the antiepileptic phenytoin (Dilantin) approximately 90% bound (see Chapter 9). Protein binding is probably not of great clinical importance if it is less than 80% (Koch-Weser & Sellers, 1976). Protein binding reduces the maximal effect of the drug, but provides a reservoir of drug and thus *prolongs* effect. Only unbound drug molecules are available for pharmacologic effects, for passage across membranes, or for participation in elimination processes.

Changes in protein binding may be dramatically induced by other drugs competing for the binding sites. For example, warfarin may be displaced from albumin by a metabolite of the sedative chloral hydrate (see Chapter 10) (Koch-Weser & Sellers, 1971). Though this may release only small amounts of warfarin, there will be a transient increase in drug effect, which may induce haemorrhagic complications by the time any new equilibrium is established.

Elimination

The term elimination is used to express the *removal of drug activity* from the body; hence, both the renal excretion of the unchanged drug and the metabolism (biotransformation) to inactive compounds are implied by the term. For most drugs one or other process predominates, but combinations of the two do occur. Most drug metabolites eventually leave the body via the kidneys, though excretion by the liver through bile into the faeces may also occur sometimes, as with the antipsychotic chlorpromazine (see Chapter 8).

RENAL EXCRETION

A small number of drugs are known to be excreted by the kidney without prior metabolism. They can be filtered at the glomerulus (e.g., digoxin), or actively secreted into tubular urine (e.g., thiazides), or may undergo both processes (e.g., penicillin).

In general it is the *water-soluble* compounds which leave the body via the kidney, for lipid-soluble molecules reaching the urine are preferentially reabsorbed back through the tubular epithelium. The pH of urine can influence the rate of excretion of a compound such as the stimulant amphetamine (Benzedrine—see Chapter 6) which is a base and which in acid urine is predominantly in the ionised and lipid-insoluble form, and thus more readily retained in the urine. Most drug metabolites are water-soluble compounds and can be excreted in the urine.

The chief sources of variation in renal excretion of drugs is impairment of renal function from any renal disease, or from dehydration which reduces glomerular filtration rate. Impairment of renal function can lead to high body concentrations of drugs excreted by the kidney and is an important source of unexpected, excessive drug effects, particularly so in the case of the potentially very toxic antimanic drug lithium (see Chapter 10).

BIOTRANSFORMATION

For most drugs, chemical alteration takes place in the body, producing a *metabolite* which is *more water soluble and so can be excreted by the kidney*. Without such a change, a lipid-soluble drug like diazepam (Valium) would be forever reabsorbed from tubular urine back to the circulation, and one dose might last a lifetime.

Metabolic transformation often, but not invariably, produces inactive compounds. Indeed, the first effective antibacterial agent prontosil has no direct action *in vitro* and has to be converted *in vivo* to sulphanilamide before therapeutic effect is obtained. Some compounds are rendered *more* toxic by metabolism, while many others have metabolites with a spectrum of action similar to that of the parent drug. For example, the antidepressant imipramine (Tofranil—see Chapter 6) is actually inert but is demethylated to an active agent desipramine, while diazepam (see Chapters 9, 10) is demethylated to form N-desmethyl-diazepam, and thence hydroxylated to oxazepam, all three of which compounds possess anti-anxiety activity.

Most metabolic transformations occur in the liver, though the organs such as lung (Briant et al., 1973) and intestinal mucosa (Powell et al., 1974) also contribute to the process.

There are four major metabolic processes: 1) *oxidation*, 2) *reduction* 3) *hydrolysis*, and 4) *conjugation*. Of these, the first and the last are quantitatively the most important. Much of this activity arises from the hepatic microsomes (fragments from cell organelles separated *in vitro* by ultracentrifugation) with several processes being available simultaneously. The metabolic transformation of any compound is largely dependent upon its structure, with the net metabolic result being dependent upon the relative rates of the various interactions. Also, metabolism can occur sequentially, for instance an oxidation reaction is often followed by conjugation.

Metabolism can reduce drug bioavailability by inactivating the drug immediately after absorption before it ever reaches the circulation beyond the liver. Propranolol, an antihypertensive agent once mooted as an antianxiety agent, is affected by this so-called *first pass* metabolism in which a proportion of an oral dose is bio-transformed in its first circulation through the liver (Johnsson & Regardh, 1976).

INFLUENCES ON BIOTRANSFORMATION

Many warnings have been issued that drug metabolism is decreased, and hence drug effect is increased, in *liver disease*. However, there is little evidence for this statement, and many studies show that patients with liver disease metabolise drugs just as efficiently as do normals (Curry, 1974).

Exogenous influences, drugs or chemicals particularly, can affect the rate of drug metabolism. The best known example is the induction of the hepatic microsomal oxidising system by barbiturates (see Chapter 9). This leads to an increased amount of microsomal protein (or enzymes) with more rapid oxidation of drugs such as warfarin. (Breckenridge & Orme, 1971). Inhibition of microsomal activity has also been demonstrated (Vessell et al., 1970).

Genetic control of drug metabolism has been shown to be of two distinct types, producing either continuous or discontinuous variation. The continuous variation is more common, and gives a unimodal curve with normal distribution. As much as six-fold individual variations in oxidation rates for the same drug are demonstrated in a series of normal individuals (Vessel & Page, 1968), although some of this variation may be related to exogenous influences. However, in twin studies, where no other drugs are taken, pairs of identical twins have virtually identical metabolism rates of the antirheumatic drugs phenylbutazone and phenazone (Vessell et al., 1971), and of the antidepressant nortriptyline (Alexanderson & Sjoqvist, 1971), while fraternal twins have widely divergent rates.

The bimodal distribution of the population as fast or slow acetylators is an example of discontinuous variation in metabolism rates. The recessive gene associated with being a slow acetylator (Price-Evans et al., 1960) has a frequency which results in a half to two-thirds of the white population being slow acetylators. Several compounds are inactivated by acetylation, and acetylator status is thus important in their use. For example, Johnstone and Marsh (1973) found that fast acetylators treated with the antidepressant phenelzine (Nardil—see Chapter 7) did no better than if they had been given placebo.

Ayd (1975) has repeatedly stressed the necessity in psychopharmacology, particularly in familial disorders such as schizophrenia and manic depressive illness (see Chapters 7 and 8), of taking a *family drug response history* as a prelude to commencing pharmacotherapy and cites studies clearly demonstrating such genetic influences. These may operate via metabolism as just described.

The Time Course of Drug Movements

Fundamental pharmacokinetic principles are based upon a simple, single-compartment model involving most of the body, which assumes uniform distribution of drug throughout that compartment. The apparent volume of distribution (V_d) *is that volume to which all the drug in the body would appear to be distributed to achieve a concentration the same as in plasma.*

$$\text{Thus } V_d = \frac{\text{Total amount of drug in body}}{\text{Concentration of drug in plasma}} \quad \ldots \ldots \ldots \ldots \ldots (1)$$

However, if a drug is actually concentrated in tissues, its V_d might be many times the actual volume of body water.

FIRST ORDER KINETICS

Most drug movements in the body are first order processes, that is a *constant fraction*, not a constant amount of drug present, is processed in unit time. There are several important consequences of first order kinetics:

1) The more drug there is in the body, the more is processed in unit time.

2) The elimination rate can be expressed by a constant (K_e), representing the fractional change per unit time. Alternatively it can be expressed by the half-life ($T\frac{1}{2}$) which is the time required for 50% completion of the process. The constant K_e is expressed in units of time^{-1} and $T\frac{1}{2}$ in units of time, and both are independent of drug load. They are related simply by the equation

$$K_e \times T\frac{1}{2} = 0.693 \quad \quad \quad \quad \quad \quad \quad \quad (2)$$

Clearance rate is the product of V_d and K_e and measures that amount of the volume of distribution cleared of a drug in unit time.

$$V_d \times K_e = \text{Clearance} \quad \quad \quad \quad \quad \quad \quad \quad (3)$$

3) Repeated drug dosing will result in drug accumulation up to the *steady state* or plateau, which is reached when the rate of drug absorption per unit time is exactly matched by elimination. The *time* taken to reach steady state is dependent upon the drug $T\frac{1}{2}$ (approximately five times $T\frac{1}{2}$ is the time required) but the *level* at steady state depends upon drug dose and dose frequency in relation to $T\frac{1}{2}$.

The $T\frac{1}{2}$ and V_d of a drug in a given situation will determine the steady state level achieved, for the other factors (dose, dose-interval) can be manipulated. The $T\frac{1}{2}$ of a drug may be fairly uniform or, as in the case of many psychotropic drugs, subject to large, individual variations. A three-fold range of $T\frac{1}{2}$ in a group of individuals taking the antidepressant nortyptiline, (Aventyl, Nortab—see Chapter 7) results in a three-fold range of steady state plasma levels when drug administration is uniform (Alexanderson & Sjoqvist, 1971) making dose/plasma level relationships most complex (see Chapter 7).

There is a *fluctuation of drug level* around the steady state concentration, the degree of fluctuation being influenced by *dose frequency* in relation to elimination rate, though the rate of absorption may be an additional variant. Thus, frequent small doses will give lesser variation about the steady state level than will a large infrequent dose. *Maintenance dose and dose intervals should be chosen to keep the fluctuations within an acceptable range* (large swings may produce toxic or sub-therapeutic levels) *while providing an acceptable schedule for the patient.* Variation of dose, or dose interval, or both, can be made to compensate for reduced elimination rate of drug in liver disease or, more particularly, renal disease.

ZERO ORDER KINETICS

There are important exceptions to first order kinetics—some compounds (e.g., ethyl alcohol) are metabolised by zero order kinetics, that

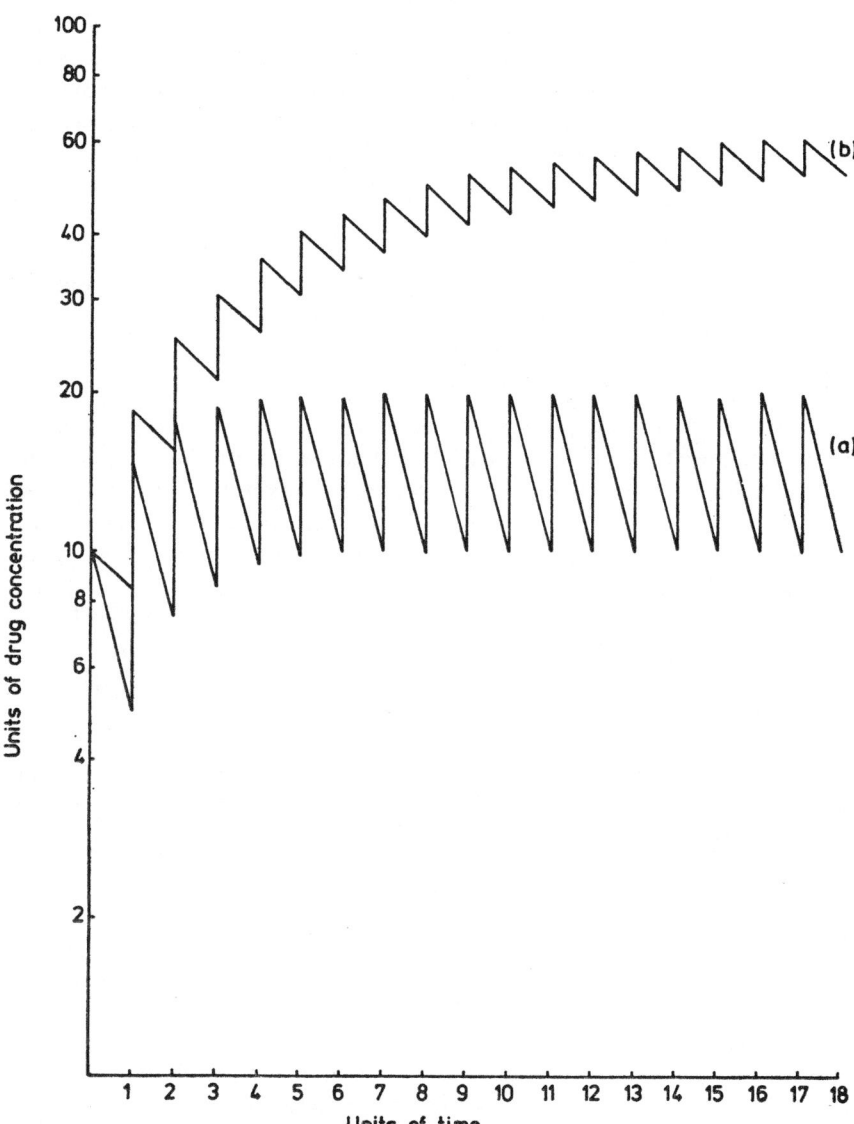

Fig. 3: The relationship between steady state plasma concentration and the plasma half life. Each curve represents the same dosing interval, but the plasma half life in (b) is 4 times as long as in (a). Thus it takes (b) 4 times as long to achieve steady state and steady state level is much higher.

is, a *constant amount* of drug is metabolised in a given time, and the rate of elimination is independent of the load. Some other compounds are handled by a complex combination of first order and zero order kinetics. For example, as discussed in Chapter 9, phenytoin in low concentration is metabolised by first order kinetics, but in high concentration, presumably because the enzyme systems are functioning at their maximum capacity, metabolism proceeds by a constant amount until reduction in body load allows the first order process to resume. An important consequence of this is that drug concentration in the body is not linearly related to dose; above a certain concentration, doubling the dose more than doubles the concentration and serious toxicity can result.

Measuring Plasma Drug Concentrations

Measurement of the plasma* concentration of drugs can in some instances be a helpful guide to therapy. It requires a sensitive, accurate and reproducible assay method *and* a recognised relationship between plasma level and effect, or plasma level and toxicity. Monitoring plasma levels is particularly useful where there is a narrow margin between therapeutic and toxic levels or where therapeutic end point is hard to ascertain, such as in the epileptic patient who has only occasional fits (see Chapter 9). There is wide individual variation in dose requirement of certain drugs to achieve therapeutic effects, and for them, too, plasma level monitoring may be a help.

For those drugs which enter saliva in a concentration which relates to the concentration in plasma (Chang et al., 1976), measuring salivary levels may prove useful. Clearly, saliva can be more easily obtained than blood, and in children, in particular, such assays would be more acceptable to patients.

Among psychotropic agents, only lithium is commonly managed with the assistance of plasma level measurements (Prien et al., 1972). A number of attempts have been made to establish a relationship between plasma level and effect of tricyclics, this being particularly difficult in a disorder like depression with such variability of presentation and high incidence of natural resolution. There seems no consensus among different workers; Burrows et al. (1972) record no relationship between levels and response, Braithwaite et al. (1972) showed a relationship, with good response at nortryptiline plasma levels above 120 ng/ml. Kragh-Sorensen et al. (1973)

---

* In this book, plasma and serum drug levels are used interchangeably. Strictly speaking, *plasma* is the unclotted, while *serum* is the clotted, blood fraction excluding red, white and other cells. As a rule, plasma occurs in vivo while serum is more conveniently used in laboratory estimations of drug concentrations.—Ed.

have shown a curvilinear relationship, with beneficial effect declining above plasma nortryptiline concentration of 175 ng/ml (see also Chapter 7).

Pediatric Variations in Pharmacokinetics

The available information about kinetics in children is sparse and provided in scattered reports and in a useful recent review by Rane and Wilson (1976). As pharmacokinetics provide a basis for drug dosage modification, more direct studies in children are needed, for as Shirkey (1972) states, extrapolation from adults to chlidren is, at best, misleading. The difficulty in obtaining accurate pharmacokinetic information because of both practical and ethical constraints on experimentation in healthy or sick children is outlined by Shirkey and in Chapter 4. As an alternative, mathematical models and computer simulations to represent drug movements in the body can and have been used where limited data are available.

A clear distinction needs to be made between the neonate and the older child. Because of immaturity of liver and kidney in the former, the potential for drug handling is quite different. Although, since psychotropic drugs are rarely indicated in neonates, this book is not particularly concerned with them, reference will be made to them in this section in terms of the process of development of full drug-handling competence.

Absorption

There are no studies specifically comparing drug absorption rates in children and adults so no comment can be made on this process.

Distribution

Variations in the constitution of the child's body as compared with the adult body lead to differences in drug distribution at different ages.

GROWING TISSUE

One such difference is the peculiarity of actively growing tissue which may alter uptake of a drug. For example, the antibiotic tetracycline is distributed to growing bones and developing enamel; this phenomenon does not in itself alter the therapeutic effect of the drug, but does represent a major cosmetic side effect, fixed for life in the teeth.

VARIATIONS IN PROTEINS

Because only unbound drug takes part in pharmacologic processes, binding of drug to plasma protein is a possible source of kinetic variation in childhood, but there is very little information about this parameter except in newborns. Aranda et al. (1976) showed reduced protein binding of the antiasthmatic drug aminophylline in the cord plasma of full-term neonates compared with adult binding of the same drug. Displacement of drug or bilirubin from binding sites by other drugs has been responsible for some drug toxicity in newborns.

FAT DEVELOPMENT

An important variation from the viewpoint of drug efficacy is the different *size of organs and tissue masses* in the developing child. Fat is an important repository of highly lipid soluble compounds, and so the total bulk of body fat will affect distribution of such drugs. Further, there is an inverse relationship between fat content and total water content in the body, due to the low water content of fat. About midway through gestation the fetus is only 0.5% fat by weight, increasing to 12-16% by the time of delivery. Thereafter, there is usually a rapid fat gain during the first year of life, and then gradual loss until the prepubertal increase.

The highly lipid soluble antianxiety agent diazepam (see Chapters 9, 10) which is frequently given to women shortly before and during labour crosses the placenta and may cause hypotonia and hypothermia in the neonate. Plasma levels of drug and active metabolite have been measured (Cree et al., 1973; Kanto et al., 1974) and found to be very high, though the actual dose received by the fetus could not be determined. Garattini et al. (1973) compared diazepam levels in premature neonates and children aged 3-6 years after a weight-related intramuscular dose. The neonates achieved higher plasma levels than did the other children. These findings might be explicable, in part, in terms of the distribution of diazepam to body fat.

BODY WATER

This has been more systematically studied than most other parameters in children and the work of Friis-Hansen (1967) remains an important contribution in this field. From measurement of total body water and extra-cellular water he was able to calculate intracellular water indirectly. Throughout growth there are changes in all these water compartments, both absolute, and relative to each other and to body weight. For instance, total body water falls throughout gestation from 97% to 76% of body weight. In the first year of life there is a further fall to 60% body weight, and by adulthood to 50%. Likewise extra-cellular water falls from 62%

An Introduction to Clinical Pharmacology

early in uterine life to 27% at age 1 year. In contrast, the proportion of intra-cellular water increases, but rather less dramatically.

If, however, one relates the distribution of body water to body surface area, a quite different picture emerges. One finds that total body water *increases* from 12.4 litres/m² at birth to 18.1 l/m² at age 12½ years and 18.6 l/m² in adulthood, and plasma volume increases to a similar degree. However, the extra-cellular water remains constant throughout development at about 5.7 litres/m². The implication of this is that those many drugs (especially ones not particularly tissue or protein bound) which are distributed throughout extra-cellular water should be dosed in proportion to body surface area, a parameter which incidentally is also related to other physiologic processes such as renal glomerular filtration. For example, Siber et al. (1975) measured the antibiotic gentamicin peak levels and V_d in children and adults after a single intravenous or intramuscular injection. The volume of distribution of gentamicin correlated well with calculated extra-cellular water volume, and peak levels were inversely related to this. Small children had a greater V_d than older ones and needed a greater weight-related gentamicin dose to achieve the same peak levels. However, when the dose was related to body surface area, the same dose would have been appropriate at all ages.

Renal Excretion

In newborns, glomerular filtration rate (per unit body surface area) is low and tubular mechanisms for secretion are immature. Both parameters increase to reach adult levels at about 6-8 months of age (Ritschel (1975). Prior to this age, drugs and metabolites excreted predominantly by the kidney will have a prolonged sojourn in the body. Cumulation and toxicity are therefore more likely in the young infant than later in childhood.

Metabolism

The most important organ involved in drug metabolism is the liver. In laboratory animals, hepatic enzyme activity is virtually absent in the fetus and neonate and, like liver weight, increases to a maximum in adulthood. In contrast, the human fetal liver has been shown by *in vitro* studies to possess some drug *oxidising* ability from 14 weeks gestational age (Rane & Sjoqvist, 1972), and these systems probably achieve adult competence soon after birth (Curry, 1974). *Conjugating* systems however are not demonstrable in the human fetus and are deficient in the neonate as the longer T½ of the antibiotic chloramphenicol and the bile pigment bilirubin indicate. Garattini et al.'s (1973) studies in premature babies and older children showed that both groups were able to *demethylate* diazepam but no *conjugated* metabolites were excreted by the premature babies.

The size of the liver, as well as enzyme activity, changes throughout infancy and childhood, both absolutely and relative to total body weight. The liver of a 2-year-old child is 40-50% greater than the adult liver, and that of a 6-year-old 30% greater, when related to body weight (Alvares et al., 1975). It would be posited, therefore, that once enzyme activity was developed the child might be a *more*, rather than less, competent drug metaboliser than the adult. Indeed, Alvares et al. (1975) have reported that a group of children aged 1-8 years had a significantly shorter T½ of both the anti-inflammatory drugs phenazone and phenylbutazone than did a group of adults, implying more rapid metabolism in this younger group, despite the fact that 8 of the 10 children studied had biochemical evidence of lead poisoning which the authors believe would, if anything, tend to decrease oxidation rates of the compounds studied.

These findings are consistent with those of Svensmark and Buchthal (1964) who found that children under 30Kg in weight needed a much larger weight-related dose of the antiepileptics phenobarbitone and phenytoin (see Chapter 9) to achieve the same steady state plasma levels as adults. Although other differences may be involved, more rapid metabolism in the children was considered the most important determinant.

The reports from Garettson and Dayton (1970) concerning phenobarbital and phenytoin, and of Pruitt et al. (1973) concerning the antihypertensive diazoxide in children, also support the contention that *drug metabolism in childhood is somewhat more rapid than in adulthood.*

Summary

The child has considerable differences in drug kinetics from both the neonate and the adult. The neonate has immature hepatic metabolising and renal excretory systems, though these all mature quite rapidly after birth. Renal excretory capacity reaches adult levels well before the first birthday. Metabolic maturation is more difficult to define as it differs depending upon the nature of the drug and the metabolic process, but for most drugs is probably optimal by the age of 1 year and thereafter may *exceed* adult capacity throughout much of childhood. Growth and development are associated with changes in absolute anatomical, physiological and biochemical characteristics and in the relative sizes of various organs and tissue masses, especialy of fat and water. These changes can have a profound influence on drug uptake and distribution, and hence upon the rate of elimination or degree of accumulation of drugs.

Dosage Modifications for Children

The choice of drug dosage for children is fraught with difficulty, not the least problem being that the standard dose for adults is empirically based in the first instance. Rather than relating pediatric dosage to adult dose, drug dose for children should be based on studies in children, but the limitations in this undertaking have already been alluded to (see also Chapter 4) and for the meantime the adult dose is the reference point.

The simplest, but from the foregoing discussion not necessarily most appropriate, scheme is to treat the child as a miniature adult and give a weight-related dose, and many formulae are available to calculate dose based upon weight or age (Reilly, 1972).

For drugs which are distributed to extra-cellular water, doses related to *body surface area*, again using adult dose as reference, are more rational (Gill & Ueda, 1976). For example, the standardization of gentamicin dosage on the basis of body area, given normal renal function, allows the same area-related dose ($60mg/m^2$) in all age groups to achieve satisfactory plasma concentration (Siber et al., 1975).

However, there are many compounds which are partly or largely concentrated in some organ or tissue, and most of the psychotropic drugs are in this category. Predictions of plasma levels or pharmacologic effect are extremely difficult considering the many variable factors involved. There would seem to be no alternative to specific studies to ascertain the correct dosage of these agents for children.

Mechanism of Drug Action

Pharmacologists use the term *drug action* to define the initial result of drug-cell interaction; subsequent changes, such as alteration of the cell's biochemical function, are termed *drug effects*.

Receptor Theory

It was postulated in the 19th century, independently by Paul Erlich and J. N. Langley that a drug produces its effect by interacting with a special part of the cell called "receptive substance" or receptor, and receptor theory remains the basis of understanding of drug action today. However, like compartments, receptors remain more hypothetical, conceptual tools than anatomical entities. They are defined by their interaction with certain drugs, while their structural features are inferred from three dimensional models of drugs that interact with them. Some receptors may be enzymes (biochemical catalysts, usually proteins) and much of the kinetic theory of drug-receptor interaction is borrowed from enzyme kinetics.

Langley believed that drug-receptor interaction was governed by the well-known law of mass action, that is, drug response relates to the number of receptors occupied, and that in turn is dependent upon the number of drug molecules available. Not all observations can be explained simply by the *mass-action or occupancy* theory and other hypotheses have been advanced to cover these variations. It is sufficient here to state that drugs have certain properties which characterise their action in relation to receptors; these properties are affinity and efficacy. High *affinity* makes drug-receptor interaction more likely (all other things being equal), while *efficacy* is a measure of the drug's ability to produce an effect once combined with the receptor. Thus, prominent drug effect will be produced by a drug with high affinity and high efficacy, while a compound with high affinity and zero efficacy will be an *antagonist* of the first drug, occupying the receptors but producing no effect.

Dose-Response Relationships

Most drug-receptor interactions produce graduated responses depending upon the concentration of drug present, that is the *dose-response* relationship. This is most conveniently expressed by plotting response against log-dose, an arbitrary manipulation which produces a sigmoid curve with a linear mid-section. The log-dose response curve can be constructed from *in vivo* or *in vitro* tests and is useful for defining the potency of a drug and its maximal effect, and for comparing the potency

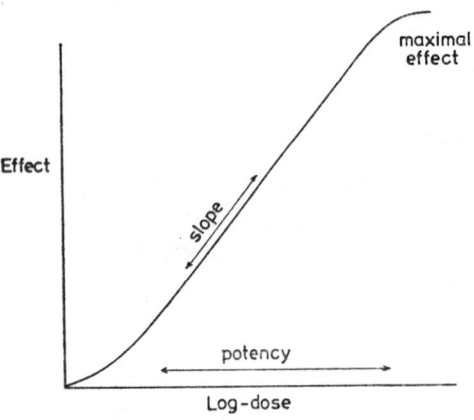

Fig. 4: The Log-Dose Response Curve

of drugs which act on the same receptor or produce the same response. The *slope* of the linear section gives an indication of *size* of drug dose necessary to cause increases in effect, and variation between individual subjects can be represented by the shape and position of the dose response curve.

Chemical Structure

Drug action bears some relation to chemical structure, again implying drug combination with structurally discrete receptor sites. Thus, a group of structurally similar compounds generally have similar actions and effects; however, apparently quite minor structural or conformational changes can be responsible for major changes in action. For instance, all phenothiazines (antipsychotics) have a similar spectrum of action, but the relatively minor manipulation of substitution of a sulphur atom by an ethylene linkage in chlorpromazine produces imipramine, which is totally devoid of antipsychotic activity but is antidepressant (see Chapters 6 and 7). Likewise d-amphetamine is a potent central stimulant while the l-form of the drug has virtually no such action (see Chapter 6).

Cellular Action and Neuronal Transmission

The cellular events involved in drug action and effect are very poorly understood. However, in the end *drug action is always mediated by a natural process, the drug either mimicking, facilitating or antagonising that natural phenomenon.*

Many drugs probably act at the cell membrane which in all living cells is the means by which they maintain the constancy of their composition. By a continuous active process, sodium ions are pumped out of the cells with concomitant inward flow of potassium ions.

Cells making up the nervous system (*neurons*) have adapted this active process for the transfer of information within the nervous system. When any point of a neuron is stimulated by any of a variety of influences, the neuronal membrane suddenly and briefly (within milli-seconds) changes its activity, permitting sodium ions to pour into the cell and potassium ions to flow out. This transient reversal spreads to adjacent areas of neuronal membrane, thus becoming a propagated *nerve impulse,* which is conducted along prolongations of the neurons (axons).

The continuous ionic pumping maintains the interior of the cell at a lower electrical potential than the outside (resting potential), usually of the order of -60 to -90mV. During the events comprising the nerve impulse (the action potential), this potential difference is reversed (*depolar-*

isation), the inside of the cell being transiently positive with respect to the outside; thereafter resting potential is soon reestablished (repolarisation). The event which initiates depolarisation must itself alter the polarity to a certain *threshold* level. The ease or difficulty of depolarisation (*excitability*) may be altered by changes in threshold, or alteration of resting potential toward or away from threshold potential.

Drugs can affect neurons by either increasing or decreasing their excitability, and do so by a variety of ways.

In the transfer of information, the initiating stimulus to depolarisation is transmitted from another neuron. Neurons may have an excitatory or inhibitory effect upon each other, the net effect of transmission to a given neuron being some sort of integration of all the stimuli impinging upon its membrane. Neurons are not physically connected together but are separated by a microscopic gap, the *synaptic cleft*, at a junction called the *synapse*. The transmission of information (*neuronal transmission*) is achieved by the release and action of minute quantities of biogenic chemical neurotransmitter substances.

Nerve endings have systems for production, storage, release, diffusion, action, reuptake and destruction of these transmitter substances, the most important of which are:

1) Catecholamines (norepinephrine and its precursor dopamine);
2) Acetylcholine (see Chapters 6, 10);
3) Serotonin or 5-hydroxytryptamine;
4) Gamma-amino-butyric acid (GABA).

Of these, the first two are probably most important for the action of psychotropic drugs, and various alterations in neurotransmitter function are attributed to these agents.

To be receptive to these chemical influences, the cells must be kept energized by a background of "tonic" impulses. This is achieved through the reticular activating system of the brain, which in turn is kept active by sensory bombardment, by feedback from cerebral processes like thinking and acting, and by the activity of the Papez circuit which is the basis of feeling (see Chapter 10).

Psychotropic drugs probably achieve their therapeutic effects in children mainly by altering the *energizing* (or activating) and *feeling* systems, though they do have widespread influence on neuronal transmission and membrane function, and their effects are thus exerted diffusely in the nervous system and on other systems as well. Like all drugs, the selectivity

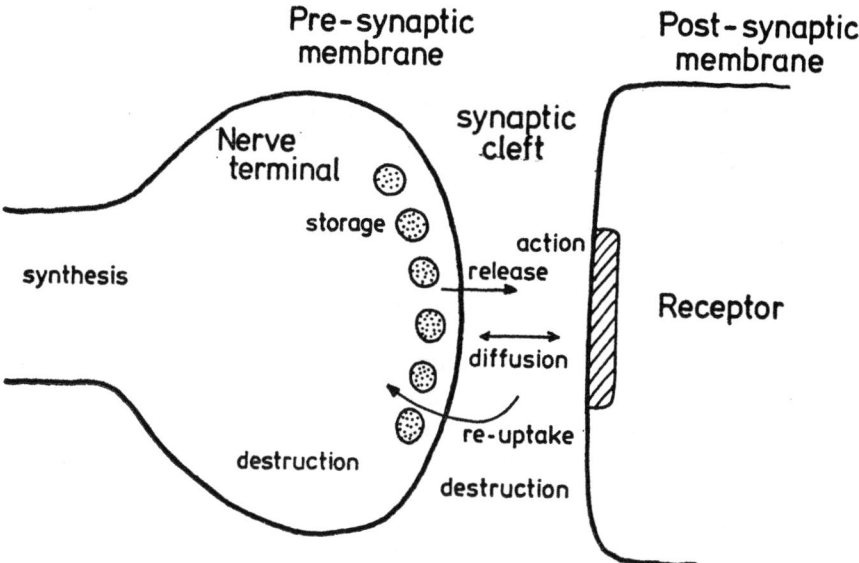

Fig. 5: Representation of the structure of a nerve ending and of the events involved in neuronal transmission.

they have depends largely upon pharmacokinetic factors and is far from ideal.

A drug is usually categorised and described by the action that seems to underlie its therapeutic effect (MAO inhibitor—see Chapter 7), or by its most prominent, desired effects (e.g., antipsychotic). However, *no drug has only one effect* and the full spectrum of effects should be used in characterisation, though no existing classification does this. Lack of selectivity of drug action is responsible for much of so-called adverse (or treatment-emergent) effects, such as dry mouth, an anticholinergic effect of the tricyclic antidepressant agents, or postural hypotension from the autonomic effects of phenothiazines. One must not be misled, then, by simplistic sounding names like antidepressant, especially in pediatric psychopharmacology where not only do names ignore much of a drug's spectrum of effects but do not even reflect their therapeutic indications! (See Introduction, p. xiii.)

Adverse Effects—Treatment-Emergent Effects

Adverse drug effects include any unwanted consequence of drug administration, trivial to fatal all falling within the scope of the term. The severity of adverse effects must be related to the severity of the condition being treated, for whereas an occasional fatal reaction to a drug used to treat an otherwise invariably fatal condition may be considered a reasonable trade-off, the same could not be said of a death in the course of treatment of a simple behaviour problem in a child.

Adverse drug effects might be divided into the classical reactions of *hypersensitivity*, that is immunologic, as in the cholestatic jaundice caused by the antipsychotic chlorpromazine; or *idiosyncrasy*, that is excessive or abnormal unexplained response to an otherwise usual drug dose, in both of which the basis is a special host factor and often unforeseen. Melmon (1971) points out that *such reactions constitute the minority of adverse effects, and far more (70-80%) are due to the extension of known pharmacologic effect* (for example dry mouth from antidepressants) *which are predictable and to a considerable extent avoidable* (Table 1).

TABLE 1

Classification of Adverse Drug Effects

1. PREDICTABLE

   A. Excess therapeutic
      e.g., hypoglycaemia from excessive insulin dose.

   B. Pharmacologic—consequences of known pharmacologic effects of the drug
      e.g., anticholinergic effects of tricyclic anti-depressants.

2. UNPREDICTABLE

   C. Hypersensitivity
      e.g., anaphylaxis from penicillin allergy.

   D. Idiosyncrasy
      e.g., haemolysis from primaquine where G-6-PD deficiency exists.

Estimates of the frequency of occurrence of adverse drug effects vary widely; one estimate on the high side, that of Melmon (1971), attributes 3-5% of hospital admissions to this cause, with 30% of these patients suffering a second reaction in hospital.

The number of deaths from adverse drug effects again is not known. In many cases the drug may simply add to an already irreversible situation and cannot be held responsible for death. However, Irey (1976) reports on 220 deaths, unexpected and unpredictable, from genuine adverse drug effects, collected over 10 years. Twenty-eight of the fatalities involved children under 11 years of age, and another 16 were in the 11-20 age group. Tranquilisers, with 18 of the 220 deaths attributed to them, were the third commonest class of drugs implicated, though they rated well below the top two contenders.

Adverse effect in children may relate particularly to size and development, for growth may be influenced by drugs, or the effects of administered drug may be influenced by the state of development. Tetracycline, for example, is actively taken up into developing bone and enamel and causes enamel staining and hypoplasia (Storey (1973) and reduction in bone growth in premature infants (Weinstein and Dalton 1968). Lengthy courses of cortico-steroid as in the management of intractable asthma retard bone growth in children, though a compensatory growth spurt may occur when treatment is withdrawn.

Incompetent metabolic systems, especially the glucuronyl transferase system in the liver, put the neonate at risk of toxicity from drugs whose action is terminated by glucuronide conjugation. For example, the well-known, but now rare, "gray syndrome" of cardiovascular collapse is caused by high levels of unconjugated chloramphenicol, an antibiotic (Weinstein & Dalton, 1968).

Drug overdose is not an adverse effect in strict definition but, whether accidental or intentional, it is another possible outcome of psychotropic medication given to a child or to some other family member. A high incidence of tricyclic overdose was noted by Brown (1975) in the 2-13 age group, coinciding with the placement of tricyclics on the free listing (1970-71) in Australia. Of the children reported, 38% overdosed with their own pills and 40% with their mothers'. Three children died.

The elicitation of side effects in children is discussed in detail in Chapter 2 while those associated with particular psychotropic drugs are to be found in Chapters 6-10. The review by DiMascio et al. (1970) is also useful reading.

Drug Interactions

Much is written about interactions between different drugs and other substances such as food; potential interactions are legion, but real and documented ones are much fewer. Interactions may occur at any point in drug administration, kinetics, action, and effect. Interactions need not necessarily be disadvantageous as long as they are controlled, and some interactions can actually be utilised to great advantage as in the treatment of hypertension.

Interaction can occur in the *gastrointestinal tract*. For example, the antibiotic tetracycline is bound in insoluble complexes with Fe^{++} from iron tablets and the absorption of both drugs is almost totally prevented. *Distributional* interactions are exemplified by competition at protein binding sites, which may lead to excessive amounts of free drug. *Metabolic interactions* involve the induction or inhibition of enzyme activity, so that the amount, and hence activity, of one drug is altered by another. For instance, the rate of phenytoin metabolism is increased by barbiturate leading to a reduction of phenytoin effect. The prevention of food-derived tyramine metabolism, ordinarily occurring in the gut wall and liver, by monoamine oxidase inhibitor antidepressants (see Chapter 7) is the basis for the hypertensive response to the combination of the inhibitors and cheese. *Renal excretion* of one drug can be altered by the renal effects of another, such as diuretic-induced low serum sodium concentration which can cause excessive retention of lithium and serious toxicity (see Chapter 10).

Interaction at *receptor sites* may involve a drug and a natural substance and may be the basis of the drug effect (for example, antipsychotics such as haloperidol may compete with dopamine for receptor sites). But drug-drug interactions also occur, such as the competition of antipsychotics and antiparkinson drugs for the same receptor sites, the ultimate drug effect depending upon relative affinity, efficacy and concentration of the competing agents.

Non-Compliance with the Prescribed Regimen

The failure of the patient to take drugs as prescribed by the doctor *probably accounts for more variability in response or lack of response to drugs than does any other factor*. It is self-evident that if a drug is not taken its beneficial effects will not be experienced. Non-compliance describes any deviation from the prescribed regimen ranging from complete failure to take the drug to varying the number of doses per day or shortening the course of treatment. Clearly, some misdemeanours are of more consequence than others.

Information about the frequency of non-compliance is hard to obtain and those studies which rely on the patient's providing the information probably detect less compliance failure than those which employ some objective measure like urine testing. Albeit, most authors give a figure of 50% or less compliance with the prescribed regimen. (Caron & Roth, 1963; Willcox et al., 1965). Even in hospital serious medication errors do occur (Wilson, 1973). Children seem to fare no better than adults at adherence to the regimen; Mattar et al. (1975) found that only 7.3% of 300 pediatric outpatients correctly completed their course of antibiotic for otitis media.

Recently Kellaway and McCrae (1977) have differentiated simple medication error from intentional non-compliance. They found the former was a problem partially eliminated by education, the latter representing a somewhat more intractable situation. Willcox et al. (1965) studying the compliance of psychiatric patients, with urine tests for drug, showed a degree of individual consistency in that repeated testing in the same individual usually gave the same result. Davis (1966) showed that, of the 37% of his adults who did not comply with their regimen, nearly half had never intended to take medication. This intention may contribute to pediatric non-compliance, for here the decisions of two people, the child and the parent, usually are involved. Reasons given by mothers for not properly dosing their child (Mohler et al., 1955) included the patient's feeling well, carelessness, lack of money (for the drug), the child's refusing the medication and the misunderstanding of instructions. Increasing complexity of dosage schedule and increasing number of doses per day may also reduce compliance (Kellaway, personal communication).

Doctors appear often to have an unrealistic vision of patient compliance ("all my patients do as they are told"), and of the therapeutic effects of drugs, and hold in low regard the self-limiting nature of much ill-health. Davis (1966) found that physicians overestimated the compliance of their patients and Charney et al. (1967) found doctors were unable to distinguish those patients who do from those who do not comply. In children, Charney found that only two factors seemed to bear any relation to compliance—the mother's perception of the seriousness of the illness and the physician's rating of the mother as "reliable" as distinct from "unreliable."

Non-compliance should be seen as an unpredictable and variable but ever-present phenomenon and a likely cause of an unexpectedly poor response to medication (Haggerty & Roghmann, 1972). Although unpredictable, it is not totally inevitable and counselling can improve patient compliance where simple errors underlie the problem (Kellaway & McCrae, 1977). Mattar et al. (1975) see certain responsibilities of physicians which patients felt were somewhat under-fulfilled. Many patients requested more information about the nautre of the illness, and more information about the drugs, including reasons for the dosage regime, possible dangers of the drug or interactions with food and other medications. Overall the requirements seem to be for *more time to talk*, to get answers to questions and to establish better rapport with the doctor. This confirms another impression (Korsch et al., 1968) that the doctor/patient relationship is very important in drug compliance; pediatric compliance was improved if the mother felt the doctor had praised her as a mother and had an easy communication with her. This concept is further supported by the compliance figure of 90% in private solo practice (Leistyna &

Macauley, 1966), 66% in private group practice (Charney et al., 1967), and only 18% in general clinic populations (Bergman & Werner, 1963).

There appears to be no study in which compliance with psychotropic medication by pediatric patients has been investigated systematically. It is likely that the various influences could have a different quantitative impact in this situation, but overall it can be assumed that somewhat less than complete reliance can be placed upon the child's taking the medication as prescribed. This has obvious implications not only for treatment of individual children but for clinical trials to establish the efficacy of a drug (see Chapter 4).

Conclusions

Modern clinical pharmacology is a rapidly developing field which offers considerable promise in attempting to develop more rational, less empirical and less tradition-bound drug treatment. It is disconcerting, however, how little is known about the cellular and system effects of psychotropic drugs, and of pediatric variations in psychopharmacology in general. While pharmacology has pretensions of an exact science, it is of interest how critical the patient-doctor relationship is to its clinical application. Without attention to this, it loses much of its exactitude. Nowhere is this more true than in pediatric psychopharmacology.

2
MEASURES IN PEDIATRIC PSYCHOPHARMACOLOGY

JOHN S. WERRY, M.D.

I. General Aspects of Measurement

Introduction

This section will review some general principles of measurement as they affect the use of psychotropic drugs in children.

In this way, readers without formal training in measurement in social and behavioral science may find Section II, where actual measures used in pediatric psychopharmacology are discussed, less strange and confusing. In particular, this section will be used to introduce terminology commonly used in measurement in the social and behavioral sciences where, because of the complexity, the *conceptual* base of measurement is considerably more advanced than in medicine where, because of generally better theory, the *technology* of measurement is much more impressive. A simple useful text for further reading in the areas covered in this section is that by Hamilton (1974).

What Is a Good Measure?

To be useful, a measure must be reliable, valid, sensitive, relevant, practicable, safe and ethical (see also Chapter 4).

RELIABILITY

This denotes *precision* of measurement—across examiners (*interobserver* reliability) or, where the datum (e.g., IQ) is considered stable,

---

Much of the author's work referred to here was supported by The Medical Research Council of New Zealand.

across time (*test/retest* reliability). There are various statistical techniques for calculating reliability of which the commonest is Pearson's product moment correlation coefficient (r), the percent agreement between observers, and so on. This is a highly technical subject beyond the scope of this book and readers are referred to books on statistics. Suffice it to say that reliability should never be assumed unless extensively demonstrated (as in some of the standard psychological tests like the WISC) *and* the examiner is properly trained in the technique. Many of the accepted measures in medicine and psychology are of unknown reliability, and their reputation is based on tradition, clinical need or status of the originator. Further, as has been shown in behavior observations, persons who do the same observation over long periods of time (e.g., long years in practice!), though initially reliable, tend to become increasingly inaccurate. This latter problem has been called, rather picturesquely, *instrument (test) drift* (Johnson & Bolstad, 1973) and seems inherent in the adaptational qualities of the human observer or examiner who tends to alter the method to his own needs or, possibly, to avoid boredom.

VALIDITY

This differs from reliability in that it refers to the inherent truth of the measure, or, put another way, *what the measure actually measures*. As with reliability, it cannot be assumed. For example, calling a rating scale a hyperactivity scale does not ensure that this is what it really measures. Indeed, there is reason to believe that many such scales measure conduct problems as much as activity level (see section on activity below). As will be seen, many of the measures and tests used in pediatric psychopharmacology have been named in *anticipation* rather than *demonstration* of validity, and, as often as not, this expectation has subsequently proven unfounded.

SENSITIVITY

A measure must also be sensitive to changes produced by the drugs. In pediatric psychopharmacology, there is already much evidence to show that, when used in appropriate clinical dosage, present drugs produce changes in behavior and function which are small compared with those produced by normal physiological events, disease processes or psychosocial circumstances. Much of the literature about drug effects on behavior and learning is contradictory, and some of this contradiction is almost certainly due to the use of drug measures of perfectly acceptable reliability and validity such as the WISC which are, however, too insensitive. Any tests such as the IQ tests, developed on the assumption of stability of the datum with time, will likely prune out minor fluctuations (of the size of drug effects) in order to achieve test/retest reliability which a concept like intelligence requires. As newer drugs are developed, the size of drug-induced changes may increase, but it seems clear at the moment that they are treatments of weak, though often quite useful, effect set in a complex interaction between the child, his physiology, and his psychosocial environment.

RELEVANCE

Though closely related, this is not quite the same as validity. For example, there is no doubt that laboratory measures of learning reviewed in Chapter 3 do indeed measure such important cognitive processes as attention as they occur in this special situation, but, so far, they do not seem to bear any relationship to academic progress in the classroom. Thus, though drug effects on learning in the laboratory may be of great theoretical interest, they have little apparent *relevance* for judgments about effects drugs will have in the classroom. However, this is not to say that the relevance of a measure must be clinical, but can involve the advance of theory or basic understanding of the drug action; it is rather more a matter of not misapplying a measure.

OTHER QUALITIES

A measure must meet other obvious requirements such as practicality, economy, safety and ethical acceptability. With children, ethical considerations (see Chapter 4) are likely to involve avoidance of pain, psychological or physical, a respect for the basic freedom of the child as a citizen and the possibility of something useful for the child and/or for many children emerging from the application of the measure. A particular problem in pediatric psychopharmacology is that, because of the weakness and restricted relevance of many measures, there is a tendency to use the "blunderbuss approach" with many hours of repeated testing which quickly exhausts the child and parent alike. Adherence to the code of ethics of the medical and other helping professions should serve as a protection against these sorts of abuse, but there is no substitute for clinical sensitivity to children's and parents' needs.

Purposes

GENERAL

Measures are of two main kinds: nomothetic or idiographic.

1) *Nomothetic* measures describe an individual child's resemblance to or difference from a group, normal or abnormal, of other children; the data they generate are assumed to be of some significance. Much of the discussion which follows is concerned, not unnaturally, with this type of measure.

2) *Idiographic* measures, however, are just as important. They are concerned with data which relate to and are likely to prove useful for this child only, and usually concern matters of some personal concern, family and social environment. This is a vital part of the management of any patient, but there tends to be a preoccupation in pediatrics with nomothetic type data and in child psychiatry with idiographic data. Child psychiatry needs to recognise that diagnosis and quantitative measurement have a useful place, and pediatrics that laboratory tests may do little to advance the actual wellbeing or social function of some patients, whereas attention to personal matters might.

SPECIFIC

The purposes for which measures may be used more specifically are several.

1) *Descriptive*: Sometimes called demographic or personal, these serve to define the population of children to which the findings of a study may apply, or to make judgments about the suitability of a particular treatment for a given child. Sex, age, ethnic group and so on are examples, as are much of the history taking in pediatrics and child psychiatry.

2) *Predictive*: Some measures are intended to be *predictive*, usually those which relate in some way to diagnosis, particular physiological, developmental, or environmental states and do, or might, predict the outcome of drug treatment in some signicant way. Since pediatric psychopharmacology is still largely an empirical science, the "blunderbuss" approach already referred to is often used in a search for predictors of drug effect. A host of measures are made before commencing treatment and a bewildering series of correlations of variables with drug response run *post hoc* on a willing but unthinking computer. To date this approach has been remarkably unproductive in pediatric psychopharmacology and suggests that better theories about causes of psychopathology, rather more closely tied to drug action, are needed.

3) *Independent Variable (treatment)*: Measures may relate to the *independent variable* or the variable which is going to be manipulated systematically by the experimenter, for example, dosage.

4) *Dependent Variable (effect)*: On the other hand, measures (usually the majority) relate to the *dependent* variable or those functions which are expected to change as the independent or treatment variable changes. These would encompass all the measures of drug effect, and it is fairly obvious that the choice of measures will limit the interpretation of effect. For example, the antidepressant drugs (see Chapter 7) have been used for well over a decade in the treatment of enuresis, but it is only recently that studies have suggested that such a use may have extra-vesical effects, including psychotropic effects (Werry et al., 1975a). Or again, the physical effects of the stimulants, such as those on weight, have only recently received any attention (see Chapter 6). It should be fairly clear that dependent variable measures in pediatric psychopharmacology ordinarily should be both physiological and psychosocial. (It could, of course, be well argued that the same rubric should apply to medical procedures with children in general, though obviously with differences in emphasis). The real enemy, however, is specialty or profession-derived tunnel vision which prevents a comprehensive view of the child as a composite of many bodily systems and a *biosocial* organism. Pediatric psychopharmacology is particularly vulnerable to this tunnel vision because of the sectarian interests and training of the various professions such as pediatrics, child psychiatry, psychology and special education, all staking a claim to behavior problems in children.

Techniques of Measurement

Measures may be *informal* or highly systematized. Both types rely on three main data collection techniques which are often combined in any one situation such as an interview. However, since their properties vary, it is important to distinguish them.

OBSERVATIONS

This term should be restricted to techniques which collect data *as they happen with a minimum of reduction of the data to underlying components or categories*. Where any reduction is done, it is numerical rather than inferential. Thus, an EEG CAT (Computation of Average Transients) would be observational whereas the electroencephalographer's interpretation of an EEG would be a rating (see below). However, in spite of its objectivity, the observational technique is not necessarily more useful in the measurement of behavior than apparently cruder techniques such as ratings, as will be seen in Section II of this chapter. While observational methods are generally somewhat easier to make reliable and situationally relevant, they may not be ethical, economic, practicable or sensitive.

RATINGS

In contrast, these require a human observer to *preprocess observational data and convert them into some qualitative judgment*. The most convenient way to elicit this sort of data is by a series of focused questions or a questionnaire. Despite criticism about reliability and validity, ratings have some clear advantages over observations in their ability to average across long periods of time and often, too, across different situations, which reduces error. Also, they are convenient, practical and more regularly drug-sensitive.

TESTS

As the term is used in behavioral science (though not in medicine), it implies the measurement of some function by actively evoking it, usually in some artificial manner. In this sense then, the WISC and the glucose tolerance test are true tests, whereas measurements of hemoglobin or height are not (they are observations). The weakness of the test as a measurement, hence, lies in its capacity accurately to simulate real life situations and to measure an adequately representative sample of the particular behavior or function. They are useful in probing for limits or unusualness of function which might take many hours of observations to elicit.

Source of Data

SOCIAL CONTACTS (INTERESTED OBSERVERS)

Much of the data used in pediatric psychopharmacology is naturalistic and gathered by the child's caretakers and other social contacts such as parents, teachers and, occasionally, peers. There has been a tendency to denigrate these sources of data, especially parents, but the empirical evidence (see below) suggests that social contacts can be surprisingly reliable and valid, particularly where the techniques of eliciting data are adequate. Data from these sources have the great advantage of relevance.

DISINTERESTED OBSERVERS

On the other hand, observers trained in a particular technique may be used. The most obvious examples would be a doctor or child psychiatrist, but increasing use is being made of persons whose sole function is to observe, not to diagnose and treat—behavior observers as they are commonly called. There is nothing magically superior in the latter who can only be as good as the observational system.

MECHANICAL

While medicine now takes for granted the value of mechanically (used here in the generic sense of derived from a machine, mechanical, electronic or otherwise) derived data, it is only recently that such methods of measuring behavior have begun to appear in the form of videotapes, actometers, polygraphs and the like. Mechanical methods have certain obvious advantages over human methods but are often expensive, cumbersome, temperamental and lack self-correcting mechanisms and creativity, so that much useful information may go unnoticed. They do, however, offer a chance to bring considerably more accuracy into some aspects of measurement of behavior, brain and cognitive function.

SELF-REPORTS

These are derived from the child himself and are among the most difficult to obtain accurately. They require an ability on the part of the questioner or the techniques to avoid production of a *response set* of conformity—"giving the right answer which makes me or my family look good or pleases the doctor"—an ability to suit the level of enquiry to the child's age, maturity, social and cultural group. This can be achieved, to a varying degree, by questionnaires or projective techniques which provide the child with a framework to describe his own feelings or opinions such as telling a story to a picture (Children's Thematic Apperception Test), or by play techniques or, more commonly, by simply interviewing the child. Many require time to build up trust and hence are error prone. Few yield usable numerical data. They have not figured greatly in pediatric psychopharmacology (Rapoport, in press) to date but deserve much closer attention.

Scope of Data

SITUATIONAL

Methods may be aimed at measuring function in quite isolated situations though more commonly the scope is much broader. One of the more recurrent problems in pediatric psychopharmacology arises when the technique of eliciting the data is inadequate for its purported scope. A common example of this is the observations of behavior made by the doctor in a hurried consultation, where a petrified child sits immobilized awaiting customary injection. The doctor is then asked to evaluate the child's behavior as a universal thing and, finding comments from the mother about the child's behavior at conflict with his own, diagnoses the child as normal and the mother as overanxious. It is a good principle, then, to assume that *the scope of the measure is restricted to the measuring situation unless proven otherwise.* A good doctor, of course, would then seek to enlarge his scope of observation by eliciting actual descriptions of the child's behavior in different environments from the mother and seeking verification from independent sources such as school.

GLOBAL/ATOMISTIC

Measures vary in the extent to which their scope is coarse or refined. Some of the best established measures in psychopharmacology described in Section II of this chapter are global in nature, telling little beyond the *direction* of the drug-induced change and shedding no light on what particular way the child has improved or gotten worse. Understandably, there is a great deal of dissatisfaction with such measures and substantial effort has been made to define behavior, brain and cognitive functions in more atomistic terms. One such time-honored concept is that of personality traits, but modern behaviorists have been even more dissecting of personality, seeing behavior as not only situation-specific but type-specific within situations (Moos, 1973). Traits have proved disappointing (Moos, 1973) and it remains to be seen whether the newer approaches do any better. Hopefully so, but it is likely that the remoteness of behavior from cellular action of drugs may sharply limit this prospect, except for measures which are closely related to discrete brain functions such as arousal or attention.

SIMILARITY V. DIFFERENCE

This is a technical issue, but certain commonly used multivariate statistical techniques such as factor analysis vary in the extent to which they look for differences or for similarity between individuals or, most notably, sources of data, examples of which can be seen in the unsuccessful search for a minimal brain dysfunction syndrome by factor analysis (Langhorne et al., 1976). Miller (1976) has argued that the failure to find communality between different types and sources of information about children's behavior or functions in some factor analytic studies may be an artifact of the underlying assumptions and subsequent mathematical solutions. This is not a trivial matter, since in pediatric psychopharmacology use is made typically of data from several different sources and one of the problems is often to reconcile conflicts between different sources. Methods which exaggerate these differences and overlook similarities can only impede development of a rational pharmacotherapy. The moral is probably to learn to distrust analytic methods unless their basic *assumptions* and *purposes* are understood, even if the mathematics or the electronics involved are too technical to comprehend.

Types of Data

The end result of measurement may be data of a purely *descriptive* kind, defying further analysis and useful only idiographically, or for generating hypotheses. This latter role must not be neglected since informal observations have a respectable history in advancing science in general and medicine in particular. However, to be most useful, whether in the clinical or the research situation, most data need to be able to be manipulated numerically. Data are of four main types, all of which are potentially numerical.

NOMINAL

Variables, such as sex, may yield only class, categorical, yes/no type data called nominal.

ORDINAL

If quantifiable, the data may be points on a scale of measurement which consists of rankings and the size of the intervals unknown, irregular or irrelevant, for example, percentiles on a height/weight chart. Much behavior cannot be measured in any strictly quantitative sense, but can be *ordered*. For example, a teacher can ordinarily rank pupils in something like troublesomeness or ability but the interval between the worst and the best child has no real quantitative meaning.

These may seem trivial points but the argument that behavior cannot be measured is true only to the extent that one insists on truly quantitative measurement and sees no value in ordinal data. For example, mothers have little difficulty in stating whether or not their child's behavior is better or worse after medication and assigning some degree to this. Yet it would be foolish to pretend that slight, moderate or great are real quantitatively, though they are valid ordinally. The point is not well appreciated in pediatric psychopharmacology where ordinal data are often treated statistically and conceptually as if they were truly quantitative.

INTERVAL AND RATIO

The third type of data is called interval, since the interval between gradations of measurement are quantitatively equal, for example, the number of crossings over a grid on a floor in unit time. Such data are of necessity nearly always *observational* or *test*-derived but by no means all data from these techniques are interval in type; they are much more likely to be ordinal or nominal. When the intervals reflect real numbers (as in the example above), the data are referred to as ratio but their occurrence is most infrequent in the measurement of behavior.

STATISTICAL TREATMENT

Each of these types of data requires different handling, especially statistically. A statement that the mean social class of a group of children was 3.55 is about as meaningful as one that says the mean sex was female and a half. Statistical nonsense is likely to be less obvious than these examples but, generally speaking, nominal and ordinal data require nonparametric statistics while interval data are best served by parametric statistics (see Chapter 4).

Which Measure Is Correct?

It is customary in pediatric psychopharmacology to collect diagnostic and drug effect measures from more than one source and, not surprisingly, discrepancies sometimes occur. The problem then arises as to which source to heed. Some (e.g., Sulzbacher, 1973) put their faith in objectivity, demonstrated or presumed, so that laboratory-derived measures or frequency counts of behavior or even doctors' evaluations are valued above those of parents and teachers (e.g., *British Medical Journal*, 1973). No measure or source is a *priori* superior to any other. The real questions are: What are the measures for, do they measure what they purport to measure, and can they detect drug effects? Accurate, theory-related measures are necessary to advance knowledge, but if the need is clinical, problems and changes in them perceived by a complainant such as a parent are likely to have a far greater significance for the individual child, or for children with similar problems. When clinically relevant information is conflicting, it is the doctor's job to decide or to determine which is the most reliable source, what is in the child's best interest, and in what environment (home or school or neither) there is the greatest need for and demonstration of change. The best *clinical* researchers in pediatric psychopharmacology are therefore likely to come from those who, in addition to their research interests, carry the responsibility for the continuing care of the child.

Conclusions

Pediatric psychopharmacology marks one of the more significant interfaces between the biological and behavioral sciences. Most doctors are reasonably conversant with measurements of biological function and recognise the need for precision and expertise within medicine in techniques like radiology and chemical pathology, but too few recognise that measurement of behavior, emotions and learning is both possible and requiring of the same kind of expertise. Non-medical scientists have been working for over a century on the development of a technology of measurement for the behavioral sciences with the same critical criteria and goals as in the biological and physical sciences. While it is true that the precision with which measurement may be made in the behavioral sciences may lag somewhat behind biology and considerably behind the physical sciences, the principles of science are the same—accurate observation as a prerequisite to hypothesis formulation and testing. Some of the methods evolved in the social and behavioral sciences are as complex and sophisticated as mechanical methods in biology. They have evolved as a way of recognizing, and attempting to deal with, the complexities of the measurement of behavior and allied functions and cannot be used intelligently without proper training. It is no longer sufficient in pediatric psychopharmacology to develop a group of *ad hoc* measures without reference to what is already known. Measurement of behavior and higher nervous system function is a formal technology essential to evaluating any drugs affecting the central nervous system, but particularly psychotropic drugs.

II. Current Measures

Bringing Order out of Chaos

Pediatric psychopharmacology is a relatively new field and, unlike adult psychopharmacology, there seem to be several competing areas—pediatrics, child psychiatry, psychopedics (mental retardation) and various nonmedical professions like special education, psychology and so on. Each seems to be going its own way and, even within the same profession, there is a tendency to do one's own thing as far as measurement is concerned. This has led to chaos which, while it has its creative aspects, makes comparison between drug studies very difficult and thus hinders the development of pediatric psychopharmacology. It is imperative, if the field is to advance, that there be some agreement on measurement techniques. Two efforts in this direction, both by U.S. Federal bodies, deserve special mention, though it should be noted that they share some contributors.

NATIONAL INSTITUTE OF MENTAL HEALTH (NIMH)

Concerned about chaos in measurement and poor methodology in adult psychopharmacology, the (U.S.) National Institute of Mental Health (NIMH) in the sixties set up an Early Clinical Drug Evaluation Unit (ECDEU now NCDEU) which set about standardizing measures. This effort which has been largely successful, so that it is now unusual to see drug studies which do not include in their principal measures those officially adopted by NIMH and set out in its drug assessment manual (ECDEU, 1976). This mission accomplished in adults, NIMH moved to do the same in pediatric psychopharmacology, culminating in publication of a battery of recommended measures (Psychopharmacology Bulletin, 1973), now incorporated in the latest manual (ECDEU 1976). This battery is not without its faults—some of the measures are untried, others too cumbersome for use outside research studies. There are serious omissions—notably, for example, the measurement of activity in an objective way. But it is a start and one which will be consistently referred to in this section.

FOOD AND DRUG ADMINISTRATION

Not surprisingly, with all the controversy around drug use in children (see Chapter 4), the (U.S.) Food and Drug Administration (FDA, in press) is in the process of publishing its own set of recommended measures and guidelines for clinical trials of drugs in children. While this is oriented to the needs of drug trials, particularly of new drugs, the reviews of the literature and the recommended measures will form a standard reference work, valuable to all interested in this area, and therefore will also be extensively referred to in this section. This work is both more comprehensive and better documented than the ECDEU manual.

CAVEAT

As noted, the FDA task force shared some of the same personnel as the NIMH one, so that investigators in psychopharmacology, while urged to use the basic measures recommended by these two agencies, should not feel entirely bound by these recommendations. Indeed, if the field is to advance, developmental work of a properly meticulous type (not simply the ad hoc throwing together of a rating scale or some such, in laziness or ignorance of the standard measures) must go on. Most of this development needs to occur in the biological and cognitive areas, in preschool age groups, and in mechanical type measures since, generally speaking, measures of behavior in children of school age and of parental attitudes have received most attention.

OTHER REFERENCE SOURCES

There are a number of useful reviews and standard works which amplify various details presented in summary form here. In addition to the NIMH and FDA sources already cited (ECDEU, 1976; FDA, in press; Psychopharmacology Bulletin, 1973), there are the series of irregularly appearing yearbooks of mental measurements by Buros (1972) which provide descriptions, sources and critical evaluations of many measures, the monographs by Frankenburg and Camp (1975) and Walker (1973) which discuss pediatric and preschool measures, and critical reviews in pediatric psychopharmacology which discuss various aspects of measurement (Barkley, 1976, 1977; Conners & Werry, in press; Safer & Allen, 1976; Sprague & Werry, 1971, 1974; Sroufe, 1975; Werry, 1977, in press a, b; Whalen & Henker, 1976).

ORGANISATION

In presenting the material here, measures have been organized by purpose for which measures are to be used since this seems to be most useful. It is not, however, a completely tidy system and there are some irregularities.

PART I. PSYCHOLOGICAL MEASURES

Background

It is obvious that any child who participates in a study or is the subject of drug treatment must be properly identified with respect to sex, age, ethnic, cultural, socioeconomic group, family structure and referral source. These are all powerful variables in influencing treatment effects. Referral source needs particular emphasis. There is now abundant evidence to show that children seen by the medical profession, whether psychiatrists or not, are biased towards overinclusion of emotionally disturbed children and obviously that the more psychiatric the treatment agency, the greater the severity of psychopathology. This may not present a problem in severe conditions like the childhood psychoses, but many of the conditions for which drugs are given are *quantitative* rather than *qualitative* departures from normality. Take, for example, the condition of enuresis for which drugs are often prescribed. A study done over 20 years ago (Halgren, 1957), showed that enuretic children referred to a clinic were more disturbed than those not referred. It is thus theoretically possible that a study done on the clinic group might find an antianxiety drug valuable, while it could be useless or even depressant in most enuretic children treated in the community.

The ECDEU Manual (1976) has a questionnaire, the Children's Personal Data Inventory (CPDI), for recording these background details though, strangely, referral data are not covered.

History

History of the present behavioral problems or disorder should include full description, age of onset, duration, severity, stability of symptoms, associated problems, prior and present treatment (especially with drugs) and response to prior treatment (FDA, in press). The ECDEU CPDI, CSH (Children's Symptom History) and PMR (Prior Medication Record) are particularly useful in this respect, covering most of the above areas in systematic, if somewhat tedious, fashion.

Eliciting past medical, perinatal and developmental history is an inherent part of pediatric and child psychiatric routine yet its reliability and utility, though widely assumed, is largely unexplored and what little data there are are not encouraging. The typical approach is often what might be called the dragnet method in which anything or everything that might conceivably be useful is recorded. An example of this can be seen in the U.S. Perinatal Collaborative Study (Broman et al., 1975) which, however, was designed as a prospective study and so items found predictive there would not necessarily be recorded or recallable retrospectively. Perhaps the most comprehensive history system in child psychiatry is that of Jenkins et al. (1966), the utility of which in studies of hyperkinetic children has been studied extensively by Loney et al. (in press). In general, empirical studies of historical items of all kinds, but particularly of the prenatal, perinatal and infancy periods, have failed to substantiate their value in drug studies (Barkley, 1976; Conners & Werry, in press; Loney et al., in press) or in childhood psychopathology in general (Werry, in press b). This is perhaps not surprising in view of the inaccuracy of mothers' recall, the inadequacy of many birth records, the unknown frequency (probably low) with which noxious events are attended by significant brain damage, the adaptability of the immature brain and the low degree of interrelatedness between behavioral characteristics in infancy and in later childhood (Bell et al., 1971). The ECDEU, CPDI and CSH include most of the common perinatal and developmental items for those who wish to record them, but do not cover medical illnesses.

Parenting and Family Environment

These would seem to be obvious areas to consider in studies in pediatric psychopharmacology, yet it is remarkable how neglected they have been (Robins, in press b). A study by Loney et al. (1975) illustrates how parenting can influence the outcome of drug treatment.

Despite the inordinate preoccupation of child psychiatry with parenting, it has produced little useful in the way of formal measures, most of which have come from child psychology. The review by Hetherington and Martin (in press) paints a rather gloomy picture of the formidable methodological problems involved in assessing parenting. They state that there has been a general disenchantment with the much used parent questionnaire type measures and a move to use observational and rating type data. The data may be behavioral, for example frequency counts of particular behaviors emitted by parents (Patterson & Cobb, 1971), or inferential judgments about such traits as permissiveness, warmth, and hostility derived from observations of parent-child interactions. These methods produce problems of their own, not the least of which relate to the artificiality of the observing situation. There appears to be no widely-accepted measure of parenting which is reliable and valid. It is likely that, as in other areas (see Conners, 1976a), simple global ratings will do as well as highly detailed instruments. For example, Loney et al. (1975) used a simple judgment of well or poorly managed children based on social and psychiatric histories, yet were able to show influences on drug effects. Similar simple judgments based on psychiatric interviews were useful in predicting long-term prognosis in hyperactive children (Weiss, 1975), but those who use such measures must check interrater reliability of such judgments.

Rutter (1976) reports the development of reliable methods of interviewing parents and codifying the data assessing family events and activities and, perhaps more importantly, marital discord. The importance of this method is that it has been shown to be reliable, independent of social class, consistent with parents' own evaluation and, most notably, predictive of both psychiatric disturbance in the children and subsequent marital breakdown. The same group also report a "malaise inventory" derived from the self reporting symptom screening device, the Cornell Medical Index, which proved satisfactory in detecting actual psychiatric disorder in parents (Rutter et al., 1976). While these instruments have not been used in pediatric psychopharmacology, their ability to predict certain states in children and certain family outcomes suggests that they might be useful in the study of parent influences upon the effect of psychotropic drugs in children.

Robins (in press b) suggests the Moos Family Environment Scale (Moos, 1974) as a comprehensive measure of the child's family environment. It is fairly reliable across time (though interobserver reliability is unknown), easily scored and discriminates backgrounds of psychiatric patients from normal populations. Its principal use, apart from an informational one, would seem to be in ensuring compatibilty of family backgrounds in clinical trials.

In summary then, this is a most difficult area which, however, deserves much more attention in attempting to predict the effect of drugs in children. It is unfortunate that those who know most about these things are often the least interested in psychopharmacology and in quantitative methods so necessary if data are to be utilizable in pediatric psychopharmacology. Anyone who wishes to use measures in this area is strongly advised to seek expert advice and to read carefully reviews such as that by Hetherington and Martin (in press), Rapoport (in press) and evaluations of specific meausres in Buros (1972). Simple ratings derived from interviews conducted by competent clinicians have proved as reliable and valid as more complex measures.

Diagnosis (Parent and Child Interviews)

Diagnostic classifications in child psychiatry are discussed in Chapter 5. There has been general dissatisfaction with existing systems, reflected in the sweeping changes in the American and International systems due to be implemented shortly. It is vital in pediatric psychopharmacology that the many vague terms like hyperkinetic syndrome and minimal brain dysfunction be tightened and subdivided (see Rie, 1975; Werry, in press b) so that comparisons between drug studies may then become possible and diagnostic indications for pharmacotherapy become more precise.

Diagnosis cannot rely on a single set of data, such as that derived solely from a psychiatric interview, but must be a composite of information gained from a variety of environments, a variety of observers and with an account of the duration of symptoms. The extent to which such data are comprehensive and reliable will influence the accuracy of the final diagnosis. The Children's Diagnostic Classification (CDC), an abbreviated version of DSM II, and Diagnostic System (CDS), a diagnostic decision tree, in the present ECDEU battery (1976) are based on just such assumptions of adequate data collection. The problem of historical data has already been discussed, and teacher and parent questionnaires and ratings, also elemental to good diagnosis, are discussed below. Suffice it to say that they are amongst the most reliable and valuable of measures available, and should should be utilised in the diagnostic process.

Since the interview of parent and child is usually considered of paramount importance in diagnosis, and since the obtaining of most of the other information needed is discussed in other sections, most of the discussion here will center on this measurement technique.

Despite the status and frequency of the interview in child psychiatry, there has been remarkably little effort either to systematize it or establish its reliability or validity. While it is not *essential* to the achievement of precision in diagnosis to systematize the interview, it seems logical that such a development might improve the chances of uniformity. The extent to which the proposed diagnostic systems set out the *necessary, sufficient and excluding criteria* for making a particular diagnosis and then proceed to define those criteria in unambiguous terms will determine the data domain to be covered in the interview. The most notable efforts to produce a standard, reliable and valid parent and child interview are those employed in the Isle of Wight epidemiological study (Graham & Rutter, 1968; Rutter, 1976; Rutter & Graham, 1968; Rutter et al., 1976). A reliable child interview technique agreeing well with other sources of data was developed. Others (Herjanic et al., 1975) have likewise succeeded but these required a considerable structuring of the interview while unstructured efforts have not proven reliable (Zrull et al. 1966). However, it is of interest that Rutter (1976) subsequently abandoned the child interview, writing as follows: "It was found that a detailed and systematic interview with the mother provided the greatest range of information needed to make a psychiatric diagnosis. This method of interview assessment proved to be reliable, to agree well with other measures and to have predictive validity. Moreover, it was shown that with the use of standardized techniques trained social scientists could make assessments of psychiatric disorder which agreed very well with those made by psychiatrists" (p. 510). However, Rutter goes on to say that their studies have also pointed out the importance of interviewer skills. It should be noted that Rutter's diagnostic system is not a comprehensive one, but directed largely to answering simply whether there is a psychiatric disorder, subdivided into only a few simple categories.

The ECDEU battery has a system for rating the psychiatric interview with the child, the Children's Psychiatric Rating Scale (CPRS). However, no interview format is specified and the CPRS is as yet untested. The extent to which it will provide the sort of information necessary for the new classifications is also uncertain.

In conclusion, then, parent and child interviews can yield reliable and valid diagnostic data, particularly if structured. Parent interviews are easier and more informative. The best-tested interviews are those of the

Isle of Wight studies, though how these will meet the needs of the new classifications (DSM III and ICD9) remains to be seen. Interview methods should be scrutinized for interinterviewer and interrater reliability and the somewhat limited scope of the child interview should be recognized.

Personality

This is a difficult concept but it differs from diagnosis in that it is a more extensive summation of the person. Typically it is defined by a number of a piori traits or dimensions, empirically-derived from multivariate statistical techniques like factor analysis. The subject and its relevance to child psychiatry have been extensively reviewed by Quay (in press) and Rapoport (in press). There are a number of well-known personality tests for children, such as the MMPI, The California Personality Inventory, Cattell's and, of course, the projective tests like the CAT and Rorschach (see Gittelman-Klein, 1978a; Rapoport, in press). Readers are referred to one of the standard handbooks such as Buros (1972) for a fuller account of all these tests. Most of the commonly used behavior rating scales discussed below are, to a certain extent, personality tests; however, with the exception of Conners Parent Questionnaire, they usually have too few underlying traits to yield comprehensive pictures of the child. To date, there has been little attempt to use personality or projective tests in pediatric psychopharmacology, partly because of the lack of interest in pediatric psychopharmacology by most clinical psychologists and partly because of some disenchantment with the whole notion of personality as a stable thing, with more awareness of the strong situational influences on behavior (Moos, 1973). In general, personality and projective tests are cumbersome, of uncertain reliability or, more often, validity, and measure stable characteristics which are unlikely to show much change with drugs. Their role in pediatric psychopharmacology remains to be defined.

Behavior

This much abused term will be used here to mean *externally observed motor, verbal or easily observable simple psychophysiological events* (such as blushing). Usually, however, these events have undergone some reinterpretation either in terms of *social evaluation* (e.g., aggressive, sassy) or inferences about internal states (anxious, depressed); but the essence of behavior is that someone else observes it. Behavior is the stuff of pediatric psychopharmacology as it is of child psychiatry and allied areas. It is because of disturbances of behavior, qualitative and quantitative, that children are brought to professionals. While the focus may shift ultimately to such things as the child's self image, it is by behavior that the world will make its ultimate judgment about the efficacy of any treatment.

Because of the importance in pediatric psychopharmacology of *motor activity* and the confusion surrounding such terms as hyperactivity, it will form a separate section where the argument will be made that this should be, as nearly as possible, a simple quantitative dimension devoid of social judgment.

Also excluded here is academic performance, cognition and learning which, while technically behavior, are ordinarily treated separately. Their importance to pediatric psychopharmacology is such that they are discussed in a chapter of their own (Chapter 3).

The various techniques of data elicitation for evaluating behavior and their general properties already have been discussed in general in Section I of this chapter.

RATING SCALES

Rating scales still form the mainstay of assessment of behavior in pediatric psychopharmacology. As noted in Section I, their essence lies in the reduction to averaged statements of a great deal of data collected often over a long period of time and in several different environments or situations. They are cheap, practical, painless (at least physically) and, despite some vulnerability to rater bias or set (e.g., Neisworth et al., 1974), a number have been shown to be reasonably reliable, valid and sensitive to drug effects. They can also be used as, or to complement, diagnostic procedures for predictive purposes.

Conners (1973a, 1976a, in press) and Quay (in press) have reviewed children's rating scales in detail. The number of such devices is legion (Buros, 1972, Conners, in press) and, as noted, such scales *seem* simple to construct, so that there is a regrettable tendency for persons unfamiliar with the literature in pediatric psychopharmacology to develop *ad hoc* scales. One of the interesting features is the extent to which rating scales of a general type all seem to share some underlying dimensions of conduct problem, neuroticism, immaturity (including distractibility) and, to a lesser degree, hyperactivity, and socialized delinquency, depending on the population studied (Quay, in press; Camp & Smerling, in press). This basic universality of children's rating scales leads this reviewer to conclude that until a scale can be shown to result in greater reliability, validity and drug sensitivity, to offer measurement of areas of behavior not presently covered or have greater theoretical interest, investigators in psychopharmacology should confine themselves to the following behavior rating scales, each of which will be discussed briefly.

1) *Teacher Scales*: The best studied by far in pediatric psychopharmacology is Conners Teacher Questionnaire (TQ) (Conners, 1973a, ECDEU, 1976), a 39-item scale which has undergone a major revision since its publication (Conners, 1969). The current version and its scoring can be found in Conners (1973a) or ECDEU (1976). While there is some variability, typically, items are scored from 1-4, "not at all" being 1 rather than 0 to avoid negative scores, and individual item scores are summed for the particular factor or dimension on which they load *and the total is then divided by the number of items loading on that factor to yield a mean factor score*. If these mean factor scores are then used to produce a mean for the group, they will then be *means of mean factor scores*. The factors or underlying dimensions of the scale are Conduct Problem, Inattention, Anxiety, Hyperactivity and Sociability.

Psychometric work on this scale (see Werry & Hawthorne, 1976; Werry et al., 1975b) has shown that while there is some variation in the factor structure in different studies (a not uncommon problem with factor analysis), this is too small to warrant any change in this widely accepted scale. Interobserver reliability data are lacking, though similar scales are satisfactory if not outstanding (Spivack & Swift, 1973) and it is subject to the practice effect described in Section I between first and second administrations independent of any treatment (Werry & Sprague, 1974), so that posttreatment scores will ordinarily be lower than pretreatment ones. If a placebo period is not used, this practice effect makes an interpretation of results difficult, since while some of the change *may* be due to treatment, it will be impossible to know how much.

No good data are available for the test/retest reliability of this scale. Some crude norms are available for U.S. Midwestern, New York City and New Zealand children (see Werry & Hawthorne, 1976; Werry et al., 1975b) if the scale is to be used diagnostically as suggested by Sprague et al. (1974). However, in contrast to its value as a measure of drug effect, its diagnostic use to predict drug response has not been particularly successful (Barkley, 1976).

One of the other areas where data are lacking is the correlation of this scale with other sources of data. In his review of this, Werry (in press a) concluded that while changes in this scale do tend to covary with changes in other treatment measures on a *group basis*, there have been few studies of intercorrelations between measures in *individual children* and, such as there are show low or little intercorrelation (Gittelman-Klein & Klein, 1975; Rapoport & Benoit, 1975).

Some persons object to individual items as vague or badly worded but, despite this, the scale seems well accepted by teachers and has been shown in numerous studies (Conners & Werry, in press) to be drug sensitive. It is highly recommended for studies involving hyperactive, inattentive or aggressive children, but could profit from further psychometric study, particularly of its reliability and validity. However, it is unlikely to be suitable in certain diagnostic groups, especially those characterized by phobias or withdrawal. The shortened 10-item version (Parent Teacher Questionnaire or PTQ), discussed in more detail under parent scales, seems a useful alternative where a simpler version is required for some particular reason.

Another good teacher scale, not yet used in psychopharmacology or widely outside England, is that developed for the Isle of Wight studies which, in a manner which could well be emulated, has been subjected to an unusually thorough testing by the originators (see Rutter et al., 1976). However, its use seems to have been restricted to epidemiological needs of diagnostic screening and it does not seem to have been used as a measure of change, so necessary in pharmacotherapy. Because of some degree of misclassification inevitable in any single source instrument, Rutter et al. advise against its use as the only diagnostic device for an individual child, though this caution would apply to any such instrument. It might well prove useful in pediatric psychopharmacology as a subject selection device (say 9 or more symptoms, as used by the originators to define pyschiatric disorder) or as a predictor of drug effect, though both these roles would have to be proven empirically.

In his review of rating scales, Conners (1973a) refers to two other American scales for teacher use, besides his TQ and PTQ—the Devereux Elementary School Behavior Rating Scale (47 items) and the Rocky Mountain Educational Laboratory Scale (80 items). However, the better known of these two, Devereux Scale, has had less psychometric study than another American scale, the Behavior Problem Checklist (BPC) (55 items) developed by Peterson & Quay (see Quay, in press) and has less predictive validity than the BPC (Proger et al., 1975). The BPC has reliability data and yields four behavioral dimensions—conduct problem, anxiety-withdrawal, immaturity-inadequacy and socialized delinquency. It is designed as a screening and predictive instrument rather like the Isle of Wight one but, unlike the latter, is suitable for use by any parent, teacher or caretaker. It, too, has considerable predictive validity in terms of prognosis or social outcome but has been used only occasionally in pediatric psychopharmacology (Weiss, 1975). Quay's (in press) extensive review is particularly recommended for further reading on this whole issue of children's rating scales. It also discusses several other scales not mentioned here.

One of the more popular simpler scales, like the equally simple Conners PTQ designed for use by teacher or any caretaker, is the Davids (1971) Hyperkinetic Scale which, as the name suggests, is more specific in scope than the previously mentioned scales which are all more or less wide range. The Davids scale has 7 items (hyperactivity, short attention span, behavioral variability, impulsiveness, irritability, explosiveness and poor school work) and appears drug sensitive (Arnold et al., 1976). However, like most rating scales, it is subject to the usual practice effect (Neisworth et al., 1974) and to rater bias (Neisworth et al., 1974). While it is simpler than the TQ, it has been much less researched and is more narrow.

Preschool children pose a particular problem since most of the above scales are unsuitable. The Children's Behavior Inventory (Burdock & Hardesty, 1973; ECDEU, 1976) discussed below is suitable for this age group. Camp and Smerling (in press), in their review of this area, suggest the Classroom Behavior Inventory (Walker, 1973) and discuss other possibilities, including an adaptation of the Isle of Wight Scale. These are all diagnostic scales with known psychometric properties though their suitability as change instruments is unknown.

Teacher information is to be particularly commended in pediatric psychopharmacology since, not only does it offer a confirmation and rounding out of data from other sources, but a teacher is more likely to be aware of drug-produced changes in peer interaction, in zest and learning, some of which, particularly with depressant drugs, might not be too conspicuous at home (e.g., Werry & Aman, 1975).

What data there are (e.g., Gittelman-Klein & Klein, 1975; Rapoport & Benoit, 1975; Safer & Allen, 1976, p. 80) suggest that, in addition to the desirable properties of drug sensitivity and interrater reliability, teacher ratings have the best correlation of any one data source with measures from other sources. However, as noted by Barkley (1976), the ability of teacher ratings to predict drug action is weak, though there are, as yet, no good predictors of drug effect and the subject has not received a great deal of systematic study.

2) *Parent Scales*: Various good reviews of this area are available (Conners, 1973a, 1976a; Conners & Werry, in press; Hetherington & Martin, in press; Quay, in press) where the problem of parents as observers has been discussed. As pointed out in these studies and in Section I, profes-

sional prejudice notwithstanding, the empirical evidence is very much in favor of the reliability and validity of parent ratings though, understandably, parents may see different facets of behavior than other raters such as teachers. Obviously, though, while this is true in general, there will be individual parents who are quite unreliable as raters.

While rating scales for parents, like those for teachers, are numerous, again only three appear to have been used at all regularly in pediatric psychopharmacology. The first is Conners Parent Questionnaire (PQ) (Conners, 1970, 1973a; ECDEU, 1976), a 93-item scale which has 7 basic dimensions or factors (Conduct Disorder, Anxiety, Impulsivity, Immaturity, Psychosomatic Complaints, Obsessionality, Antisocial Problem). Rating and scoring are similar to the TQ with the ultimate scores being mean factor scores. According to Conners (1970, 1973a) the scale discriminates well between psychiatric and normal children, and has an interparent reliability of .85; however, it has not been the subject of studies of test/retest reliability, nor has its relationship to other commonly used measures such as the TQ, particularly with drug induced changes, received much attention. What little data there are are not supportive (Gittelman-Klein & Klein, 1975; Rapoport & Benoit, 1975). As far as sensitivity to drug effects is concerned, although Conners (1973a) found in his own studies that the first 2 factors (conduct problem and anxiety) showed drug changes, other investigators have not found the scale very sensitive (Gittelman-Klein & Klein, 1975; Gittelman-Klein et al., 1976b; Werry & Sprague, 1974). Gittelman-Klein and Klein (1975) claim that this is because the scale is too heterogeneous, so that some items which can change only with unwanted side effects tend to obscure the effect of others which reflect improvement. It is also susceptible to the practice effect between first and second ratings mentioned above in TQ; in fact, this effect is somewhat more marked with this questionnaire (Gittelman-Klein & Klein, 1975; Gittelman-Klein et al., 1976b; Werry & Sprague, 1974). It is also extremely cumbersome with its 93 items. Thus, despite its adoption by ECDEU and its wide use in pediatric psychopharmacology, this measure does not seem to meet the requirements of a good scale so clearly evident in the Conners TQ. It may yet prove to have diagnostic or predictive capacities, though the evidence to date in this respect is conflicting (Barkley, 1976). However, its insensitivity and cumbersomeness vitiate its use as a measure of drug effect.

Conners was obviously aware of the problems with the PQ and produced a simplified version, the PTQ (mentioned above), of 10 items common to both TQ and PQ (see ECDEU, 1976). One study (Werry et al., 1975b) showed this scale to correlate well with the larger TQ and others suggest that it is drug sensitive (Conners & Werry, in press; Lerer & Lerer, 1976; Sleator et al., 1974). Thus, it looks like a good scale, but needs further investigation.

A third scale, the Clinical Global Impressions, used commonly and most effectively in adult psychopharmacology where the rater is ordinarily the psychiatrist or physician (Lipman et al., 1965), has also been used in pediatric psychopharmacology, with parents and teachers as well as doctors as raters (Conners, in press; Gittelman-Klein et al., 1976b; Werry & Sprague, 1974). Of all the *parent* utilizable rating scales, this would appear to be the simplest and most drug sensitive. This consists of a simple 7-point scale in which the parent (or other rater) is asked to rate the degree of overall change about a nodal point of 4 (unchanged), with the 3 points either side ranging from minimal to much through very much. Criticism may be offered that this scale yields no information about the *nature* of any drug-induced changes, and this is a valid objection. However, it can be used, most valuably, as a detector of drug effects and their overall social direction. It is particularly useful in making the decision as to whether to continue medication or not.

The Davids Hyperkinetic Scale, discussed under Teacher Scales above, might also be a useful parent scale to specify change areas in hyperkinetic children (Arnold et al., 1976), as might that developed by Arnold and Smeltzer (Arnold et al., 1972, 1973, 1976) which is drug sensitive though it exhibits the typical practice effect.

Other scales are the Devereux Child Behavior Rating Scale (Conners, 1973; ECDEU, 1976), the Isle of Wight Parent Scales (Rutter et al., 1976; Rutter, 1976) and the Behavior Problem Checklist (Quay, in press), all of which have a significant amount of psychometric study, but none has been used much in pediatric psychopharmacology and, as with teacher use or equivalents, their principal use seems to be diagnostic. As such, they might well have a role to play in subject selection or prediction of drug effects.

For children of preschool age, Camp and Smerling (in press) recommend the Louisville Behavior Checklist (Miller, 1976) and the Home Behavior Inventory (Schaefer & Aaronson, 1966). The Child Behavior Inventory (Burdock & Hardesty, 1973; ECDEU, 1976) is also suitable for, though by no means restricted to, this age level. While there are a certain amount of reliability and validity data for these scales, none seems to have been designed as other than a screening or prognostic instrument and their suitability as measures of drug-induced change is unknown.

In *summary* then, the role of parent scales in demonstrating psychopathology is well established and acceptable scales for children at all ages exist, though few of these scales have been used as measures of drug effect. Of those that have, most have shown that, given a suitable instrument, parents can be reliable and sensitive detectors of drug-induced changes in their children's behavior and, while doctors tend to give them less credence than teachers in their final assessments (Gittelman-Klein & Klein, 1975), they have a useful role as raters in pediatric psychopharmacology.

3) *Physician Scales*: Since all children on medication must be assessed regularly by a physician who must also make decisions about further treatment, physician-based estimates of indications for and effects of drugs are of paramount importance. Diagnostic rating scales based on physician *interviews* have been discussed above (see Diagnosis). The 63-item Children's Psychiatric Rating Scale (CPRS) (ECDEU, 1976) mentioned above has not been used extensively to date as a measure of drug effect. In one study, Gittelman-Klein et al. (1976b) found only 17 items occurred, of which half showed drug changes.

A variety of other physician-based measures have been reported (Arnold et al., 1972; Hoffman et al., 1974; Weiss et al., 1971a; Werry et al., 1966) and there seems to be a regrettable lack of standardization in this area, with one exception and that is the Clinical Global Impression (ECDEU, 1976). The use of this scale by the physician differs from that by parents or teachers in that data from all sources (parent, teachers, child, etc.) are used and there are two scales in addition to the 7-point improvement scale. The first is an *efficacy index*, a two-dimensional classification of 4 points each, one dimension being therapeutic effect and the other a global rating of the degree of side effects. The second additional scale is for global rating of the severity of the psychiatric disorder.

The CGI scale then has some distinct advantages as a measure in that it allows for the weighting of data from a variety of sources which may well be in conflict and takes account not only of good effects, but of side effects, both of which are critical to decisions about overall benefit and continuation of medication.

Other physician-based measures deserve mention. Two are from Rapoport et al. (1971, 1974b) and are really observations, one from a playroom situation and one from parent diaries, but these require a physician's judgment at the end to convert the results into ratings. They are described in the subsection on observations below.

The third (Arnold et al., 1972) is unique and ingenious in that it attempts to provide idiographic or individual data within a nomothetic framework to suit both individual patient and research needs. Parents are asked to state the 4 to 5 most pressing problems which are then shaped into reasonably clear terms by the interviewing physician. At each reassessment, the physician records on an index card comments from interviews with parents, children, or anyone who is in contact with the child, in a manner analogous to rating the Clinical Global Impressions. At the end of the study (or treatment), the cards are sorted into a rank order of change independently by two or more physicians. These rankings can then be combined for all the children and treated by non-parametric statistics to test for drug effects. This method, which has been proved drug sensitive in the originators' hands, would seem to have much to commend it, particularly if children get rather similar assessment since, if a crossover design is used, it combines the needs of clinical practice and of research and helps deal with individual variation in symptomatology.

In *summary* then, the role of the physician-based estimates of problem behavior and drug effects (including side effects) would seem to be most unique and valuable when they attempt a *synthesis of all the available information* to arrive at a global estimate. Their value will obviously be only as good as the extent and reliability of data from other sources and the doctor's clinical skill in eliciting data from parent and child. They will also be liable to distortions inherent in his expectations of a particular treatment and hence will be best when he can be kept blind, though if he has to monitor for side effects this will not be easy (Cole, 1968; Werry & Aman, 1975; Werry et al., 1975a).

4) *Other Professionals*: Perhaps because children are hospitalized only infrequently for psychiatric problems, there are no inpatient nurse rating scales (like the ECDEU's adult NOSIE). However, the Children's Behavior Inventory (ECDEU, 1976) is eminently suitable for such purposes. It consists of 139 items in developmental clusters so that progressively more items are added with each age level up to 13. It is of demonstrated interobserver reliability (Burdock & Hardesty, 1973; ECDEU, 1976) though some training of raters is necessary, and a minimum of 8 hours exposure to the child during different activities on each rating occasion is recommended. Scoring is simplified by the use of 9 subcategories of items, but the differing numbers of items at two-year intervals would make comparisons between children difficult. No data are available as yet on its sensitivity to drug effects. Other nurse or child care worker measures useful in inpatient or day-patient settings are discussed under Observations.

Since psychologists frequently have to administer tests in the course of a drug study, it is not surprising that there are a number of rating scales which utilise this particular observational setting. One such is that used by Gittelman-Klein and her colleagues (Gittelman-Klein & Klein, 1975; Gittelman-Klein et al., 1976b) which yields 10 ratings (gross motor activity, distractibility, cooperation, frustration tolerance, mood, attention to work, aspiration level, attention seeking devices, interest in tasks and anxiety about failure) rated from 1-5. This measure was drug-sensitive in the originators' hands (Gittelman-Klein & Klein, 1975; Gittelman-Klein et al., 1976b) but has not been used by other investigators. Also worth attention is the scale recording frequency of events like intrusions by the tester and overall activity level by Rapoport et al. (1974b) which correlated somewhat with other measures (Rapoport & Benoit, 1975) and was drug-sensitive.

In short then, administration of psychological tests like the WISC offers a common and relatively standardized observing situation in which drug effects can be detected.

Loney et al. (in press) have developed a reliable rating system yielding 8 categories of symptoms (negative affect, aggression, hyperactivity, inattention, judgment deficits, incoordination, fidgetiness, and lacks self esteem) which can be applied to case history material to produce initial ratings when these data are available but only in anecdotal form. This would be particularly useful for retrospective or informal studies.

5) *Peer Ratings*: This type of measure uses the child's peers—nearly always classmates—as raters. In their recent review, Pekarik et al. (1976) point out that, in addition to the advantages of rating scales discussed above, this type of measure is stable, independent of sex or age of raters, agrees well with other (adult) raters and behavior observations and can predict maladjustment. These measures have an additional advantage in that they tend to be free of the prosocial embellishment found particularly in child self ratings but also, to some extent, in parent ratings. Added to the teacher rating, they improve discriminative and predictive power. However, most extant peer evaluation methods, in their view, are too narrow in scope or target population to be very useful. Building on previous scales and data relating to them, they developed a 35-item Pupil Evaluation Inventory in which each child in the class rates each other child. The scale, which had 3 factors (aggression, withdrawal, likeability) was stable, had a high interrater reliability and correlated well with teacher ratings. In short, it was psychometrically robust.

Because of criticism by civil rights groups of authority-based judgments leading to the overuse of behavior modifying drugs in children, peer assessments have a certain attractiveness. However, the fact that the whole class or a large portion of it would have to be involved makes them too cumbersome and disruptive for routine use in pediatric psychopharmacology. Also, their sensitivity to drugs would have to be established if use were to be extended beyond diagnosis. Perhaps their greatest value would lie in validating teacher and parent judgments.

OBSERVATIONS

As noted in Section I, observations record behavior as it happens with a minimum of inference or data reduction and, ordinarily, in the child's natural environment. Jones et al. (1976) have suggested the term *naturalistic* to encompass all these features. There has been a great increase in the popularity of this measurement technique coincident with the rise of behavior modification and the behavioral approach to childhood psychopathology, but to date, there have been few applications in pediatric psychopharmacology (Werry, in press a). This method has been extensively reviewed (Jones et al., 1976; Johnson & Bolstad, 1973; Werry, in press a).

The advantages of this technique are objectivity, freedom from observer bias and direct relevance to the child's actual problems but there are real disadvantages too, namely the logistical difficulties and clumsiness of the technique, the expense, the objection of professionals to being observed, the boring nature of the task when repeated over long periods, leading to a loss of interobserver reliability (Johnson & Bolstad, 1973; O'Leary et al., 1975) (initially generally high in this technique), and the difficulty of getting sufficiently long runs of behavior and data from several environments. To date, its greatest defect as a measure in pediatric psychopharmacology where it has been used is its somewhat variable sensitivity to drugs.

Unlike rating scales, there is also somewhat of a shortage of good general scales applicable to groups of children since most of the behavioral work has been oriented toward custom-based measures for a particular case, though even this has been used to advantage by converting individual behaviors to common categories such as negative interactions (Rapoport & Benoit, 1975) or using changes in the ranking of target behaviors (Arnold et al., 1972, 1973, 1976).

Since it is difficult—short of videotaping—to record *everything* that happens as it happens and even more difficult to utilise such an amorphous mass of data, most behavior observations delineate categories of behavior to be observed. Where this is not done, as in the running record (see below), the recorder will usually do it in lieu to some extent.

There are three main ways of doing behavior observations: 1) the running record; 2) time sampling, and 3) mechanical recordings.

1) The *running record* in which *all* the occurrences of one or more behaviors are recorded over a period of time as, for example, in the recording of the number of wet nights in the treatment of enuresis or the number of temper tantrums in a day. An example of this is the parent diary method (Rapoport & Benoit, 1975; Rapoport et al., 1971, 1974b) in which parents record all the events involving the child over a specified number of days, usually two weekends and two weekdays. The data have, of course, to be reduced substantially by ratings into various categories (activity shifts, negative interactions and a global rating of problem behavior) which makes this less than a typical behavior observation. Greater use could be made of this technique in the treatment of individual children, by selecting behaviors pertinent to that child and getting the mother to note them as they occur during a pre, intra or post drug and, preferably, placebo period. The diary method has proven drug sensitive in the originator's studies (Rapoport et al., 1971, 1974b).

2) *Time sampling*: Instead of recording all the time, however, most investigators resort to sampling behavior, assuming, of course, that their time sample is a valid indicator of the whole. The necessary proportion of a given behavioral situation (such as the classroom) to observe, or the *reliability of data sampling*, as it is called (Patterson & Reid, 1970), is a poorly researched question. Most seem to opt for a manageable but arbitrary interval around 30 minutes (e.g., Patterson, 1969; Werry & Quay, 1969), though Rapoport & Benoit (1975), in their home observation technique, used one hour. Children's behavior is highly variable, even in a basically similar situation like the daily arithmetic session (Werry & Quay, 1969), and this is no doubt one of the reasons that rating scales, with their averaging power, are more drug sensitive than time samplings.

Available methods which have been used in drug studies and found to be drug sensitive at least one, though, unfortunately, often not more than that, even with the originators, are: 1) the classroom techniques of Gittelman-Klein et al. (1976a, b), Werry & Quay (1969), Wolraich et al. (in press); 2) the very simple playroom technique of Rapoport et al. (1971, 1974b; Werry & Sprague, 1974); 3) the 3-minute-per-hour daily check for inpatients, easily utilisable by nursing or child care staff with minimum disruption of their work, of Alderton and Hoddinot (1969); 4) the nursery school techniques of Schleifer et al. (1975); and 5) the psychologist counts of her limit-setting intrusions during tests (Rapoport et al., 1976b) described in the rating section (under Other Professionals). A number of other attractive methods have been tried but have not proven drug sensitive, such as the play/peer interaction methods of Ellis et al. (1974). As a general rule, *free field* methods in which the child is left to his own devices have proven less drug sensitive than those in which demands are made on the child; this has been noted as a general principle in pediatric psychopharmacology (Whalen & Henker, 1976). There is only one good method for studying family interactions, that of Patterson (Jones et al., 1976; Patterson & Cobb, 1971). Though this has not been used in pediatric psychopharmacological studies, it covers such an important area that it deserves a mention (Werry in press a).

3) *Mechanical Recordings*: These are discussed in the section on activity since it is there that they have received greatest use.

In *summary* then, behavior observations have many attractive features for pediatric psychopharmacology, both as diagnostic and effect measures, but they are not lacking in difficulties and disadvantages. As yet, their potential has not been fully exploited.

SUMMARY OF MEASURES OF BEHAVIOR

There are a wide variety of measures of behavior suitable for use in pediatric psychopharmacology though most are considerably better at detecting drug effects than at predicting which children will respond to medication. All methods have advantages and disadvantages, with teacher-based ratings probably the best established and most studied. However, the correlation between different measures and different observers or raters is, at best, modest (Whalen & Henker, 1976). Some of this discrepancy is inevitable since behavior is highly variable across environments (Moos, 1973), and some may be an artefact inherent in the statistical method, such as factor analysis, used to score the results (Miller, 1976). This means that no one method or one person has a premium on truth and best results will come when a combination of methods is used and data are synthesized into a meaningful clinical statement or decision. Numerical or statistical techniques may help in this, but some global clinical judgment will be necessary in the end.

Activity

This behavioral dimension occupies a place of central importance in pediatric psychopharmacology since one of the prime indications for psychotropic drugs in children is hyperactivity. There has been much well deserved criticism of the latter notion as vague and variously interpreted (e.g., *British Medical Journal*, 1973; Rie, 1975; Werry, in press, a, b). As suggested by Cromwell et al. (1963) and reiterated at intervals since (e.g., MacKeith, 1974; Routh & Schroeder, 1976; Routh et al., 1974;

Werry, 1968a), activity should be regarded as a purely quantitative dimension of behavior. Unfortunately, it has been used promiscuously to include any kind of socially undesired act, like aggression, which is executed motorically (e.g., Huessy & Cohen, 1976) and/or disorders of attention (see Chapters 3 and 5). When a strictly quantitative definition is applied and proper measures used, many children diagnosed clinically as hyperactive prove to be no more active motorically than coevals, though a substantial minority are (Barkley & Ullman, 1975; Routh & Schroeder, 1976; Sprague et al., 1974; Werry, in press a, b). This has led to modification in the proposed classifications of children's psychiatric disorders discussed in Chapter 5.

While the term *activity* as used here will carry a purely quantitative connotation, since that is not sufficient reason for pharmacotherapy, the term *hyperactivity* will include an assumption that the level of activity is not only raised above normal, but that this increase results *of itself* in undesirable social consequences or is the source of complaint. Useful comprehensive reviews of measures of activity and of hyperactivity can be found in Cromwell et al. (1963), Sprague and Werry (1971, 1974) and Werry (1968a, in press a, b).

INTERVIEWS

Judgments by physicians or other professionals about activity and hyperactivity based on interviews with the child are, of course, one of the sources of data by which diagnoses and estimates of drug effects are made. When they conflict with parent or teacher judgments, they are sometimes accorded a superior validity (e.g., Kenny et al., 1971). However, considering the ordinarily brief time of observation and the strong dependence of behavior upon the situation (Moos, 1973, see below) which, in this case, is highly atypical of the child's real world, *observations on activity level from clinical interviews would seem among the least likely to be valid*, particularly when interviews are informal and do not follow one of the methods of established reliability (see Behavior).

RATING SCALES

Nearly all the rating scales discussed in the previous section on Behavior also yield measures of activity; however, because they are clinically oriented, these measures are mostly couched in terms of hyperactivity or, occasionally, other evaluative facets such as fidgetiness (e.g., Loney et al., in press).

There is only one currently popular rating scale which claims to be a measure of activity alone, namely, the Werry-Weiss-Peters Activity Scale (Werry, 1968a). It can be used by parents and other caretakers such as nurses or child care workers who see most of a child's daily behavior but, apart from a small section, is unsuitable for teachers because of their unfamiliarity with much of a child's domestic routines. This scale was developed at the request of the CIBA pharmaceutical company as an amplification of a reliable and drug-sensitive psychiatrist's rating scale based on a semi-structured interview with a parent (Werry et al., 1966). However, instead of the psychiatrist's global ratings for each category, a series of objective, situation-specific questions about motor behaviors, such as those occurring during meals or TV, were substituted and it became, in essence, a parent questionnaire. Because of its sponsorship, it began to be used in pediatric psychopharmacology but without any formal examinations of its psychometric properties. It certainly proved drug sensitive (Conners & Werry, in press; Gittelman-Klein & Klein, 1975; Rapoport et al., 1971), but recent studies have revealed some significant shortcomings. It does not correlate well with objective measures of activity (Barkley & Ullman, 1975; Gittelman-Klein & Klein, 1975; Routh & Schroeder, 1976; Routh et al., 1974; Shaffer et al., 1974) or with teachers' estimates of hyperactivity (Gittelman-Klein & Klein, 1975; Gittelman-Klein et al., 1976b) and correlates with estimates of conduct disturbance rather than activity (Shaffer et al., 1974). However, if a *group* of children defined as hyperactive by the scale is compared with normal children as a whole, the hyperactive group will score more highly on objective measures of activity, like grid crossings. A factor analytic study (Routh et al., 1974) revealed that instead of a single, homogeneous dimension of activity, the scale consists of 7 discrete factors, some specific to the kind of behavior (e.g., verbal) and some to the situation (TV behavior).

In summary then, the Werry-Weiss-Peters Scale is drug-sensitive, but appears to be less a measure of activity than of various kinds of motor behavior with an emphasis on those which are socially unacceptable. It is thus as much a "problem child" defining measure or measure of *hyperactivity* as we have defined it here as an estimate of activity level. Its failure to correlate well with other estimates of activity (or even hyperactivity), while no doubt due, in part, to the secondary complications of being overactive, suggest that *activity level as a unitary quantitative dimension of behavior which transcends all environments is too simplistic a notion* and perhaps that one of the characteristics of hyperactive children is their relative, rather than absolute, inability to inhibit motor behavior, or, as suggested in DSM III, the defect lies in attention not motor activity.

Again, this raises the problem discussed in Section I as to what is the correct measure, or what is the real problem? The scale certainly measures what the parent sees as a problem in the motor area and what presumably thus becomes a problem for the child. Whatever the true nature of this problem, the scale can detect drug changes in it.

These validity problems have been discussed at some length because they would appear equally true of all the general behavior rating scales discussed above under Behavior, as far as the measurement of hyperactivity is concerned. Even the purer, factored scales like Conners TQ and PQ have items loading on the hyperactivity factors which are obviously conduct type and which, in fact, in subsequent factor analyses, sometimes load on conduct problem factors (see Werry et al., 1975b). One of the purer-looking, more recent scales containing hyperactivity items is that by Loney et al. (in press), but its validity is still to be confirmed. The simple Davids Hyperkinetic Scale, which likewise contains some activity items, has a marked vulnerability to rater bias (Neisworth et al., 1974), though this is likely to be a bias common to most rating scales—it is just that this one has been investigated!

OBSERVATIONS

Again, most of the methods described under Behavior include self-evident activity measures. As with rating scales, too, in the clinical situation of diagnosing problem behaviors or estimating drug effects, general measures are likely to prove more useful overall than those restricted to motor activity. As a result, observational measures of activity alone are uncommon, being combined usually with other measures, notably of attention. A typical technique (Barkley & Ullman, 1975; Cromwell et al., 1963; Klaverboer, 1975; Pope, 1970; Rapoport et al., 1971; Routh et al., 1974; Routh & Schroeder, 1976; Shaffer et al., 1974; Werry, in press a; Wolraich et al., in press) consists of putting the child in a room in which toys are distributed in various sectors, with the floor marked off in squares for easy counting, though it can be used in naturalistic situations such as nursery schools, too (Schleifer et al., 1975). It is important to distinguish between free-play and restricted (by instruction not to move or sedentary task requirements) situations since results are quite different; it is only in the latter that hyperactive children most typically differ from normals (Barkley & Ullman, 1975; Routh & Schroeder, 1976; Schleifer et al., 1975) and drug effects may differ accordingly (Hutt et al., 1961).

The advantages and disadvantages of observational measures have been discussed in detail under Behavior and will not be repeated except to note that despite their objectivity they are, in general, of variable sensitivity to drug effects.

MECHANICAL AND ELECTRONIC METHODS

Since activity is a quantitative dimension of behavior, it would seem to be eminently suitable for automated measurement. Indeed, there has been some effort in this direction (see Cromwell et al., 1963; Sprague & Werry, 1971, 1974; Werry, in press a), though only modest and with some surprising omissions, such as relatively infrequent use of videotape and movie cameras (e.g., Ellis et al., 1974; see also Sprague & Werry, 1971, 1974). It is probable that expense of the equipment, the tediousness of data analysis and obtrusion into the observing situation have acted as deterrents though the development of cheap, portable video equipment should have reduced some of these problems.

The most popular mechanical device is the actometer, a modification of the self-winding wrist watch, developed by Schulman and Reisman (1959) and now marketed commercially by the Timex Watch Company (Barkley & Ullman, 1975). Ordinarily, it is placed upon wrist or ankle. The device has some inherent problems (Johnson, 1971), namely, it responds to *acceleration* more than to *degree* of movement and it is uniplanar, a defect which can be minimised by the placing of two devices in planes at right angles. It is also obviously sensitive only to movement in that part of the body to which it is attached. Surprisingly, in contrast to its use in recording activity (Barkley & Ullman, 1975; Kaspar et al., 1971; Pope, 1970; Schulman et al., 1959), it has been used only infrequently in measurement of drug effects (Millichap & Boldrey, 1967; Millichap & Johnson, 1974) where it proved drug sensitive.

Other less frequently used devices are light grids focused on photo-electric cells, ballistographic devices (Ellis & Pryer, 1959), pressure sensors in the floor (Cromwell et al., 1963; Montagu & Swarbrick, 1975), pedometers (Rapoport et al., 1971), telemetric instruments (Sprague & Werry, 1971) and the ingenious ultrasonic devices. (Montagu & Swarbrick, 1975) which are similar in principle to the burglar alarm. All these devices have been used occasionally to detect drug effects and have been successful to a varying degree. Most of them, however, are complicated, expensive, restricted to a laboratory situation, present problems in measuring sedentary activity, or have other defects (see Werry, in press a). Further, since someone must supervise the child when the apparatus is being used, they are considerably disadvantaged with respect to simple observer-based counts which can measure much more behavior such as sedentary activity and shifts in attention at the same time.

Two other devices deserve mention. The first is the stabilimetric chair of Sprague (Sprague & Toppe, 1966) which is inexpensive to construct, unobtrusive, produces simple numerical data and, in the originators' and the author's hands, is highly drug-sensitive with intratask type motor overflow (Sprague & Werry, 1971, 1974; Werry & Aman, 1975; Werry & Sprague, 1974; Werry et al., 1975 a, b).

The second is not strictly an activity device but measures a derivative of it, namely noise (Montague & Swarbrick, 1975). It appears drug-sensitive and would seem to have distinct possibilities for this particularly aversive aspect of activity.

In summary, while mechanical devices have many attractions and appear drug sensitive, a word of caution is necessary. Their intercorrelation with each other and with other objective measures such as grid crossings is at best modest, though considerably better than with rating scales. Like all objective activity measures, they are highly influenced by the testing situation. Restricted or demand-type conditions produce quite different results from the free play situation (Barkley & Ullman, 1975), usually magnifying or exposing differences between hyperactives and normals. With the exception of the actometer and the less useful pedometer (not suitable for anything except true locomotion—see Barkley & Ullman, 1975), they are mostly cumbersome and unsuitable for naturalistic observations.

SUMMARY OF ACTIVITY MEASURES

Activity measures suggest that activity level is only partly a stable personality characteristic, most being determined by the demands of the situation. It is not surprising then that ratings of activity level by parents and teachers do not correlate with situation specific, often highly artificial, objective measures, and are contaminated by qualitative social judgments. From a *clinical* point of view this is surely an advantage since it focuses attention on *problem areas* which are the proper targets of pharmacotherapy. However, from the research point of view, particulraly in examining the pharmacological properties of psychotropic drugs and for the study of activity, objective methods have considerable advantages.

Mood and Self-Image (Self-Ratings)

Here we will be concerned only with inner feeling states and self-image as *reported by the child*. This area of measurement has recently been reviewed by Rapoport (in press) who points out that, in contrast to adult psychopharmacology, self-ratings have scarcely been used in pediatric psychopharmacology because of the difficulties of applying these largely pen-and-paper tests to children. She points particularly to the problems of translating adult concepts into a form comprehensible to, acceptable to, and, as in the case of depression, valid for children. A further difficulty lies in the discrepancies reported (Herjanic et al., 1975; Montgomery & Finch, 1974; Morena & Litrownik, 1974; Wordarski et al., 1975) between self-reports and others' estimates, though, as was seen in the sections on history and diagnosis, this is not an invariant characteristic of child-derived data, but only more intimate material.

The problem of discrepancy between observers, so recurrent in this review, must in the end be accepted as one of the inescapable differences produced by information processing mechanisms as individual, flexible, and sensitive as human beings. The notion of which observer or reporter is right is, to some extent, sophistic; the question should be, rather, what is the goal in treatment? Surely one of the goals should be improvement of the inner state of the child where this is distressed. As noted, pediatric psychopharmacology has been less than zealous in studying drug-induced changes in inner comfort and, despite methodological difficulties, this must be rectified (Rapoport, in press; Werry, 1977; Whalen & Henker, 1976). Rapoport makes the important point that some adaptation of strict self-reporting may have to be made with younger children, such as reading the questions and taking oral answers or, as employed by the reviewer and his colleagues, pre-recording the questions on tape, which has the added advantage of standardization of presentation.

There are three types of self-report: 1) global change; 2) self-image; 3) inner feeling states.

GLOBAL CHANGE

Despite its simplicity and success with parents, teachers and physicians, the Clinical Global Impressions Scale (see above) has been used only occasionally with children (e.g., Gittelman-Klein & Klein, 1971) but can be drug-sensitive with them just as with reporters on their behalf. It merits further consideration, though the reviewer has not found it particularly sensitive with hyperkinetic children who tend to deny any change or simply report expected improved conduct.

SELF-IMAGE

This means simply how one feels about oneself as a person. The most popular and best—though scarcely adequately—studied device is the Piers-Harris 30 Yes/No Item Scale which is modestly valid in its ability to differentiate clinic from normal children and underachievers from normals (Piers, 1972). Rapoport found hyperactive children resistive to this test but this has not been the experience of this author and his colleagues who use the tape-recorded method of administration. Its use as a predictor or a measure of drug effect is unexplored except in one instance (Rapoport et al., 1974b) when it was insensitive to drug effects.

INNER FEELING STATE (MOOD)

Two mood states predominate in adult psychopharmacology—anxiety and depression-elation. The measurement of anxiety in children has attracted much more interest than depression, perhaps since mania and depression are disputed entities in children (see Rapoport, 1976 and Chapters 5, 7 & 10). According to Rapoport (in press) there is as yet only one mood instrument for children—an unpublished one by Kovacs and Beck, which showed a surprising number of depressive-type symptoms in a group of junior high school students; this instrument has yet to prove its utility in pediatric psychopharmacology.

There are a few prominent anxiety scale for children. The first is the Children's Manifest Anxiety Scale (Castaneda et al., 1956) which is the child equivalent of the Taylor Manifest Anxiety Scale derived from the well-known personality test, the MMPI. It consists of 42 anxiety items and 11 lie scale items to detect invalid responses. This scale is reliable, and seems to discriminate well between emotionally disturbed and normal children (see Montgomery & Finch, 1974), but it is not homogeneous, consisting of at least three kinds of anxiety—oversensitivity (or cognitively perceived anxiety), somatic anxiety symptoms and impaired concentration (Finch et al., 1974).

The long-held suspicion that anxiety is not homogeneous led Spielberger (see Montgomery & Finch, 1974) to develop the State-Trait Anxiety Scale which consists of two independent 20-item scales designed to measure *state* or here-and-now feelings of anxiety and *trait* or the tendency to generate anxiety as a stable personality dimension. Though still under study, it seems to have some degree of reliability and validity (see Bedell & Roitzsch, 1976; Montgomery & Finch, 1974). The interest of this scale for pediatric pyschopharmacology is that, as posited by the originator, the State Scale appears sensitive to stress, while the Trait Scale is not (see Bedell & Roitzsch, 1976). It thus has potential as both a diagnostic and a drug-effect measure.

An 11-item school-related self-rating scale developed by Loney et al. (1975, 1976, in press; Whaley-Klahn et al. 1976) for elementary school children was reasonably reliable, discriminated well between hyperactive and normal children, and has crude norms. It seems of potential value in pediatric psychopharmacology, since it gives information about the child's perception of teacher attitudes to him, as well as his about school, and also has mood indicators. However, as yet, it has not been used in actual drug studies.

SUMMARY

Self-reports are a neglected and potentially important data source in pediatric psychopharmacology, particularly if, as Rapoport (in press and Chapter 7) suggests, interest is to be extended beyond behavior disordered to emotionally distressed children. Global change measures, self-image and mood measures all merit considerations as selective, predictive and effect measures, with the development of alternatives where the existing instruments reviewed here are found wanting.

Intelligence, Cognition and Learning

Because of the complexity and importance of this area, it is covered separately in Chapter 3.

Motor Coordination and Development

See Part II (Motor Function).

II. PHYSICAL MEASURES

Physical Examination (Excluding Neurological)

Physical examination is part of the tools of trade of every doctor and so will not be discussed in detail. The fullness and frequency of the physical examination required will depend partly on response of the individual patient, partly on the pharmacology of the drug concerned, and partly on the state of knowledge about the drug, with early (Phase I) type studies obviously requiring much more vigilance than routine clinical use.

Two points are worth noting:

> 1) Almost all psychotropic drugs can cause idiosyncratic toxic responses such as blood and liver disorders at any time, but particularly near the beginning of treatment; their long-term use has not infrequently revealed unanticipated, special physical effects such as growth inhibition (stimulants), tardive dyskinesias (antipsychotics) and pig-

ment metabolism disturbances (chlorpromazine) in *some* patients taking the drugs. Thus, even when a drug is well established, periodic physical examinations and a properly vigilant attitude are necessary. Children are developing organisms and thus in some ways potentially more vulnerable to pharmacotherapy, with particular attention needing to be paid to physical development, as the recent history of the stimulants illustrates (see Chapter 6).

2) Despite its respectability, the physical examination as conducted clinically is a rough and ready affair, applied with varying degrees of thoroughness. For example, initial reports that the stimulants had no effect on cardiorespiratory function were subsequently shown to be erroneous when the precision of measurement was tightened up (e.g., Aman & Werry, 1975a; Ballard et al., 1976; Boileau et al., 1976; Greenberg et al., 1975). Thus the standard of the routine physical examination without further specification may be neither systematic nor fine enough for pediatric psychopharmacology, particularly in clinical trials, so that some properly detailed and systematized scheme is then desirable.

A particular facet of the physical examination not ordinarily done routinely, which has attracted interest in various childhood psychopathological disorders such as psychoses, learning disabilities, hyperkinetic and aggressive disorders (Goldfarb, 1960; Rapoport & Quinn, 1975; Steg & Rapoport, 1975; Waldrop et al., 1968), is that of minor congenital anomalies or malformations. These are scored in a systematic manner (see Rapoport & Quinn, 1975; Waldrop et al., 1968), are thought to represent minor anomalies of development in the first 12 weeks of intrauterine life and may have biochemical relationships with the monamines involved in the action of many psychotropic drugs (Rapoport & Quinn, 1975; Rapoport et al., 1976a, 1977). Rapoport and her colleagues suggest that minor physical anomalies may have major implications for distinguishing between subgroups of hyperkinetic children and hence for predicting drug action. This interesting area deserves further attention, particularly since the examination for these anomalies is painless, easily incorporated into the routine physical examination, and takes very little time to learn or to execute.

Laboratory Investigations

Modern medicine relies greatly on laboratory tests to supplement physical examinations. It is always a problem to know how much to investigate either preventively, as in a drug trial, or symptomatically when giving a drug clinically, since children abhor "needles" and many tests have other unpleasantness and even risks. The FDA (in press) and the

American Academy of Pediatrics guidelines set out a series of investigations which, as might be expected in trials of new drugs, are most extensive, covering particularly hematologic, hepatic, renal, cardiovascular and endocrine nervous system. Since the investigation of new drugs will ordinarily be covered by stringent governmental regulations, such as those of the FDA in the U.S., this is less of a matter for discussion than the procedures required in the continuing monitoring of a drug and in routine clinical use. Generally speaking, the use of special investigations in the monitoring of psychotropic drugs once their initial safety has been established has not been particularly useful and, indeed, all the important long-term effects so far appear to have been detectable by astute clinical observation and simple physical examination.

In recent years, there has been a great upswing in biochemical psychiatry, the tocsin of which in child psychiatry was sounded by Wender (1971). Indubitably, much of the impetus to this has come from the advent of the psychiatric drugs which, discovered serendipitously and applied empirically, have led to systematic study of their biochemical actions and to the induction of etiological hypotheses about various psychiatric disorders. Buttressed by observations of psychiatric disorders caused as side effects of medical drugs such as l-dopa and antihypertensive agents, and by animal models of psychiatric disorders such as the hyperkinetic syndrome (see reviews in Werry, 1977, in press b), all these hypotheses seem convergent on neural transmission by biogenic monoamines, acetylcholine and membrane physiology. Most of the psychiatric drugs useful in children act in this way (see Chapters 1, 6-10). It seems likely, then, that biochemical tests will assume an increasing role in prediction of drug-responsiveness. There have been some beginnings of this in pediatric psychopharmacology, though nothing of clinical significance has yet emerged (see Werry, 1977, in press b). One thing appears clear, however—any such biochemical predictors will not come from current laboratory procedures but from those that somehow can estimate brain or, more probably, localized transmitter and membrane states.

Neurological Examination

The neurological examination occupies a place of special interest in pediatric psychopharmacology because of the so-called minimal brain dysfunction syndromes such as the hyperkinetic syndrome, which are considered particularly suitable for pharmacotherapy, and because the psychotropic drugs all act on the nervous system and can produce neurological symptoms. The neurological examination thus has roles to play in diagnosis and treatment alike.

Many children with psychiatric disorders are considered to show *soft* neurological signs, not detectable by the routine neurological examination, and, therefore, special systems of examination are deemed necessary in child psychiatry and behavioral pediatrics. This is a most contentious area which has been reviewed at length elsewhere (Rutter et al., 1970; Werry, in press b). The conclusions seem to be that most of the so-called soft signs are, in fact, not bona fide neurological signs but immaturities or what Rutter et al. (1970) call *developmental signs*. They are more properly called developmental since they are abnormal only in a chronological sense, being found normally in younger children, and disappearing with age (Peters et al., 1974). They are soft in the sense that their significance in terms of etiology and of nervous system function is unknown. They could reflect learning or environmentality-based defects as much as inherent central nervous system (CNS) defects—many involve sensorimotor coordination, an age-dependent and, at least partly, learned skill.

There are several systems of examination which, in addition to the standard neurological examination, search for soft signs. The best studied by far (for reliability and validity) is that of Rutter et al. (1970), developed for the Isle of Wight studies. Others are Close's Physical and Neurological Examination for Soft Signs (PANESS) (ECDEU, 1976) which has not stood up well to validation studies (see Camp et al., 1977; Werry & Aman, 1976), those of Peters et al. (1974) and Werry et al. (1972) which have some reliability, validity and outcome data, and various others which have not been properly assessed or specified (Lerer & Lerer, 1976: Millichap, 1975; Paine & Oppe, 1966; Schain, 1972). For school age children, the method of Rutter et al. (1970) seems the best available. Developmental screening tests for preschoolers which often have a large neurological component are discussed in Frankenburg and Camp (1975).

The ECDEU (1976) Abnormal Involuntary Movement Scales (AIMS) is a special abbreviated neurological examination to screen for extrapyramidal symptoms (EPS), especially the tardive dyskinesias. It is systematized, takes less than 5 minutes to execute and is highly recommended where EPS producing drugs (see Chapter 8) are to be exhibited for long periods.

Motor Function

This is clearly allied with the neurological examination and developmental signs but is often approached in a somewhat different way. It is also one of the more frequently drug-sensitive of the neurological functions (Lerer & Lerer, 1976; Spring et al., 1976; Wade, 1976). The approach is sometimes that of a simple developmental type test which tries to establish a motor age or a percentile position. The best known test for this purpose is the Oseretsky Motor Development Scale for school age children (for preschool children, see Frankenberg & Camp, 1975). It has undergone various modifications (Bialer et al., 1974; Rutter et al., 1970; Sloan, 1955) mostly with a view to shortening an originally cumbersome test. It is important to stress, as pointed out by Rutter et al., that *this test does not give any qualitative neurological information, simply a developmental age.* The shortened versions appear reasonably reliable, agree well with judgments of neurological abnormality (unspecified) and are sometimes drug-sensitive.

Another test battery which deserves mention is the adaptation for children of the Halstead Neuropsychological Battery for children by Reitan, Klove, & Matthews (Reitan & Davison, 1974). Unlike the Oseretsky test, this is a true neurological type test which, through psychological-test type standardization of proceedings, seeks to refine and extend the standard neurological examination. Unlike psychological tests, however, it was developed in neurosurgical units with consequent rather better medical advice and validation. It includes tests of higher CNS function which are better classified as tests of cognitive function (see Chapter 3), but a self-standing section called the *motor performance battery* contains a group of motor tests which can yield both qualitative (e.g., unilateral muscle weakness) and quantitative results. Although unsuitable probably for routine clinical use, individual components such as maze tracing have distinct possibilities for use as measures of drug effect (including side effects) affecting the motor system (see ECDEU, 1976; Sprague, in press).

Electroencephalographic and Psychophysiological Measures

This is a most difficult area and at the outset it must be stated, in unequivocal terms, not one for the amateur or occasional operator. Both types of measures require expensive equipment, generate large quantities of data which often require computer anlaysis, are subject to serious artefacts from movement, electrode, machine and patient state factors. None of these problems is as great, however, as is the interpretation of the findings. Readers are referred to various reviews particularly relevant to children and pediatric psychopharmacology (Barkley & Jackson, in press; Ellingson, 1954; Millichap, 1975; Sroufe, 1975; Werry, in press b). The role of EEG abnormalities in the diagnosis and management of childhood psychopathologies is also discussed in Chapter 9.

The ordinary EEG is, at the moment, useful only as diagnostic instrument for serious neurological disorders like epilepsy. While children with psychiatric disorders, especially those subsumed under the rubric of minimal brain dysfunction, seem to have a higher frequency of abnormalities on the routine EEG, like the neurological findings, they are mostly of a *developmental* kind, in the form of slower basic rhythms or arrhythmias (Millichap, 1975; Werry, in press b) found normally in younger children with only a minority showing disturbances of the type suggestive of major brain dysfunction.

Specialized EEG techniques such as averaged evoked potentials (EP) which apply stimuli (usually auditory or visual) and record EEG changes have attracted interest lately in child psychiatry and, to a lesser extent, as possible predictors of drug response. Often they have been combined with other non-neurological psychophysiological measures such as the galvanic skin response, pupillography, myography and cardiovascular tone (Barkley, 1976; Conners, 1975a; Douglas, 1974; Halliday et al., 1976; Montagu, 1975; Montagu & Swarbrick, 1975; Porges et al., 1975; Satterfield, 1976; Satterfield et al., 1974; Zahn et al., 1975) aimed at evaluating arousal or attentional levels. While these measures show distinct promise as predictors and measures of drug response, a great deal more work is necessary before they can be accorded the status of useful measures in pediatric psychopharmacology.

Side Effects (Treatment Emergent Symptoms)

There are two principal kinds of side effects or, following official parlance (ECDEU, 1976), treatment emergent symptoms (TES). The first simply reflect the normal actions of the drug on systems other than the one of immediate concern. Thus, when imipramine (see Chapter 7) is given for treatment of depression, its inhibition of bladder action is called a side effect whereas in the treatment of enuresis this is the therapeutic action and any psychotropic effect is considered a side effect (Werry et al., 1975a). It is seldom possible to produce a therapeutic effect with psychotropic drugs *without simultaneously producing some unwanted effects* or TES. The second kind of TES, usually called *toxic effects*, is due to an idiosyncratic sensitivity to the drug, for example, the depression of bone marrow or production of jaundice with chlorpromazine (see Chapter 8). There are only a limited number of ways the body can react in this fashion and most of them are already well described, involving particularly bone marrow, liver and kidney, and not peculiar to psychotropic drugs. To be marketed, unless for a life-threatening condition such as cancer, a drug ordinarily has to be *relatively* free from serious and from toxic TES in normal clinical dosage, but these still do occur occasionally. In contrast, because they are multisystem (or dirty) drugs, most psychotropic drugs regularly produce minor annoyances in many systems. For a comprehensive coverage of possible range of TES with psychotropic drugs, see the monograph by Shader and Di Mascio (1970) and chapters on specific types of drugs elsewhere in this volume. A shorter, more readable review is to be found in Winsberg et al. (1976).

In the ordinary course of pharmacotherapy, it is these milder TES that are of principal concern and the role of the prescribing physician is to determine whether or not the therapeutic response is vitiated by the level of discomfort of TES. Occasionally, however, serious TES such as tardive dyskinesias, epileptic seizures and cardiac arrhythmias will occur, especially in higher dosages.

To detect TES it is necessary to look for them and not to be lulled into complacency because of the comparative safety of psychotropic drugs. The ECDEU Dosage and Treatment Emergent Symptoms Scale (DOTES) includes a systematic review of all body systems, part inquiry and part simple physical examination, with provision for special investigations, such as EKG or hematology, if these are felt necessary. The author uses this system of interrogation of the parent at each drug review, adding items derived from the physical examination, such as weight loss, later. Its great virtue is that, if followed, it leaves no important area uncovered or forgotten, but it has the detraction of generating a lot of pseudo side effects or false positives. For this reason, it is important to administer it first, *before drug treatment is started,* so that a baseline level of symptomatology can be established. It is important in ascertaining TES for physicians to remember psychotropic type side effects like tearfulness and irritability, covered in DOTES. A good knowledge of the pharmacological action of the drugs being used will also help to elucidate particular symptoms and relate them to treatment or incidental illness.

Other side effect screening devices are the AIMS for abnormal movements (see Neurological Section above and ECDEU, 1976), and those described in FDA guidelines (in press), Greenberg et al. (1975), Saraf et al. (1974) and Winsberg et al. (1974b). All except that by Greenberg et al. consist of a series of items, some behavioral and emotional and some physical, obtained partly by systematic interrogation of parents and partly by physical and laboratory examinations.

In summary, the most important thing about side effects is to look for them in a systematic but not overzealous way. Serious effects are rare in normal clinical dosage but minor annoyances are easily overlooked in children where most of the dialog tends to occur between doctor and parent, where children are often shy or afraid of the doctor, and where the side effects may be behavioral rather than expressed complaints.

Pharmacokinetic Measures

See Chapters 1, 6-10. In general, apart from antiepileptic and antimanic drug therapy, pharmacokinetic measures have no established place in clinical practice, though their research value is considerably more promising.

Summary of Physical Measures

Physical and neurological examinations in pediatric psychopharmacology are necessary for proper assessment and to monitor the physiological effects of medication. The frequency and extent of these examinations should be adjusted to the stage of treatment, to the risks of and state of knowledge about any particular drug, and to the child's symptoms. Special medical investigations need be done only in exceptional circumstances. While their research potential is high, their clinical utility at the moment is minimal.

CONCLUSIONS

In Table 1 are set out the reviewer's recommendations for measures to be used in pediatric psychopharmacology. In general, these are measures with which he has had personal experience, which are widely accepted, especially by official bodies such as NIMH or the FDA, and, if possible, which also have established reliability, validity, and drug sensitivity. Readers are referred to specific sections of the text for alternatives or additions and for substantiating comments or references. While in many areas there is no dearth of measures, in others, such as in self-reports and predictors of drug responsivity (see Barkley, 1976), there is a grave deficiency.

Most of the discussion has centered on non-biological measures. This is partly because physicians are more familiar with biological measures, but also because, apart from the detection of side effects, the role of biological measures in pediatric psychopharmacology to date has been disappointing. However, this situation is not likely to continue. *A priori*, since this type of measure is closer to the site of action of the drug, it must prove better ultimately as a measure of drug responsivity and efficacy than those based on behavior or feelings which are the algebraic sum-

TABLE 1
Recommend Measures

I. PSYCHOSOCIAL

Area	Data Source	Rater	Measure[1]	Use (C=Criterion[3] E=Effect I=Informational)	Reliability[3]	Validity[4]	Prediction[5]	Sensitivity[6]
A. Background/ History	Parent	Interviewer	1. CPDI & CSH (ECDEU 1976)	I/C	?	?	?	NA
			2. (Jenkins et al 1966 Loney et al—in press)	I/C	+	±	—	NA
B. Prior Treatment	Parent	Interviewer	1. CPDI (ECDEU 1976) 2. PMR (ECDEU 1976)	I	?	?	NA	NA
C. Family Function	Parent	Interviewer	1. Isle of Wight Scales (Rutter 1976) 2. Family Environment Scale (Moos 1974)	I/C I/C	+ +	+ +	? ?	? ?
D. Diagnosis	Parent Child	Physician Physician	1. Isle of Wight Scales (Rutter et al 1976) 1. Isle of Wight Scales (Rutter et al 1976) 2. CPRS (ECDEU (1976)	C/E C/E C/E	+ + ?	+ + ?	? ? ?	? ? ?
E. Personality			No recommendations					
F. Behavior (Ratings)	General Parent	Parent	1. Isle of Wight Scale (Rutter et al 1976) 2. Behavior Problem Checklist (Quay—in press) 3. Conners PQ (ECDEU 1976) 4. Conners PTQ (ECDEU 1976)	C/E C C/E C/E	+ + ? ?	++ ++ + +	? ? — —	? NA ± +

TABLE 1 (Continued)

Area	Data Source	Rater	Measure[a]	Use (C=Criterion[a] E=Effect I=Informational)	Reliability[a]	Validity[a]	Prediction[a]	Sensitivity[a]
			5. Hyperkinesis Scale (Davids 1971)	E	+(?)	+(?)	?	+
			6. Preschooler Home Behavior Inventory (Schaefer & Aaronson 1966)	C/E	+	+	?	?
	School	Teacher	1. Conners TQ (ECDEU 1976)	C/E	?	+	—	++
			2. Conners PTQ (ECDEU 1976)	E	?	+	—	+
			3. Isle of Wight Scale (Rutter et al 1976)	C/E	+	++	?	?
			4. Hyperkinesis Scale (Davids 1971)	E	+(?)	+(?)	?	+
	All	Physician	1. CGI (ECDEU 1976)	E	++	?	NA	+++
	Parent	Physician	1. Target Behaviors (Arnold et al 1972)	E	++	?	NA	++
	IQ Testing	Psychologist	1. Gitelman-Klein et al (1976b)	E	?	++	?	+?
	Inpatient Setting	Nurses, etc.	2. Rapoport et al (1974b)	E	?+	++	?	?
	Peers	Peers	1. CBI (ECDEU 1976)	C/E	+	+	?	?
			1. Pupil Evaluation Inventory (Pekarik et al 1976)	C	+	+	?	+
G. Behavior (Observations)	Home	Parent	1. Diary (Rapoport & Benoit 1975)	C/E	+	+	?	+
	Inpatient Setting	Observers	1. Patterson & Cobb 1971	C/E	+?	+?	??	?+
		Nurses, etc.	1. Alderton & Hoddinot (1969)	E	+	+	?	+
	School	Observers	1. Gitelman-Klein et al (1976)	C/E	+	+	?	+

TABLE 1 (*Continued*)

Area	Data Source	Rater	Measure[1]	Use (C=Criterion[2] E=Effect I=Informational)	Reliability[3]	Validity[4]	Prediction[5]	Sensitivity[6]
			2. Wolraich et al (in press)	E	+	?	?	+
H. Activity (see also Behavior)	Playroom	Observers	1. Rapoport et al (1971)	E	+	+	?	±
	General	Parent/Nurse	1. Werry-Weiss-Peters Scale (Werry 1968a)	C/E	±	±	?	++
	Playroom	Observers	1. Grid-crossing (e.g. Routh et al 1974)	C/E	+	+	?	±
		Mechanical	1. Ultrasonic etc. (Montagu & Swarbrick 1975)	C/E	+	+	?	+
	Anywhere	Mechanical	1. Actometer (see Barkley & Ullman 1975)	C/E	+	±	?	+
	Sedentary Task	Mechanical	1. Ballistographic Seat (Sprague & Toppe 1966)	C/E	+	+	?	++
I. Self Image	General	Child	1. How I Feel About Myself (Piers 1972)	C/E	+	+	?	−(?)
J. Mood (see also I)	School	Child	1. Loney et al (1975, 1976)	C/E	+	+	?	?
	General	Child	1. Depression Scale Kovacs & Beck (see Rapoport—in press)	C/E	No Information			
			2. State-Trait Anxiety Scale (see Montgomery & Finch, 1974)	C/E	+	+	?	?
II. PHYSICAL								
K. Minor Anomalies	Child	Physician	1. Rapoport & Quinn 1975	C	+	+	+(?)	NA
L. Neurological Status	Child	Physician	1. Rutter et al 1970	C/E	+	++	?	?
	Child	Physician	2. Peters et al 1974	C/E	++	++	−	−

TABLE 1 (Continued)

Area	Data Source	Rater	Measure[1]	Use (C=Criterion[2], E=Effect, I=Informational)	Reliability[3]	Validity[4]	Prediction[5]	Sensitivity[6]
M. Motor Function	Child	Psychologist	1. Modified Oseretsky Motor Development Scale (Rutter et al 1970; Bialer et al 1974)	C/E	+	+	−	±
			1. Motor Performance Battery (Reitan & Davison 1975)	C/E	+	+	?	±
N. EEG	Child	Electroencephalographer	1. Evoked Potentials (Conners 1975a, Halliday et al 1976)	C/E	+	+	±	+
			2. Resting (see Halliday et al 1976)	C/E	±	±	−	+
O. Psychophysiological State	Child	Psychophysiologist	1. See Conners (1975a) Montagu & Swarbrick (1975) Satterfield et al (1974)	C/E	±	±	±	±
P. Side Effects	All Systems	Physician	1. DOTES (ECDEU 1976)	E	?	?	NA	+
			2. Saraf et al 1974	E	?	?	NA	++
			3. Winsberg et al 1974b	E	?	?	NA	?
			1. AIMS (ECDEU 1976)	E	?	?	?	?
	Extrapyramidal System	Physician	2. Motor Performance Battery (Reitan & Davison 1975)	E	+	+	?	?

NOTES:

1. ECDEU (1976)—most can be found also in Psychopharmacology Bulletin (1973). The measure may not have been used as specified but would seem possible.
2. Criterion = for selection or classification of subjects or prediction of drug effect.
3. Reliability = Interobserver and/or test-retest.
4. Validity = discriminates psychiatric/nonpsychiatric groups and/or correlates with other measures and/or predicts outcome in other than drug studies.
5. Prediction = of drug responsiveness. See also Barkley (1976) for review.
6. Sensitivity = to drug effects.

mation of a wide variety of psychosocial and biological factors,* though obviously not to the exclusion of psychosocial measures which must serve as the final arbiters of pharmacotherapy.

A point frequently reiterated throughout this review has been that the measurement of behavior, emotions, cognition and so on is a highly specialized area, now in its second century, with a set of canons and a technical vocabulary which befits any applied science. To refuse to admit the expertise or to dismiss the technical vocabulary as jargon (as editors of medical journals are wont to do) is an hallmark of ignorance of the needs of scientific study appropriate to the interface between biology and the social and behavioral sciences, an interface nowhere more manifest than in pediatric psychopharmacology. This is no field for amateurs.

Another reiterated point is that data from different sources must be elicited and of the sources available the presently most useful are from parents, teachers and, to a lesser degree, the child himself.

It is the doctor's job to integrate all this information, weighing the importance, reliability and validity of each, and to reach a conclusion in the child's best interest. To the extent that the doctor takes the trouble to be informed on pediatric psychopharmacology, takes the trouble to elicit the requisite data properly, and is a good, sensitive clinician, so will his pharmacotherapy be in the best medical tradition.

---

* Contrarily, Whalen and Henker (1976) argue that psychosocial measures are potentially the best predictors, but only if they are addressed to as yet unresearched socio-cognitive concepts of etiology and medication held by the child and those in his social environment. This view, of course, minimises any direct drug-induced changes and is reminiscent of past psychodynamic explanations of antidepressant and antipsychotic drug activity in adults.

3

DRUGS, LEARNING AND THE PSYCHOTHERAPIES

MICHAEL G. AMAN, M.A.

INTRODUCTION

It has been aptly stated that the work of the young is to learn (Werry, 1968a, b). In pediatric psychopharmacotherapy the objectives of treatment often include improved learning in school. In other instances, while improvement in learning may not be an immediate consideration, it is of considerable importance to ensure that such medication does not impede normal learning. Thus, when children are treated with psychotropic drugs, any effects on learning are of paramount importance and must not be ignored when evaluating the overall effectiveness of drug therapy. Learning is the end but continuing result of a complex set of cognitive processes and while the global end result is the ultimate area of interest, it is likely to be heuristic to try to study its antecedents as well as learning itself.

Yet the study of drug effects on such cognitive processes associated with learning has been spasmodic and disjointed thus far. Although the actual *number* of drug studies investigating learning variables may initially appear large, when examined closely these studies often lack the qualities to enable firm conclusions to be drawn.

Since this is a most complex area, this review will first examine the cognitive deficits seen in the types of children to whom psychotropic drugs are given and the ways these deficits are measured. This will be followed by a look at drug effects on these deficits with a simultaneous examination of drug-sensitive measures of learning and other cognitive functions. Then the few empirical studies which look at drug effects on actual academic achievement and the even fewer which study the interaction between other psychological treatments and drugs will be examined. Finally, there will be a brief look at state dependency and its implications in the pharmacotherapeutic treatment of children, followed by overall conclusions.

Particular tests of cognitive function mentioned in the sections are generally readily commercially available throughout the English-speaking world through suppliers to psychologists who ordinarily administer them. If tests mentioned are not yet commercially available, reference sources are given. A useful general reference source with descriptions and evaluations for many of the tests is Buros (1972).

Cognitive Deficits in Different Diagnostic Groups

Before attempting to assess drug effects on specific learning variables, it makes good sense to examine what aspects of learning are deficient in the particular patient populations in which psychotropic drugs are often used. Despite voluminous research, because of naive concepts and poor methodology, answers to this question have been slow in coming, though there has been some improvement recently. This is not intended as an exhaustive review of the areas of cognitive deficits in exceptional children, but focuses on areas of particular interest in pediatric psychopharmacology.

Hyperactivity

Among the key clinical features of hyperactivity, certain cognitive ones have long been recognized: short attention span, distractibility and poor academic performance. This has been so much the case that, as can be seen in Chapter 5, the proposed new American diagnostic system shifts the primary criterion from hyperactivity to an Attention Deficit Disorder. However, the clinical impression of inattention and distractibility was not actually tested formally until recently. In a now classic study, Sykes et al. (1971) compared matched groups of hyperactive and control subjects on an experimenter-paced Continuous Performance Test. Essentially, this is a test of attention in which a random sequence of letters is presented and the subject is instructed to make a specified response (usually a lever press) when a target letter appears and to refrain from responding when the other letters appear (Sprague, 1973, in press). As compared with controls, hyperactive children detected fewer of the significant letters and made more incorrect (impulsive) responses to nonsignificant letters or were more inattentive. Surprisingly, the presence or absence of an auditory distractor had no influence on either group of children, suggesting that hyperactives were not necessarily more *distractible* in the laboratory situation.

In a related experiment which compared children with specific learning disabilities to controls on a vigilance task, Anderson et al. (1973) found that the learning disabled subjects performed at a deficit, making fewer correct detections and more false alarms. The learning disability group was further subdivided into hyper-, hypo-, and normoactive subgroups. It was found that the hyperactive learning disability children were most susceptible to attentional deficits, the hypoactive children showed some deficit but not as much, and the normoactive children manifested near correct performance.

Sykes et al. (1972) further investigated this area of attentional deficits in another comparison study employing hyperactives and controls. On this occasion several types of attentional measures were used including subject-paced and experimenter-paced tasks. The hyperactive subjects performed at a deficit only on the experimenter-paced task, suggesting that the attentional deficit is of a momentary and unpredictable nature and that these subjects can compensate for this when pacing themselves. *Thus, brief attention span has consistently emerged as a major area of difficulty with hyperactive children* and this has been perceived as an explanation for many of the other problems encountered by these children.

PERCEPTUAL FUNCTION AND COGNITIVE STYLE

Douglas (1974) has summarized a series of studies which examined other cognitive deficits in hyperactive children. Included in this battery was a large number of tests which assess abilities ranging from motor development to perceptual processes and academic achievement itself. Out of this battery of tests, the hyperactive-normal comparisons yielded two findings of import: The hyperactive children showed more scatter on the subtests of the Wechsler Intelligence Scale and they did more poorly on a group of tests usually considered measures of perceptual motor functioning (the Bender Visual-Motor Gestalt test, the Goodenough-Harris Draw-a-Person test, and the Frostig Developmental Test of Visual Perception). However, Douglas queried whether these results might simply reflect a basic attentional deficit, and not be of much diagnostic value in this group of children.

The study of *cognitive style* has become increasingly prevalent in recent years. Cognitive style refers to a child's characteristic manner, largely unrelated to IQ, of dealing with learning situations. Cognitive style has been used to refer to such dimensions as the amount of time a child takes before committing himself to a solution (this dimension is dubbed reflection-impulsivity) and also to his ability to ignore peripheral or distracting cues irrelevant or counterproductive to solution of the problem (field dependence-independence). One popular test of cognitive style, the Matching Familiar Figures (MFF) task (Kagan, 1965), requires the subject to select from an array of six line drawings that which is identical to the standard. Both accuracy and decision time are relevant measures. It has been argued that knowledge of a child's cognitive style can be useful not only in understanding the child, but also in customizing an educational program for the child (Satterly, 1976).

Campbell et al. (1971a) investigated differences of cognitive style between hyperactives and carefully matched controls, using a test of reflection-impulsivity (this test also has a strong perceptual element) and one of field dependence-independence. The former test showed that the hyperactives tended to be more impulsive in their responses and to make more perceptual errors of an unusual nature. The results of the latter test (field dependence-independence) suggested that hyperactive children have greater difficulty in isolating embedded figures from more complex designs, a finding which also could be interpreted as suggestive of a visual perceptual deficit.

In summary, the hyperactive child suffers from well-documented attentional problems, perceptual difficulties of a visual nature, and a tendency towards high levels of impulsivity when confronted with a task requiring a complex solution, particularly when tasks have to be performed at a rate which is other than one of the child's choosing. Since these deficits are common targets of drug treatment, they would seem to have an important role in pediatric psychopharmacology. Many other areas, including memory and discrimination learning, have not been well-studied in this group of children but deserve attention.

Specific Learning Disabilities

The term *specific learning disabilities* refers to a condition in which there is a substantial deficit in academic achievement in children of normal or superior IQ which cannot be reasonably attributed to emotional, motivational or educational problems. Some researchers prefer to use the term educational retardation to refer to a specified degree of deficit in achievement with respect to mental age (e.g., Rutter & Yule, 1973). Still others prefer the term learning backwardness to refer to an academic deficit of a certain number of months relative to chronological age (Pilliner & Reid, 1972). Clearly, there is a great deal of overlap regardless of which of the above terms is employed. While at the moment learning disability *per se* is not an indication for pharmacotherapy, it is frequently found in conjunction with bona fide indications like hyperactivity. There is also some experimental work (e.g., Gittelman-Klein & Klein, 1976) underway to see if learning disability does constitute any indication.

Laboratory tests have revealed some elemental skills or processes in which learning disability children appear to be deficient. Kirchner and Knopf (1974) tested high- and low-achievement children on a vigilance task and it was found that high achievers made more correct detections and fewer false responses, suggesting attentional difficulties in the low attention group. However, the attention study of Anderson et al. (1973), described above, relating findings to subgroups based upon activity level, should warn against too ready a generalization regarding learning disabled children as homogeneous, though attention deficits would seem to be a problem for this group.

Birch and Belmont (1964) have devised a test of auditory-visual integration which seems to discriminate between learning disability and control groups. The essential feature of this test is that it requires an active coding or translation of a stimulus from one sensory dimension (e.g., sound patterns) to another (e.g., light patterns) (Blank & Bridger, 1966). When compared to normal controls, children with specific learning problems show a substantial difficulty with this task. Thus, a deficit in *mediational capacity* seems to be characteristic of children with severe learning problems. This task has been refined (Blank & Bridger, 1966; Rudel & Denckla, 1976) and quite extensively used (Birch & Belmont, 1964, 1965; Blank et al., 1968). Though it does not seem to have been used to study hyperactives or drug effects in any diagnostic group, it would seem to be worthy of study in pediatric psychopharmacology. A related task *has* been employed with some success to study the mediational functioning of hyperactive children and stimulant drug treatment (Butter & Lapierre, 1974, 1975).

One of the major areas within specific learning disability is that of reading. The Matching Familiar Figures (MFF) task, developed by Kagan (1965) as a test of impulsivity and perceptual accuracy in children and discussed under hyperactivity above, has proved useful in differentiating good from poor readers and also in predicting reading performance one and two years later.

In a recent study (Aman, 1977), children with severe reading disabilities (2 years or more below both chronological and mental age) were compared to controls matched for age, sex, IQ and parental education. The reading disability children were shown to have deficits in attention, mediational capacity, and visual perception, but not on a test of short-term memory and on reflection-impulsivity as measured by the MFF task.

SUMMARY

Children with specific learning difficulties clearly have a number of cognitive problems. An attentional deficit is common, particularly in the more hyperactive of these children. They also exhibit difficulties in coding sensory input and in visual perception. Psychopharmacological studies then should take cognizance of these areas when dealing with learning disability children.

Mental Retardation

While mental retardation is not an indication for pharmacotherapy, commonly associated behavior problems (see Chapter 5) are, so that as a group the retarded are probably the most medicated in pediatric psychopharmacology (see Chapter 8).

Comparison studies which investigate differences between retarded children and controls face special problems of matching. Groups can be matched on chronological age (CA), or on mental age (MA) by comparing the retarded to much younger normal children of equivalent MA. When matched for CA, the study essentially investigates whether the retarded group suffers from a given deficit as a function of mental age. When matched for MA, however, the study enquires whether the retarded group suffers from a deficit, over and above that due to lowered mental age. Ideally, such comparison studies should use two control groups, one matched for CA and one matched for MA.

ATTENTION OR DISTRACTIBILITY

Like the hyperactive child, the mentally retarded child has long been considered clinically to suffer from brief attention span and a high level of distractibility (Crosby, 1972) and, to some extent, this has been borne out in the research. Semmel (1965) compared retarded and control subjects, matched for CA, on a test of vigilance. The retarded subjects had substantially lower vigilance scores, indicating an attentional deficit. In addition, Semmel found that the performance of the retarded tended to decay much more rapidly over time than did that of the controls. In an elegant study which included both CA and MA controls (as well as a non-institutionalized retarded groups), Crosby (1972) found that the attentional behavior of non-brain-damaged retarded children differed from that of normal children matched for CA, but not from that of normal children of the same MA. Additionally, although the retarded children had more lapses of attention, their performances were not more affected by *distraction* than normal subjects. Interestingly, these findings are identical to those obtained with hyperactive children (Sykes et al., 1971).

Zeaman and House (1963) have stated that the mentally retarded suffer from an extreme difficulty in picking out the relevant stimulus dimensions or distinctive characteristics when faced with a discrimination task involving the presentation of a group of common objects from which the subject must select that object which is representative of a given concept. The objects may differ along a number of dimensions, such as color, shape, size, and so on. Once the subject attends to the appropriate dimension, learning usually reaches criterion quite rapidly, regardless of intellectual ability. Zeaman and House concluded that it is the ability to select the appropriate stimulus dimension which distinguishes the mentally retarded on this task and this selection facility they labeled, somewhat confusingly, attention, since it seems more cognitive than simple vigilance or attention span.

However, Stevenson (1963), citing other research in this area, questions whether the retarded do suffer from an *exaggerated* disability of attention or stimulus selection; he questions whether it can be reliably demonstrated when the groups are matched for MA. Klugh and Janssen (1966) were unable to demonstrate a deficit in discrimination learning using such a matching procedure. However, they did discover that the retardates were frequently unable to *verbalize* the rule by which they solved the problems, a finding suggestive of a mediational deficiency, and confirming the cognitive rather than attentional nature of the task.

MEDIATION AND MEMORY

Das (1972) conducted a comparison study in which retarded children and controls were matched for MA. Reliable differences were demonstrated in reasoning ability, shorter memory and intermodal integration (mediational ability), suggesting exaggerated deficits in the retarded group. Of particular note here is the finding that this last category was the best discriminator of group membership. Thus, as noted above, this test of *cross-modal coding* may be a very useful tool for the study of cognitive effects of drugs, not only in the mentally retarded but in the learning disabilities as well. Winschel and Lawrence (1975) have reviewed the area of short-term memory (STM) in the retarded. They concluded that the mentally retarded do not perform at a level commensurate with their mental age, suggesting a specific memory deficit.

It may surprise the reader to learn that the evidence for other specific cognitive deficits in the mentally retarded is not striking. When comparison studies match the groups on the basis of CA, though reliable differences are generally found between retardates and controls, they are quite small. Further, when matching for MA is done, it is generally very difficult to demonstrate a deficiency in the retarded which could be interpreted as evidence for a *specific* disability. Lipman (1963) has reviewed studies of rote verbal learning (e.g., paired associate learning), perceptual motor learning, and classical conditioning in the retarded. Generally the group differences on these measures are very modest indeed and when groups are equated for MA, differences often disappear completely. None of these measures by themselves can account for the extensive academic differences between the retarded and control subjects. Lipman questions whether any single major area of cognitive deficit exists among the retarded. Instead he suggests that the retarded may suffer from multiple cognitive disabilities, which collectively produce a profound learning impediment.

SUMMARY

Thus, comparison studies suggest that the mentally retarded suffer from difficulties in mediation and short-term memory (and possibly attention as well) over and above that attributable to their lowered mental age. It is not known whether they also suffer from difficulty in selecting relevant stimuli in discrimination learning. Some of their deficits are qualitatively similar to those of hyperactive and learning disabled children and suggest a common core of interest as far as possible drug indications and effects on cognitive function are concerned.

Implications for Measures of Drug Effects

Studies which employed simplified mechanistic and preferably automated types of tasks have been emphasized in the above review. There are several reasons for this: 1) The simpler a task is, the easier it is to interpret from a *task analysis* persepctive. For example, the Continuous Performance Task quite clearly measures the rather simple function of concentration or attention span. 2) Such tests can often be dissected into or compiled stepwise into fundamental psychological processes. For example, Douglas (1974) queries whether the observed deficits of hyperactive children on certain popular pencil-and-paper perceptual tests might be due to a simple basic *attentional,* rather than the commonly assumed perceptual, problem. 3) Such mechanistic tests are more objective, yield numerical scores and minimize bias results from interaction between examiner and examinee. These three features make them particularly attractive as measures of cognitive function for use in pediatric psychopharmacology.

The major disadvantages are: 1) Automating such tasks is expensive and limits their application. However, some tests such as the Matching Familiar Figures and Auditory-Visual Integration task can easily be administered in either automated or manual fashions. 2) These cognitive processes are not synonymous with learning in the real world and their validity as measures of this cannot be assumed. Learning in its more traditional sense should be assessed too (see below).

Recommended measures of cognitive functions for pediatric psychopharmacology will be discussed after an examination in the next section of drug studies in which such tests have been used.

DRUG EFFECTS ON COGNITIVE FUNCTIONS AND TESTS

In this section only cognitive functions prerequisite to learning will be examined rather than the terminal goal of learning or academic achievement which is covered in a separate section below. Further, tests which qualify unequivocally as measures of cognitive processes elemental to learning will be reviewed, whereas others more peripheral to learning will not be treated. For example, tests of motor performance undoubtedly have a learning component (Knights & Hinton, 1969; Wade, 1976) but these and many others are not treated here as they contain large task components unrelated to learning and are therefore not amenable to unequivocal interpretation. They are discussed in Chapter 2.

When viewed against the backdrop of areas of cognitive deficit outlined earlier, it will be seen that there are grave shortcomings in the research in pediatric psychopharmacology as it affects tests of cognitive function. First, there has been a failure in many instances to direct the research to the specific areas of deficit. Second, only a very narrow range of drugs, principally the stimulants (see Chapter 6), have been studied for their cognitive effects (see also Chapters 6-10). Third, most of the good research has involved only hyperactive children, so that there is a noticeable lack of information about other diagnostic groups.

Attention (CPT, RT)

1) *Stimulants*. Both the Continuous Performance task (CPT) and reaction time (RT) tasks are widely recognized indices of attention. Using these tests, the stimulants (see Chapter 6), particularly methylphenidate (Ritalin) and dextroamphetamine (Dexedrine), have been found consistently to enhance attention in hyperactive children (Cohen et al., 1971; Conners & Rothschild, 1968; Douglas, 1974; Porges et al., 1975; Sykes et al., 1971; Werry & Aman, 1975; Yepes et al., 1977). Methylphenidate has

also been shown to be effective in improving attention in learning disability children, but the number of investigations is much smaller (Gittelman-Klein & Klein, 1976; Lewis & Young, 1975). There is at least one report that deanol (Deaner) tends to improve attention in children with specific learning problems (Lewis & Young, 1975).

2) *Antidepressants.* The effects of the antidepressants (see Chapter 7) on these tests of attention are less clear at present. When administered to behaviorally disordered (further unspecified) children, amitryptyline (Elavil) resulted in a significant improvement on the CPT (Yepes et al., 1977). When enuretic children were treated with imipramine (Tofranil), there was a slight nonsignificant improvement in attention (Werry et al., 1975a). The only available report on lithium (see Chapter 10) indicated that it was ineffective in improving the reaction time of hyperactive children (Greenhill et al., 1973).

3) *Antipsychotics* (see Chapter 8). Chlorpromazine (Thorazine) has been found to have no significant effect on attention in hyperactive children (Werry et al., 1966); haloperidol (Haldol, Serenace) has been shown to improve attention at lower doses and possibly deteriorate it at higher doses, also in hyperactive children (Werry & Aman, 1975), and to cause significantly longer reaction times, suggesting attentional impairment in high doses (Cunningham et al., 1968). The balance of evidence is thus in favor of depression of attention by antipsychotics in hyperactive/aggressive nonretarded children, but only at higher doses.

Verbal Learning (PAL)

Paired associate learning (PAL) requires the subject to learn a series of pairs such that when the first member (the stimulus) of the pair is displayed, the subject must try to anticipate its mate (the response). Thus, the paired associate task is primarily a test of memory.

1) *Stimulants.* Methylphenidate generally facilitates performance in behaviorally and learning disordered groups (Conners & Eisenberg, 1963; Conners & Rothschild, 1968; Conners et al., 1964; Gittelman-Klein & Klein, 1976). Of interest was the observation that children of low and average IQ in Conners' studies displayed greater gains from the drug treatment than did those of high IQ. It will be recalled that a memory type deficit has been posited to exist in the retarded.

2) *Antipsychotics.* Helper et al. (1963) studied the effects of chlorpromazine on an analagous task, rote memory, in emotionally disturbed children. Chlorpromazine resulted in a decrement in performance, especially

in the later learning trials. In addition, the slower learning subjects were more affected by the drug. Once again, there appears to be an interaction between subject characteristics (possibly related to IQ) and drug effects on learning.

Thus this test, though used infrequently, has generally been drug-sensitive.

Cognitive Style (MFF)

It was noted earlier that both hyperactive and learning disability children suffered deficits in areas of learning collectively called cognitive style, measured by the Matching Familiar Figures Test (MFF) and field dependence-independence tests.

1) *Stimulants.* When administered to hyperactive children, methylphenidate has generally been found to result in significantly increased *decision times* on the MFF, suggesting a reduction of impulsivity (Campbell et al., 1971a; Rapaport et al., 1974b) but not always (Yepes et al., 1977). A reduction in *errors* on this task would be suggestive of enhancement of visual perception. Campbell et al. obtained such an improvement, but this was not replicated by Rapoport et al. and Yepes et al. On a test of field dependence-independence, which presumably also taps certain perceptual skills, methylphenidate failed to enhance the performance of hyperactive children (Campbell et al., 1971a).

2) *Antidepressants* (amitryptyline and imipramine) have not yet been shown to have any effect on reflection-impulsivity as assessed by the MFF (Yepes et al., 1977; Rapoport et al., 1974b).

The MFF is thus one of the more drug-sensitive tests, especially to stimulants, and has the advantage of measuring deficits seen in target diagnostic groups.

Short-Term Memory (STM)

Short-term memory (STM) is defined as memory over a few minutes or a few seconds (Winschel & Lawrence, 1975) and can be assessed using pictures, numbers, words, and so on. An automated method for assessment of STM, described by Scott (1971), involves the presentation of a varying number of cartoon characters, followed a few seconds after by a single character, and the child must decide whether it was a member of the preceding group.

1) *Stimulants.* Methylphenidate has generally been shown to facilitate performance on this task, increasing accuracy levels and often decreasing

decision time or latency (Sprague, 1972; Sprague et al., 1970; Sprague & Sleator, 1973; Werry & Aman, 1975), but not always (Yeyes et al., 1977).

2) *Antidepressants.* Amitriptyline and imipramine have not been shown to differ from placebo in their effect on STM (Werry et al., 1975a; Yepes et al., 1977).

3) *Antipsychotics.* Thioridazine (Melleril) has been shown to depress accuracy on this task and to increase decision time (Sprague et al., 1970). Haloperidol tends to have a dose-related effect, resulting in unchanged performance at lower doses and in slight deficits at higher doses (Werry & Aman, 1975).

Two points are relevant here. First, while the STM task is fairly drug-sensitive, it has not been shown to discriminate between hyperactive and control subjects (comparison studies simply have not been done), so it may not be of particular relevance to the cognitive deficits of exceptional children.

Second, studies with the STM task suggest a complex dosage effect as follows: The greatest improvement with methylphenidate is generally found at 0.3 mg/kg and improvement is less pronounced as the dose is made smaller or greater (Sprague et al., 1970; Sprague, 1972; Sprague & Sleator, 1973, 1975). Haloperidol in low doses (.025 mg/kg) does not tend to influence performance on this task but higher doses (.050 mg/kg) probably impair STM (Werry & Aman, 1975).

Intelligence (WISC)

Many studies have examined drug effects on IQ as measured by tests such as the Wechsler Intelligence Scale for Children, presumably because such tests are well-known, readily available and predictive of academic performance.

1) *Stimulants.* A number of studies of the stimulants (methylphenidate or dextroamphetamine) in *hyperactive children* have failed to demonstrate any drug effect on the WISC (Finnerty et al., 1971; Quinn & Rapoport, 1975; Rapoport et al., 1974b; Weiss et al., 1975). On the other hand, other studies show improvements in IQ scores, some attributable to changes on the verbal subtests (Weiss et al., 1971a; Weiss et al., 1968) and others to improvements on the performance scale (Epstein et al., 1968; Hoffman et al., 1974). Thus while the *stimulants* do not appear to have a unitary effect in *hyperactive* children, on the whole their effect is mildly facilitative. This is probably due, as Sroufe (1975) has observed, to nonspecific effects of the medication such as enhanced attention span or even heightened motivation.

The effects of stimulants on the WISC in children with *learning disabilities* is also unclear. Some studies have found no changes (Conners & Rothschild, 1968; Conrad et al., 1971; Rie et al., 1976), whereas a number of others have demonstrated improvements in IQ, largely attributable to changes in the *performance* scales as a result of methylphenidate treatment (Gittelman-Klein & Klein, 1976; Knights & Hinton, 1969; Lewis & Young, 1975). Enhancement on the performance scales has also been demonstrated in response to the stimulant-like acetylcholine analogue deanol (Deaner) (Lewis & Young, 1975) (see Chapter 10). It may be that stimulants have a more specific effect directed to functions assessed by the performance scale in this group of children.

2) *Antidepressants.* Studies investigating imipramine have been unable, as yet, to demonstrate changes in IQ, though they are few in number and from only one investigator (Rapoport et al., 1974b; Quinn & Rapoport, 1975).

3) *Antipsychotics.* Chlorpromazine has generally been observed to have no immediate effect on performance on the WISC (Weiss et al., 1968, 1971a), though there is one follow-up study reporting improvement in verbal IQ over time (Weiss et al., 1971b). Similarly, when compared to placebo, haloperidol seems to have no effect on IQ in emotionally disturbed children (Wong & Cock, 1971).

4) *Antiepileptic Drugs.* There is one report of the use of an antiepileptic drug in learning disability children with mixed EEG records (Smith & Weyl, 1968). Ethosuximide (Zarontin) was reported to have dramatic effects on both the verbal and performance subscales of the WISC, but the conclusions are weakened by an almost complete lack of experimental controls. This area is discussed in more detail in Chapter 9.

Thus the WISC is sometimes sensitive to effects of various drugs, though the relationship of the effects to classroom learning remains to be demonstrated.

Perceptual Function (Various Tests)

This section was included with some reluctance, since the tests in this group are difficult to understand from a task analysis point of view. Additionally, the value of some of these instruments is open to question. For example, Larsen et al. (1976) conducted a study which challenges two of the most popular, the Illinois Test of Psycholinguistic Abilities (ITPA), and the Wepman test of Auditory Discrimination, but upholds a third, the Bender-Gestalt, as valid tests of learning difficulties. There are many other tests on the market, developed out of clinical demand and/or potential profitability, which are of little or of unproven value as measures of cognitive deficits. However, this group of tests still constitutes one of the commonest measures of drug response in children.

The following tests are discussed together because they all appear to have or claim to have a large perceptual component, that is, the ability to recognize and organize sensory input. In the summaries below, results were presumed statistically nonsignificant if an investigator reported that a measure was given but did not report it further as having been influenced by the drug trial.

BENDER VISUAL MOTOR GESTALT TEST

Since there appear to be no marked differences in their patterns of response, studies of hyperkinetic and learning disability children are reported together here.

1) *Stimulants.* Methylphenidate and dextroamphetamine have generally been found to have no significant effect on this assessment of visual-motor perception (Friedman et al., 1973; Garfinkel et al., 1975; Knights & Hinton, 1969; Millichap et al., 1968; Rapoport et al., 1974b; Rie et al., 1976; Weiss et al., 1968, 1971a, b). Only two reports suggest significant improvement, both as a result of methylphenidate (Lewis & Young, 1975; Seger & Hallum, 1974) but the latter study was uncontrolled. Thus, methylphenidate and dextroamphetamine probably have no direct effects on performance of the Bender Gestalt.

One study (Lewis & Young, 1975) suggests that deanol (Deaner) may facilitate the performance of learning disability children on this test.

The only study of caffeine which investigated such performance found no change as compared to placebo (Garfinkel et al., 1975). Thus the test is relatively drug-insensitive, as far as it has been tested.

2) *Antipsychotics.* Chlorpromazine has generally been found to have no effect on the performance of hyperactive children as measured by the Bender Gestalt (Weiss et al., 1971a, b).

3) *Antidepressants, etc.* No data are available on other classes of drugs.

FROSTIG TEST OF VISUAL PERCEPTION

Evaluation of drug effects on the Frostig is difficult owing to the number of subtests comprising this instrument. Only the stimulants appear to have been studied. Two studies have found significant improvement on *some* of the subtests as a result of methylphenidate and dextroamphetamine (Hoffman et al., 1974; Conrad et al., 1971) and two nonsignificant improvements (Conners & Rothschild, 1968; Weiss et al., 1971a). One (Friedman et al., 1973) was unable to detect any effect of the stimulants on this instrument. Thus this test does not seem to be particularly drug-sensitive, at least to stimulants.

ILLINOIS TEST OF PSYCHOLINGUISTIC ABILITIES (ITPA)

Once again, assessment of this test as a measure of drug effects is complicated by a large number of subtests.

1) *Stimulants.* After first validating the ITPA as discriminating between controls and hyperactives, Butter and Lapierre (1974) then noted that methylphenidate improved performance on the *auditory* modality, a specific effect which was later replicated in a sample of learning disability children (Rie et al., 1976). Another study suggests more general improvements on the ITPA as a function of methylphenidate (Butter & Lapierre, 1975). Lewis and Young (1975) found no effect of methylphenidate or deanol on the Visual Sequential Memory subtest of the ITPA. Also, it should be mentioned that others have been unable to demonstrate a deficit in hyperactives on this task (Douglas, 1974). The status of this test in pediatric psychopharmacology is thus uncertain although conceptually this is a promising instrument.

WEPMAN TEST OF AUDITORY DISCRIMINATION

The only studies using this popular test which could be located found no effects of either methylphenidate or dextroamphetamine (Friedman et al., 1973; Weiss et al., 1971a).

PORTEUS MAZES

The Porteus Maze Test is considered by its originator to be a test of planning capacity and intelligence, but it clearly also has large perceptual components relating to the organization of visual stimuli. In addition, Conners and Rothschild (1968) consider it to be a sensitive indicator of impulsive responding.

1) *Stimulants.* Methylphenidate and dextroamphetamine generally result in significant improvement in the test age score (Conners et al., 1964; Gittelman-Klein & Klein, 1976; Hoffman et al., 1974; Rapoport et al., 1974b), the one exception occurring with mentally retarded children in which no change was observed (Blacklidge & Ekblad, 1971).

Table 1
EFFECTS OF VARIOUS DRUGS ON COGNITIVE TASKS AND TESTS

TASK[2]	Stimulants[1]		Deanol	Antidepressants[1]		Chlorpromazine	Antipsychotics[1]	Thioridazine
	Methylphenidate	Dextroamphetamine		Imipramine	Amytriptaline		Haloperidol	
1. Attention (CPT & RT)	7 improved	1 improved	1 improved	1 non-sig. improved	1 improved	1 non-sig. improved	1 improved 1 non-sig. worse 1 worse	
2. Verbal Learning (Paired Associates)	3 improved 1 non-sig. improved					1 worse		
3. Cognitive Style MFF (Impulsivity)	2 improved 1 non-sig. improved			1 no change	1 no change			
MFF (Accuracy)	1 improved 3 no change			1 no change	1 no change			
4. Short Term Memory	4 improved 1 no change				1 no change		1 (dose related) low dose no change, possible deficit at high doses	1 worse
5. Intelligence (WISC)	4 no change 1 improved in Verbal scale 4 improved in Perf. scale	3 no change 2 improved in Verbal scale 1 improved in Perf. scale	1 improved in Perf. scale	2 no change		3 no change 1 improved in Perf. scale	1 no change	
6. PERCEPTION								
6.1 Bender	2 improved 1 non-sig. improved 6 no change	3 no change		1 no change		2 no change		
6.2 Frostig	2 improved 1 non-sig. improved 1 no change	1 improved 2 no change						
6.3 ITPA	1 improved, subtest unspecified 2 improved (auditory subtest) 1 general improved 2 no change		1 no change					
6.4 Wepman	2 no change	1 no change						
6.5 Porteus	4 improved 1 no change	2 improved		1 non-sig. improved 1 no change — (long term)		1 worse		

Note: 1. See also Chapters 6-10. Antianxiety (sedative) drugs are covered in Chapters 9 and 10.
2. See text and Buros (1972) for descriptions and availability of tests.

2) *Antidepressants.* Imipramine has been found to result in a nonsignificant improvement in hyperactive children (Rapoport et al., 1974b) and no change over a one-year follow-up period (Quinn & Rapoport, 1975).

3) *Antipsychotics.* Chlorpromazine, when administered to emotionally disturbed children, resulted in a significant deficit on the Porteus Mazes (Helper et al., 1963).

The Porteus Maze test is thus one of the more drug-sensitive measures of cognitive function, though the nature of changes is difficult to interpret.

Summary of Drugs and Cognitive Tests

For the reader's convenience Table 1 summarizes the effects of the drugs used most commonly in pediatric psychopharmacology on the previously discussed measures of cognitive function. The most striking feature of this table is the large number of empty spaces, which is an apt reflection of our current level of knowledge so far as cognitive effects of these drugs are concerned.

In Table 2 the emphasis is on *measures* used in the assessment of drug effects on cognitive function. A *Drug Sensitivity Index* of the various measures has been developed on the basis of total number of studies, irrespective of subject, population, dose, type of drug or time of drug. Thus, it can be only the crudest of indices, intended to give some indication of the potential usefulness of that particular measure.

It is important to realize that discussion to this point and the data in Tables 1 and 2 do not extend to measures of or effects on learning or academic performance (see next section).

Measures of Achievement

These tests are used to assess an individual's present level of knowledge, skill, or performance in a test situation which hopefully simulates the ordinary academic situation.

Wide Range Achievement Test (WRAT)

There are a number of versions of standardized achievement tests but only one, the Wide Range Achievement Test, has been employed extensively in drug studies to assess achievement in basic school skills: reading, mathematics, and spelling (Rapoport et al., 1974b; Quinn & Rapoport, 1975; Gittelman-Klein & Klein, 1976). This instrument tends to be widely used as a follow-up measure, probably because it can be applied over a

Table 2
VARIOUS TESTS OF COGNITIVE FUNCTION AS MEASURES OF DRUG EFFECTS

Task	Cognitive Capacity Presumed Measured	Drug Sensitivity (% Studies Showing Sig. Changes)	Comments	Major References
Continuous Performance Task (CPT)	Attention span.	78% (9 studies)	Perhaps the best behavioral test of attention, due to the low priority placed on motor response (see below). The "Vigilance" task is operationally the same as the CPT but requires much longer test time.	Sykes et al, 1971, 1972. Source: Rosvold et al, 1956.
Reaction Time (RT)	Attention or concentration span.	67% (6 studies)	A major difficulty in assessing cognitive function is the obvious motor component inherent in this task. Since drugs affect motor function (e.g. Knights & Hinton, 1969), it could be difficult to interpret changes as due solely to attentional processes.	Sykes et al, 1972; Cohen et al, 1971.
Verbal Learning (Paired Associates)	Ability to memorize rotely and to retain over moderate to long intervals.	80% (5 studies)	Not extensively studied in drug research. Provides two measures of import: rate of initial learning and level of recall after some specified time interval.	Helper et al, 1963; Conners et al, 1964. Methodology: Battig, 1965.
Short Term Memory Task (STM)	Recognition memory over brief intervals.	67% (6 studies)	Not yet assessed as possible discriminator of hyperactivity; established as a useful tool in mental retardation.	Sprague et al, 1970; Sprague & Sleator, 1973. Source: Scott, 1971.
Discrimination Learning	Ability to select and learn relevant concept or stimulus from a stimulus complex.	50% (2 studies)	Virtually unstudied in drug research. Of particular relevance in the mentally retarded.	Breitmeyer in Sprague & Werry, 1971. Source: Zeaman & House, 1963.
Auditory Visual Integration (Mediation)	Ability to code stimuli from one dimension and translate into a different one. Temporal discrimination necessarily involved.	No drug studies to date.	This task has been included because it appears to tap a new sphere of cognitive function. Although not used in drug studies, comparison studies suggest it could have considerable usefulness.	Blank & Bridger, 1966; Rudel & Denckla, 1976. Source: Birch & Belmont, 1964.

Table 2 (continued)

Test	Description	Results	Comments	Source
Matching Familiar Figures (MFF)	Visual perception; also the ability to withhold from responding until consideration has been given to all aspects of the stimuli (Reflection/Impulsivity).	Accuracy 33% Impulsivity 67% (3 studies)	Renders two measures: Accuracy of response, a reflection of the child's perception and decision time, an indication of impulsivity.	Campbell et al, 1971. Source: Kagan, 1965.
Wechsler Intelligence Scale for Children (WISC)	Intelligence as assessed by ability on a number of discrete subtests.	Not listed here due to the large number of subtests potentially involved. See preceding text.	Composed of 12 subtests assessing a broad spectrum of abilities. With the exception of the mazes section, a specific effect due to drugs has yet to be identified. Any possible drug effectiveness is more likely due to nonspecific effects on arousal, motivation, and attention.	Sroufe, 1975; Sprague & Werry, 1971; Sprague, in press b.
Bender Visual Motor Gestalt Test	A maturational test of the child's ability to respond to a constellation of stimuli as an integrated whole.	20% (10 studies)	A large motor component involved in this test. As mentioned in RT (above), it is difficult to determine whether drug-determined change is a function of altered *cognitive* or *motor* functioning. Other non-specific factors could also be major factors (see WISC).	Lewis & Young, 1975; Douglas, 1974. Source: Bender, 1946. Scoring: Koppitz, 1964.
Frostig Test of Visual Perception	Visual perception. Eye-hand coordination.	40% (5 studies)	Suffers from the same problems of interpretation mentioned above: Obvious motor involvement and possibility of improvement due to nonspecific factors.	Douglas, 1974.
Illinois Test of Psycholinguistic Abilities (ITPA)	Receptive and expressive functions and their integration.	75% (4 studies)	Some dispute regarding ability of this instrument to discriminate normal from exceptional groups (see text). Composed of a broad spectrum of subtests.	Douglas, 1974; Butter & Lapierre, 1974.
Wepman Test of Auditory Discrimination	Auditory discrimination.	0% (2 studies)	Relatively unstudied in drug research. Subject to many of the qualifiers outlined above.	Friedman et al, 1973; Weiss et al, 1971a.
Porteus Mazes	A. Planning capacity and intelligence. B. Perceptual components. C. Impulsivity.	71% (7 studies)	Although a sensitive indicator of drug effect, this task has the difficulties of determining just what abilities are being affected. Perhaps its greatest use is as an index of whether drug improvement (unspecified) does occur.	Conners & Rothschild, 1968. Source: Porteus, 1967.

Note: See also Buros (1972) for details and evaluation of some tests.

broad age range (from kindergarten to college) and in a brief time period. However, as pointed out by two test reviewers (Courtney, 1949; Sims, 1949), it is obvious that in order to cover such a broad age range in restricted time, the test must give up something. Since the number of items per grade is limited, the *sensitivity* of this test is necessarily reduced. Additionally, this test has been criticized for failing to differentiate adequately between intelligence and achievement (Payne, 1974). Consequently, this is probably *not* a good test for monitoring drug effects over a brief drug trial, although it may be satisfactory for long-term follow-up studies which often span a number of years.

Given that there usually is limited time for assessment procedures, investigators might do well to use single subject-matter tests or selected subtests from the better documented achievement batteries such as the Metropolitan Achievement Test, the Stanford Achievement Tests, or the Iowa Tests of Basic Skills. Diagnostic tests for the basic subjects (such as the Gray Oral Reading Test and the Neale Analysis of Reading) may prove to be useful achievement measures. Additionally, Clay (1975) has devised an observational technique (the Running Record) which results in a detailed linguistic breakdown of the actual behavior during oral reading tests. Such an analysis can provide both qualitative and quantitative information not ordinarily available in achievement tests.

Behavior Observations

Behavior observations are timed samples of observable behavior (see Chapter 2). They employ explicit categories of behavior, either adaptive or maladaptive, and they result in a frequency count for each of the various categories. As has been pointed out in Chapter 2, where various types of measures have been discussed extensively, behavior observations ordinarily measure behavior in the naturalistic situation and have the virtue of high reliability and obvious relevance.

Of course the *process* of learning cannot be observed but activities which are either compatible or incompatible can. For example, Sprague et al. (1970) found that "on task" behavior increased as a result of methylphenidate but thioridazine had no effect.

Additionally, behavior observations offer one way of validating impressions gained through performance tests and rating scales. Kupietz and Richardson (in press) found that "off task" behavior bore a strong relationship to performance measures of attention but only a modest relationship to teacher ratings of attention span.

Work Output and Effectiveness

Work output and effectiveness collectively refer to concrete measures of academic productivity and accuracy and they can encompass any of a wide variety of activities. For example, Wolraich et al. (in press) assessed the effects of methylphenidate and behavior modication on the accuracy of copying a paragraph, measured by the number of letters copied correctly and the number of correct responses made during the individual work period. Similar assessments have been employed to measure children's retention for educational films by the provision of comprehension questions afterwards (Christensen & Sprague, 1973).

Such measures of work output and effectiveness are uncommon but they strike at the very heart of the matter. Since they can be employed in classroom or pseudo-classroom settings, and since they use materials similar to those of the classroom, these measures tend to be more representative of real life learning situations.

The above indices of achievement have not been extensively used in drug research although, as a group, they show great promise. Although the WRAT has not been very sensitive to drug effects, there are other standardized tests which may prove superior. Direct measures such as behavioral observations and work output have been sensitive and have the advantage of anchoring research to real life situations.

To this point, discussion of drug effects has centered on the component cognitive processes presumed to underly learning rather than on learning itself. This is because most of the effort has been centered there.

DRUG EFFECTS AND ACADEMIC ACHIEVEMENT

Although many drugs (particularly the stimulants) have repeatedly been shown favorably to affect attention, memory and perception in the laboratory situation, the evidence for benefit on academic performance, particularly in the long-term, is not overwhelming.

A number of follow-up studies have been conducted assessing the effects of methylphenidate, imipramine, and chlorpromazine, separately or in some cases assessing a variety of drugs, when drug treatment has been customized to suit the individual child's needs. When compared to an untreated control group of children with similar diagnoses, treated children generally show no gains in academic performance (Weiss et al., 1975). Other studies which compare the performance of treated hyperactive children to *normal* controls also generally present discouraging results. The hyperactive children continue to repeat more grades, to show deficits on achievement tests (Mendelson et al., 1971; Riddle & Rapoport,

1976; Weiss et al., 1971a, b), and occasionally even demonstrate academic deterioration (Riddle & Rapoport, 1976). Thus, any improvement in the educational problems of hyperactive children is difficult to demonstrate in children who have been maintained for some period on the commonest drugs (methylphenidate, dextroamphetamine, imipramine, and chlorpromazine) used in this condition.

These findings are subject to two qualifications. First, follow-up studies are faced with an apparently insurmountable problem. Due to clinical, if not also ethical considerations, occasioned by the obvious behavioral benefits of these drugs (see Chapters 6 & 7), it is difficult to withhold treatment and *randomly* assign subjects to no-treatment subgroups. Consequently, to date, control or no-treatment groups have been largely self-assigned by dropout or treatment refusal and are likely to be less severely impaired or have different family backgrounds from their drug-treated counterparts. Had these control subjects experienced identical levels of hyperactivity, learning difficulties, social maladjustment and so on, it is likely that their families and schools would have insisted upon some form of intervention, medical or otherwise. The second problem is that even if defective learning processes are rectified as a result of drug treatment, these children may have no academic *foundation* on which to build. For example, basic skills such as reading are ordinarily not formally *taught* after the first 2 or 3 years in elementary school. Thus, a child with a reading problem would be faced with a hopeless task in trying to cope with his *other* school work, even if cognitive skills were greatly enhanced by drug treatment.

Long-term prospective studies emphasizing educational rather than behavioral measures are uncommon. Rie et al. (1976) examined the effects of methylphenidate in a mixed group of children composed largely of hyperactive and learning disability subjects. The authors concluded that no substantial drug effects on achievement were found and that methylphenidate should not be used to treat learning disorders. However, scrutiny of their results suggests that there tended to be general, although not significant, improvements on a number of achievement tests. Gittelman-Klein and Klein (1976) studied the effects of methylphenidate in a very carefully defined group of children with reading disabilities. Their findings were generally negative except for transitory initial gains in arithmetic and oral reading, which were no longer present after 12 weeks of treatment.

As already noted, these studies may be falsely negative unless some effort is made to build basic skills simultaneously. Only two studies could be located which specifically measured drug effects when combined with prescriptive remedial education. Friedman et al. (1973) examined the effects of medication (methylphenidate and dextroamphetamine) against combined drug-educational treatment. The children in the combined group showed no gains, as measured by perceptual tests, over the drug-only group. In a very carefully designed and well-executed study (Conrad et al., 1971), hyperactive children were assigned to 1 of 4 treatment combinations: placebo/no tutoring, placebo/tutoring, dextroamphetamine/no tutoring and dextroamphetamine/tutoring. The results indicated that the drug improved performance on a number of perceptual motor subtests and that tutoring produced gains on some WISC subtests. However, neither condition influenced academic attainment as measured by achievement tests.

In summary, then, it seems best to agree with Barkley and Cunningham (in press) who, in a comprehensive review of the effects of stimulants on the academic performance of hyperactive children, concluded that stimulants seem to have little effect on actual academic achievement. They attributed most instances of reported improvement *to enhanced attention during testing rather than heightened scholastic ability* and concluded that, in cases where school performance is a problem, it is necessary to ensure that *remedial educational assistance is provided* and management not left simply to stimulant treatment.

Before dismissing drugs as potentially useful in the management of learning problems, it should be noted that treatment of such handicaps by remedial education is not very impressive either (Lovell et al., 1963; Carroll, 1972). A treatment such as stimulant pharmacotherapy which can decrease impulsivity and improve attention, not only on laboratory tests but also as measured directly in the classroom (e.g., Sprague et al., 1970; Wolraich et al., in press) and as consistently reported by teachers (Barkley, 1977; Conners & Werry in press, see also Chapter 6), may well operate to the child's benefit if only in making school a more agreeable place resulting in more praise and less censure. However, this is not the same as saying that medication *must* be given long-term preventively as some claim, but only where parent, child and teacher perceive substantial benefit in school-related behavior.

PSYCHOTHERAPY, BEHAVIOR THERAPY AND DRUG TREATMENT

Psychotherapy and behavior therapy can be viewed as learning processes in which adaptive *behaviors* are strengthened or learned and maladaptive behaviors are weakened or discarded (extinguished). Changes that are ordinarily attributed to *personal growth or emotional insight* can also be viewed as resulting from cognitive, emotional, and social learning (Alexander, 1963; Murray & Jacobson, 1971). That the learning experience in this case does not deal with academic matters is immaterial. The key point is that during psychotherapy the patient is asked to explore social and emotional relationships and it is the *reorganization* of these relationships which constitutes the learning experience. However, whether one accepts that psychotherapy constitutes a special form of learning experience or not, the empirical data regarding interaction between psychological therapies and drug treatment are of importance.

Traditional Psychotherapy

Cytryn et al. (1960) tested the effects of meprobamate (Equanil, Miltown), prochlorperazine (Compazine, Stemetil), and placebo, in combination with psychotherapy, in neurotic and hyperactive children. Far more of the neurotic than the hyperkinetic children responded to psychotherapy, but neither drug had any facilitative effect. The same group (Eisenberg et al., 1961) examined the effects of brief psychotherapy in conjunction with perphenazine (Trilafon) and placebo in neurotic and hyperactive subjects. Again it was found that the majority of the neurotic children responded to psychotherapy whereas the hyperactive children were resistant to such treatment. However, perphenazine *in combination with psychotherapy* did appear to benefit the hyperkinetic subjects, but not the neurotic patients.

It is noticeable and perhaps a sad commentary that despite the popularity of psychotherapy and of pharmacotherapy there have been no further studies since these, which were done almost 20 years ago.

Behavior Therapy

Behavior therapy is a form of psychological treatment which is explicitly based upon learning principles which have been demonstrated in the laboratory. Learning in this case is defined as a relatively permanent change in behavior as a result of experience. Behavior therapy is made up of several techniques using either operant or classical conditioning (Werry & Wollersheim, 1967). Operant conditioning posits that actions undertaken by a person are eventually controlled by the reinforcements (rewards and punishments) consequent to those actions. Classical (or respondent) conditioning posits that responses once under the control of unconditional stimuli which cause reflexive responses in the organism can become contingent upon other stimuli which occur in temporal proximity to the unconditional stimuli. A number of papers have recently been published demonstrating how behavioral principles might be incorporated as an adjunctive treatment in pediatric practice (Murray, 1976; O'Leary et al., 1976; Werry & Wollersheim, 1967).

As with psychotherapy, studies examining the interrelationships of behavior therapy and drug treatment are scarce but increasing. Young and Turner (1965) investigated the effects of dextroamphetamine and methylamphetamine (Methedrine) in enuretic children to determine whether the drugs would enhance the bed-buzzer conditioning treatment which all subjects received. It was found in this less than rigorous study that significantly more subjects who received conditioning treatment alone dropped out than in two drug-conditioning groups. Also those groups which received the combined therapy attained success in treatment more quickly than the conditioning-alone group. However, when followed up one year later, it was found that the dextroamphetamine/conditioning group had a significantly higher relapse rate than the other groups. This is a result possibly suggestive of state dependency, a topic which will be discussed later in this chapter.

Christensen and Sprague (1973) examined the effects of operant conditioning and methylphenidate treatment in a group of emotionally disturbed children from special education classes. Both the conditioning procedure and the drug treatment reduced activity when used independently. More important, however, is the fact that these effects tended to be *additive* and the greatest benefit accrued from *conditioning in combination with methylphenidate.*

Christensen (1975) further investigated the combined effects of methylphenidate and a reinforcement program, this time with hyperactive retarded children. The results indicated that the behavior modification procedure produced increases in work-oriented behavior and decreases in disruptive behavior; medication had only minor behavioral effects probably owing to the marked success of the conditioning procedure, not uncommon when exceptional children are placed in unusually felicitous classroom situations (see also Glavin et al., 1971; Wolraich et al., in press). Deviant behavior was decreased to such an extent by the conditioning treatment that it was improbable that the drug could have any further beneficial effects on these behaviors. Notably, however, neither the active drug nor the conditioning procedures improved academic productivity or academic accuracy.

Gittelman-Klein et al. (1976a) also investigated the relative merits of behavior modification, methylphenidate, and their combination in treating hyperactive children, but in rather more natural circumstances. Their results suggested that all 3 treatments were effective, but that the *com-*

bination treatment resulted in the greatest improvement, followed respectively by methylphenidate alone and behavior modification alone.

Wolraich et al. (in press) investigated the effects of behavior modification (a token program) in hyperactive children with and without concomitant methylphenidate treatment, as with Christensen (1975), in a highly favorable special classroom. During the initial group study period only one behavior, fidgeting, was decreased by the medication, whereas behavior modification was very successful. However, during the subsequent individual study period the results were essentially reversed, with significant reductions resulting in a number of behavioral categories from the stimulant but not the conditioning procedure. Although both treatments resulted in some improved academic output measures, only behavior modification caused a *significant* improvement. Of particular interest in this study is that while both treatments worked, they tended to be effective in different settings and on different functions. Again there was no facilitative action of medication on behavior modification.

The studies by Christensen (1975) and Wolraich et al. (in press) show greater effect on the whole with behavior modification whereas that by Gittelman-Klein et al. (1976a) suggests greater efficacy of stimulant therapy. Two studies (Christensen & Sprague, 1973; Gittelman-Klein et al., 1976a) suggest that the greatest improvement would typically be expected to come from a synergistic combination of stimulant and conditioning therapy, but the studies by Christensen (1975) and Wolraich et al. (in press) show no such advantage, and that by Young and Turner (1965) only a short-term advantage (in enuresis). Some of this conflict seems related to the learning situation and some to the behavior concerned. In general, when learning is optimized, as in small special classes with an enthusiastic behavior modification backup team, behavior modification works quickly and well. In the child's real, more difficult world, drugs act more strongly and synergistically with behavior modification.

These empirical data are in keeping with earlier speculations by Werry (1968b) as to how conditioning and drug treatments might interact in the context of day-to-day activities in the hyperactive child. In arguing against simplistic medical models of drug treatment, he advanced the idea of a catalyzing role. Drugs provide a useful and relatively simple way of promoting non-hyperactive and reducing hyperactive behaviors or, in short, *making socially acceptable behavior more probable*. Improved adjustment on the part of the child should therefore result in greater positive reinforcement from the significant persons in the child's environment though this is more likely to happen if such reinforcement is properly programmed in a contemporaneous behavior modification program. Ultimately, drugs (and then behavior modification) could be faded out. This catalytic view seems more sensible than current antagonistic views which would opt for drug or behavior therapy to the exclusion of one another.

STATE-DEPENDENT LEARNING AND ITS IMPLICATIONS

Within the last few years a phenomenon observed in animal learning studies has raised questions with respect to the use of psychotropic drugs in man, particularly in children. Overton (1964) in a classic series of experiments in animals showed the existence of *state-dependency* or *dissociation of learning*, a phenomenon in which material learned under a given drug condition is most readily elicited or recalled only when the same drug condition is reinstated. Overton drew 2 important conclusions from his animal studies. First, virtually complete dissociation (failure to transfer learning) could be produced in these animals when *heavy* doses of a sedative drug were used. Second, only partial dissociation of learning occurs when drug states are not sufficiently different from each other or the non-drug state. Thus, dose is an important consideration when trying to demonstrate state dependency.

Overton (1968) has reviewed the studies pertinent to state dependency in both animals and man. Among his observations are the following. State-dependent learning can be: 1) task specific, that is, demonstrable with some learning measures and not with others; 2) asymmetrical, meaning that transfer will sometimes appear in one direction (non-drug state to drug state) but not the other (drug to non-drug). Additionally, Overton concluded that very little information is available on state-dependent learning in man.

The issue of state-dependency is of more than theoretical interest to the area of pediatric psychopharmacology. If clinical doses of psychotropic drugs cause dissociation of learning, then the treatment of exceptional children with such medication may actually work to the ultimate detriment of their academic performance when these children are eventually taken off medication. Furthermore, if psychotherapy is viewed as a learning experience, then gains made during drug treatment may not transfer optimally to the off-drug state (Kamano, 1966; McCabe & McCabe, 1972).

The issue of state-dependency has been virtually ignored in pediatric psychopharmacological research. Aman and Sprague (1974) reported on a collection of 3 independent studies which evaluated methylphenidate, dextroamphetamine and thioridazine for possible state-dependent effects on a variety of learning tasks. None of the results was suggestive of state-dependent effects. It was concluded that these drugs, given in reasonable doses, do not cause dissociation.

A subsequent report (Swanson & Kinsbourne, 1976) evaluated methylphenidate for its possible state-dependent effects upon rote verbal learning in a group of hyperactive children responsive to stimulant medication and in a control group of children who had previously been found not to respond favorably to medication. It was found that the stimulant responders also demonstrated state-dependent effects, whereas the nonresponders were insensitive to a change in drug state. This is a particularly serious finding, as this is the very subgroup which is most likely to be placed on long-term medication, and, according to this report, to suffer learning dissociation when treatment is discontinued.

It appears that the issue of state-dependency is far from settled, even with stimulants, the most commonly studied psychotropic drug in children. For his part, the clinician should be aware of the problem and opt for the smallest possible effective doses. Furthermore, it might be advisable slowly to phase out a given medication rather than to precipitously take a patient off a drug (McCabe & McCabe, 1972).

Conclusions

1) The whole area of cognitive functioning including that of exceptional children and the relevant effects of drugs upon it is grossly underresearched. The reviewer was repeatedly struck by the paucity of methodologically sound, comparative work in the various areas of exceptionality. The number of studies examining the deficits of hyperactive, learning disabled, and retarded children is small and replication is required even here. Much more must be known about the learning difficulties these children exhibit if they are to be treated knowledgeably with medication.

2) Drug research should not be conducted in a theoretical vacuum or confined to one area of function such as social behavior. Yet, when viewed against the structure of what is *known* about exceptional children, the research has been haphazard indeed. More investigators should initiate their studies by first examining all the areas of difficulty and only *then* trying to ameliorate these through treatment regimens. Certainly today, the cognitive effects of most psychotropic drugs except perhaps the stimulants are largely unknown because of insufficient or inept study. While measures of cognitive function leave a great deal to be desired in validity and drug sensitivity, there are enough good ones to establish basic effects and justify inclusion of cognitive function as a necessary part of clinical assessment of drug effects in children.

3) A further area of difficulty is the trend in research to investigate drug effects in mixed populations with no further analysis regarding the subpopulations. Although the value of diagnosis in assisting treatment remains largely untested (Barkley, 1976; Werry, 1973; Sprague, 1973b; see Chapter 5), the practice of studying mixed populations seems likely to lead to false or misleading conclusions. This review has shown that different types of disorders have different cognitive deficits and respond differentially to medication.

4) Another problem is that of dosage. Sprague and Sleator (Sprague, in press a; Sprague & Sleator, 1975) cogently argue that different realms of behavior may respond differently to given dosages in the same individual. Thus, a child's *learning* may be optimally improved at one dose and his *social* adjustment may asymptote at another dose. Viewed in this light, the common practice of establishing dosage by titrating until optimal *social* improvement occurs may be disadvantageous or misleading from a learning point of view. Clinical improvement may be at the expense of the optimum learning performance (Werry & Sprague, 1974). Such dose-response studies employing mg. per kg. drug administration are cumbersome and not popular in pediatric psychopharmacology, but the research relating particularly to short-term memory would suggest that they do have merit, especially in studying effects on cognition.

5) There is a conflict between laboratory and educational measures of drug effects. It must also be acknowledged that, viewed from the perspective of educational achievement, drugs have not proven to be terribly effective, although some minor facilitation probably does accompany drug treatment. Nor have long-term studies been able to establish continued benefit. This must be a very qualified statement, however, since ethical considerations rule out a conclusive experiment on this question. However, the results do call for extreme caution in extrapolating laboratory or test based studies of cognitive function to classroom learning.

6) The number of investigations examining the interaction between other treatments and drug treatment is inexcusably low. The most favorable ways of treating disordered children must be sought. Yet three of the most obvious ways of attempting to do this—combining drug treatment with psychotherapy, behavior therapy or remedial education—have hardly been tested at all. We simply do not know what benefits (or disadvantages) are likely to accrue from the various forms of therapy in conjunction with drug treatment.

7) Finally, the issue of state-dependency serves to complicate the area of drugs and learning further. To date there is little conclusive evidence

indicating that this is a serious problem in pediatric psychopharmacology. However, since state-dependency is a dose-related phenomenon, the lowest useful doses should be employed when treating children.

All of the above suggests that we have barely scratched the surface insofar as the cognitive effects of drugs are concerned. It has been said that "Nature is not malicious." Applied to the current topic this means that if an agent is facilitative in several instances, then that agent is probably *generally* facilitative. However, we cannot afford to take this for granted and much more study is imperative, taking the different areas of exceptionality, different cognitive functions, and different drugs into account.

4

PRINCIPLES OF CLINICAL TRIALS AND SOCIAL, ETHICAL AND LEGAL ISSUES OF DRUG USE IN CHILDREN

ROBERT L. SPRAGUE, Ph.D.

Current Frequency of Psychotropic Drug Use

Stimulants

Stimulants are used with tens of thousands of children in the United States although the *percentage* of children receiving such medication is quite low. The best estimate of school children receiving *stimulants* (see Chapter 6) is that by Krager and Safer (1974) who surveyed Baltimore County (excluding City), and found 1.73% of the 50,000 children were receiving stimulant medication. In more recent surveys of special education populations covering most of Illinois, Gadow (1975, 1976) reported that about 8% of preschool special education students, age 3 to 5, were receiving psychotropic medication. These surveys and other data have been reviewed (Sprague & Gadow, 1977), and on the basis of population census figures, it is estimated that about 600,000 school children in the United States are receiving stimulant medication during any one year.

Antipsychotics

The usage patterns of antipsychotic (neuroleptic) medication which, as pointed out in Chapter 8, are used largely as behavioral depressants, are quite different. Lipman (1970) surveyed institutions for the mentally retarded, and reported that about 50% of the institutional population were receiving psychotropic medication, often at very high dosages and for

---

The preparation of this review was supported in part by USPHS Grant No. MH 18909 from the National Institute of Mental Health.

very long periods of time. The picture has not changed much in the past 7 to 8 years according to Cohen and Sprague (1977)—if anything, the percentage may have increased somewhat to around 60%, though the length of time the residents are on medication seems to have declined (Sprague & Baxley, in press). Data from one New Zealand institution indicate about 40% of the retarded residents there were receiving psychotropic drugs (Sewell & Werry, 1976). In contrast to children in institutions, Gadow (1977) found that of 3,300 children in trainable special education classes in Illinois, about 7.5% were receiving antipsychotic medication. Projecting the 7.5% prevalence to the 1,350,000 retarded children in public schools in the United States would amount to about 101,000 on antipsychotic (neuroleptic) medication.

Current Issues and Attitudes

The Public

Public concern about the use of psychotropic drugs in children has continued unabated since 1970 (Maynard, 1970), when it was alleged on television and in national newspapers that large numbers of children (as high as 25%) in the Omaha school district were receiving stimulant medication for treatment of learning disabilities. Such unsubstantiated reports were later proven to be wrong (Sprague, 1972), but the stories were sufficient to result in a Congressional Hearing called by Representative Gallagher in September just prior to the Fall Congressional elections. During these hearings, Lipman (Gallagher, 1970) gave the first estimate as to the number of children in the United States receiving psychotropic drugs, an *estimate* which has been quoted repeatedly as if it were established *fact*. Despite its sensationalism, the Congressional enquiry faded before expert evidence and there is reason to believe it may have been politically motivated in the first place (Alpern, 1976; Sherill, 1973).

These sensational reports in the media and the Congressional hearings were sufficient to encourage a number of like stories for the next few years. One of the more prolific freelance writers, Divoky (1973), has written a number of articles and co-authored a book (Schrag & Divoky, 1975) which is extremely critical of a wide range of programs for exceptional children, particularly those affiliated with the public schools, and of the disorder of hyperactivity (see Chapter 5) which the authors seem to assume is a myth developed by a conspiracy of authoritarian physicians, school administrators, and teachers in cooperation with parents, to control difficult children (Schrag & Divoky, 1975). Evidence of continuing interest can be seen by a recent article by Bell (1977) dealing with the issue of hyperactivity and stimulant drugs centered on description of a lawsuit arising from one school district in California.

The Schools

Public schools have always been involved in the diagnosis and treatment of the hyperactive child because it is primarily the environment of the classroom with its necessary constraints that led to the recognition of the problems of the hyperactive child. But public focus on the role of the public schools in the diagnosis and treatment of such children has arisen only in the last few years. Perhaps the single most influential article was that by Grinspoon and Singer (1973) which appeared in the prestigious *Harvard Educational Review*. Unfortunately, this comprehensively referenced article contains numerous *interpretations* of data that many researchers in this area, including this author, seriously question. Interest in the role of the public schools continues to grow as evidenced by a recent publication of a monograph (Robin & Bosco, 1976) which was subsequently reissued as a book (Bosco & Robin, 1977). These authors have been interested in the sociological analysis of the process by which children are identified as hyperactive. In a chapter in their book, Freeman (1977) exhaustively traces how many professions dealing with children have been drawn into the hyperactivity business by diagnosing and/or proposing their own brand of treatment for the difficulties of these children.

Another indication of public school interest was discernible in 1977 when the Council on Exceptional Children, one of the largest organizations of special education in the U.S., with about 60,000 members, started a series of credit institutes on a variety of topics, including the issue of psychotropic drug medication for exceptional children in the school. Further, many state educational regions, for example, the northern district of Iowa, have sponsored their own in-service seminars for training in the area of diagnosis and management, as well as examining the role of the public school in the treatment of hyperactive children.

The Institutions

Public, and for that matter private, institutions have been plunged into the controversy by numerous lawsuits initiated primarily in the 1970's. Although the history of these suits will be covered in more detail later in this chapter, it is worth mentioning here that the most famous one, *Wyatt v. Stickney* (1972), set the pace for other litigation. In this, a resident of Partlow State School in Tuscaloosa, Alabama, sued the State Commissioner of Mental Health, Dr. Stonewall B. Stickney, demanding many changes in the program of institutional care for the retarded including the use of psychotropic drugs. Judge Johnson issued an order that residents of such public facilities have a constitutional right to treatment which he then defined by a number of standards. He also ruled that residents have a right to be free of excessive medication and that behavioral effects of the medication must be noted in the medical records. This suit was followed quickly by other suits. Perhaps the most extensive set of court standards has been issued in Minnesota in the case of *Welch* v. *Likins* (1976) (see below).

The Government

REGULATORY SYSTEMS

In the United States there are several agencies and levels of government which have authority to regulate the use of psychotropic medication. Ultimately, most of this regulation is handled at the nationwide or Federal level, but more and more of the State governments are becoming involved. Usually the Department of Mental Health or Hygiene in a state has extensive control and influence over the services provided in that state for children, through the issuance of regulatory guidelines. These usually control the public institutions in that state directly and private facilities indirectly through reimbursements and other payments.

However, regulation need not stem from without. For example, one pace-setting institution for the mentally retarded, the Georgia Retardation Center in Atlanta, Georgia, has developed its own set of policies regarding the use of psychotropic drugs under the leadership of superintendent, Dr. James Clements.* Perhaps the most dramatic innovation in the Georgia Retardation Center policy is the requirement for team prescription of psychotropic drugs. Under this policy the physician cannot by himself prescribe drugs, but it must be a prescription consented to by a team representing a variety of disciplines and reviewed by other committees.

U.S. FEDERAL AGENCIES

Under national law in the United States, the *FDA* (*Food and Drug Administration*) has the final authority over certifying drugs for ship-

---

* Dr. Clements is a nationally recognized leader in the care and treatment of the mentally retarded as evidenced by his presidency of the American Association on Mental Deficiency, his active role in numerous lawsuits regarding the care and treatment of the mentally retarded, and his membership on the President's Mental Retardation Committee.

ment across state boundaries—which means that ultimately this agency determines what drugs will be approved for national marketing. The history of the FDA is most interesting because it reflects three legislative efforts arising out of crucial problems in the country related to medication. A more complete account of the FDA history and activities will be given subsequently.

Another Federal agency intimately involved, particularly in the development and testing of drugs for children, is *NIMH (National Institute of Mental Health)*. Although the FDA controls and regulates the testing and use of drugs in the United States, it does not provide funds for conducting research into the effects of medication. The comomnest source by far of funds for research with psychotropic drugs is NIMH. The funds are granted after critical peer review evaluation, i.e., a committee of peers— other experts in the speciality—thoroughly review the research applications and make recommendations to NIMH. A brief history of the important role of NIMH in the development, and especially the testing, of certified drugs for use with children has been written by Lipman (1974), who reported that the first grant to study pediatric psychopharmacology was awarded to Dr. Leon Eisenberg at Johns Hopkins University in 1958. Subsequent to this initial award, 12 other research grants have been awarded (up to the time Lipman's article was written) to investigate a wide range of topics from neurochemical actions to long-term effects. A total of 12 research projects is a relatively small number of investigations considering the large numbers of children actually receiving such medication and the complexities of the problems involved in a thorough understanding of the why, when, how, and for how long psychotropic drugs should be given to children; but of course, a certain amount of the knowledge about the effects of these drugs in adults and animals where the number of grants made by NIMH is legion, is applicable to children. Some of this paucity is due to a lack (until very recently) of interest, and, as a consequence of this, of trained investigators in pediatric psychopharmacology (Werry, 1977).

ETHICS OF RESEARCH WITH CHILDREN

The above discussion of the control and regulation of psychotropic medication for children has involved in some forms the matters of *safety* and *efficacy*, but in the 1970's serious questions have begun to be raised about the *ethics* of conducting research with children, particularly studies investigating the effects of drugs (Experiments, 1975; Katz, 1972). This concern was formalized when the *National Commission for the Protec-*

tion of Subjects of Biomedical and Behavioral Research was established (Hershey & Miller, 1976). The Commission, composed of 11 individuals from medicine, law, ethics, and lay people, was given the mandate of establishing recommendations for the ethical use of subjects in such research.*

The problem of research with children has been particularly complex and difficult (Koocher, 1976). At the time of writing this (mid-1977), the Commission has prepared only a preliminary draft of its recommendations in this area, which obviously may be changed before they become national regulations for the United States. But it is clear from the drafts that research with children, particularly research that is considered *at risk*, defined as any increased possibility of harm above the probabilities ordinarily encountered in everyday life to the subjects, such as in psychotropic drug research, will be much more tightly controlled. It is likely that the Commission will recommend that any research involving children may be conducted only if 1) the research has scientific merit; 2) appropriate studies have been first conducted in animals and adults; 3) the risk of harm or discomfort is minimized; 4) children across different groups (probably meaning racial and ethnic groups) will be selected in an equitable manner; and 5) provisions will be made to protect the privacy of the children and confidentiality of the data.

Where research involves a risk greater than that of ordinary life, which automatically involves all drug research, it is likely that the Commission will recommend that such research may be done only if additional criteria can be met, namely if 1) the experimental interventions are likely to lead to direct benefit for the individual subjects participating in the study; 2) the benefit/risk ratio is as favorable in the planned experiment as in other available alternative approaches; and 3) adequate, informed consent has been obtained from the parents or guardians of the children. In order for studies categorized *at risk* to be conducted on children, they must be approved by a human subjects committee (Institutional Review Board at each university or hospital) which will determine if: 1) risks encountered are tied to treatments being given for direct benefit to individual subjects;

---

* The members of the Commission are: Kenneth John Ryan, physician, Boston Hospital for Women; Joseph V. Brady, psychologist, Johns Hopkins University; Robert E. Cooke, physician, University of Wisconsin; Dorothy I. Height, president, National Council of Negro Women; Albert R. Jonsen, professor of bioethics, University of California; Patricia King, attorney, Georgetown University; Karen Lebacqz, professor of Christian ethics, Pacific School of Religion; David W. Louisell, attorney, University of Virginia; Donald Wayne Seldin, physician, University of Texas; Eliot Stellar, psychologist, University of Pennsylvania; and Robert H. Turtle, practicing attorney.

2) adequate monitoring for the well-being of the children has been established; 3) anticipated benefits are greater than the anticipated risks; and 4) provision has been made for the informed cooperation of the children, i.e., the children understand as best they can and are willing to participate in the study. It is likely that a national ethics board will be established to handle those few projects which appear to have merit but cannot be approved on the basis of the above criteria at the local level.

By history and precedent in American law, *consent* for children requires that their parents(s) or legal guardian(s) give permission for a number of procedures including medical treatment, school trips, etc. But the Commission has introduced the concept of *assent* which means the willingness on the part of the child to cooperate with the procedures suggested although it is recognized that such assent would not be legally binding. Assent or informed cooperation on the part of the child actively involves the child in the consent process which is the goal of the Commission. The age or level of psychosocial development at which a child can reasonably be expected to give his approval is a complex question. In other Commission documents it was suggested that the cutoff age would be 7 years of age based, apparently, on religious tradition. Many people interested in this area vigorously objected to such a fixed age cutoff, and the Commission has now established a flexible age cutoff based upon vague criteria. It seems that this problem of the child's approval has not been clarified but may become even more complex and difficult.

Whatever the outcome of the deliberations of the Commission, it is clear that the mood of the government, at least in the United States, will no longer tolerate giving researchers studying children a free hand to develop whatever designs they deem necessary and ethical for their investigations. Restrictions and regulations have arrived and more are coming. A few nationally publicized cases of highly questionable research practices such as the injection of live cancer cells in geriatric patients in Brooklyn or the deliberate withholding of treatment for syphilis of people in Alabama have led to a climate of suspicion and distrust reflected in the development of regulations such as those discussed above (Barber, 1976). However, a counterreaction pointing out that, in some cases, a failure to conduct important research would be equally unethical (Haywood, 1977) may be beginning and help to affect excessive control.

REGULATION OF CLINICAL TRIALS

Clinical trials are of course tests of the characteristics, efficacy and safety of a drug and as such are primarily experimental rather than therapeutic, though many clinical trials can be beneficial to individual participants if properly designed (Werry & Sprague, 1972). They are subject to governmental regulation in most countries. Most of the discussion will center on the U.S. which has one of the tightest systems of controls, but other countries have basically similar systems.

FDA *(Food and Drug Administration)*

A brief history of this, the main regulatory agency in the U.S., is encompassed by a summary of 3 laws (Sprague, 1977a). For a more detailed account of the history and function of the FDA than is given here, an excellent book by Silverman and Lee (1974) or a shorter account by Ray (1972) is suggested. At the beginning of the twentieth century, the United States faced a number of public health problems including a significant number of people addicted to opiates and extremely unhealthy conditions in the food industry, notably meat packing. One of the main causes of opiate addiction lay in the fact that over-the-counter medicine routinely used by many people contained opiates, and there was no indication on the label to warn people that narcotics were ingredients. After several sensational series of stories on various food and drug topics in popular magazines and books, such as Sinclair's *The Jungle,* Congress passed the Pure Food and Drugs Act of 1906 which required that medicine had to be accurately *labeled*. The next major law came in 1938 with the passage of the Food, Drug, and Cosmetic Act requiring that drugs be *safe* which Congress passed in reaction to the death of 107 people after an oral sulfa drug was placed on the market without prior testing for safety. Finally, in 1962, after extensive hearings by Senator Kefauver regarding profits of pharmaceutical firms and the thalidomide scandal in Europe, Congress passed the Kefauver-Harris amendments of 1962 which added the third and final legislation, namely a statutory requirement that a drug had to be proven *effective* before it could be marketed. In summary the 3 laws involved first, labeling of the ingredients, second, testing for safety, and finally, testing for efficacy prior to marketing.

The FDA is organized into bureaus. The primary division of concern to readers of this book is the Bureau of Drugs. Functioning under the Bureau of Drugs are a number of committees which are advisory to the staff of the FDA. In response to much criticism (Silverman & Lee, 1974) the FDA now presents many of the issues concerning medication to the appropriate advisory committee prior to making a decision. The committee dealing with psychotropic drugs in the United States is the Psychopharmacological Agents Committee consisting of experts who are usually faculty members of Universities throughout the nation selected from various academic disciplines.

A subgroup of this Psychopharmacological Agents Committee is the Pediatric Subcommittee now consisting of 10 members (Sprague, 1977b). This Subcommittee was formed July 1, 1974 after many problems had arisen in the area of psychotropic drug usage with children. Since the Psychopharmacological Agents Committee usually had only one or two pediatric members, it was decided to appoint a full Subcommittee specialized in these problems to handle the numerous questions and controversies which were gaining attention. One of the first issues brought before the Subcommittee was the issue of extensive use of neuroleptic medication with the institutionalized mentally retarded (Hayes, 1975; Lehr & Tatel, 1975).

Regulations for New Drugs

As evolved by the mid 1970's, there is a maze of complicated regulations concerning steps necessary to approve a new produce for marketing in the United States (Cavers, 1969). The reference file containing all available information for certifying a new compound for use within the United States is known as the NDA (New Drug Application). Typically, an NDA is filed by a pharmaceutical firm for a compound it has developed. The documentation involved in filing an NDA is massive, e.g. an NDA may be supported with 200 to 400 volumes each containing several hundred pages. The author has been involved in reviewing NDA's for the pediatric field, which has led him to ask his secretary, "How many feet of mail today?"

The addition of the psychotropic agents to the treatment of the mentally ill has been termed a "pharmaceutical revolution" (Lasagna, 1969), but questions are now being raised about the true extent of such a revolution. Goddard (1973), a former Commissioner of the FDA, has written that the peak number of NDA's was reached in 1958 with 253, but many of these NDA's involved merely fixed combinations of two products previously marketed. In fact, as is pointed out in the Introduction to this book, the number of newly synthesized drugs peaked in 1959 at about 60 and has steadily declined since, until during the 1970's on the average only 15 to 20 new entities were approved as NDA's (Fulda, 1976). However it has been suggested that some of this decline is due to delays within the FDA and the cumbersomeness of its requirements (FDA, 1975).

The long, complicated process of preparing an NDA with its extensive documentation and inevitable delays is not without its advantages. In 1961 a drug manufacturer, Richardson-Merrell, had an NDA for thalidomide, but Dr. Frances Kelsey, a physician-pharmacologist on the FDA staff, delayed the NDA for further information and it was never issued. Obviously, with the severe teratogenic effects of thalidomide (Lesser, 1974), this delay has been lauded as an extremely wise action (Goddard, 1973).

Another stage in the process of approving a drug for marketing is the IND (Claimed Investigational Exemption for a New Drug) (Finkel, 1973). After a compound is chemically produced and tested in the chemical laboratory, it is, obviously, necessary to test it first in animals and then in humans. The IND involves 9 items (Goddard & Allan, 1970): 1) pharmacological information, 2) results of preclinical animal studies, 3) acute toxicity data in two animal species, 4) complete description of the planned study, 5) qualifications of the investigators, 6) copies of informational material for the experimenter, 7) an agreement that the investigators will notify the FDA of adverse reactions, 8) certification that informed consent will be obtained from prospective subjects, and 9) agreement to submit annual reports.

There are 3, perhaps 4, distinct steps or phases through which the compound must proceed sequentially before it can be approved for marketing (Guidelines, 1974).

1) Phase I involves *safety*, pharmacological effects, and dose-related side effects. These are obtained in normal volunteers and are based upon open studies (no fixed time or required number of subjects is set) of a single dose and some time-limited multiple doses. Evidence for the drug absorption, distribution, excretion, and metabolism is usually obtained during this phase.

2) Phase II involves evidence of *clinical efficacy* in appropriate patient groups. The studies usually start with *single-blind* studies (the patient consents to be uninformed of drug conditions until the study is completed) on small numbers of patients and proceed to more well designed *double-blind* studies (both patient and physician uninformed as to the drug conditions).

3) Phase III provides the final step for extensive studies with larger samples and methodologically complete experiments. This phase is designed to confirm the tentative evidence obtained from patient groups in Phase II.

4) Phase IV. Up until the recent years, a drug only had to pass through these three phases before being certified for use with the general population under the care of a medical practitioner. However, there has

been great dissatisfaction with the lack of continued monitoring after introduction on to the market and with the slow, cumbersome method, fraught with many legal roadblocks, of removing a drug from the market once it had been certified (Mintz, 1969). The concept of post-marketing surveillance, known as Phase IV, has been proposed and is being accepted, at least by the advisory committee. It involves placing limitations on the certification of the NDA, contingent upon the manufacturer continuing to monitor for specified effects of the drug and producing required information at intervals after the introduction of the drug on the market. For the pediatric psychopharmacology area, an example of a Phase IV requirement is that relating to the stimulant pemoline (Cylert) (see Chapter 6).

FDA Pediatric Psychopharmacology Guidelines (see also Chapter 2)

In spite of the extensive documentation required for the NDA and the series of formal phases described above, the FDA had not developed a specific set of rules and standards by which a firm would be expected to plan its research on a psychotropic NDA intended for use with children. The absence of such guidelines produced criticism on one hand that the FDA was too lax scientifically and politically in applying standards of scientific rigor to NDAs and, on the other hand, (mainly from the drug firms) that the FDA was capricious and confused as to what it really wanted. One of the tasks assigned to the Pediatric Subcommittee was the development of such a set of guidelines.

In a 28-page document entitled "Guidelines for Evaluation of Psychoactive Agents in Infants and Children" plus several hundred pages in nine appendices which define concepts and procedures and amplify discussion of techniques, the Pediatric Subcommittee has developed a set of standards for pediatric psychopharmacology. The stated goals of the guidelines are, "... *intended to help those who design and conduct investigations of psychopharmacologic agents in children. They will be utilized in the review of IND protocols designed to conduct such studies, and in the evaluation of safety and efficacy of psychoactive substances claimed in new drug applications.*" When safety data are lacking for Phase I studies, it is recommended that these data be obtained on adult volunteers before beginning Phase I studies with children. The type of research facility and kind of experimenters are specified, "... *studies ... should usually be conducted largely in or in cooperation with pediatric research units ... by experienced multidisciplinary teams comprised of clinicians, psychopharmacologists and behavioral scientists.*"

Selection criteria for patients are recommended to include specification of the target behavior and the context in which it occurs plus other important variables: 1) age of onset, 2) age of entry into the study, 3) severity of symptoms, 4) duration of symptoms, 5) associated symptoms, 6) sex, 7) sociocultural-environmental context, 8) study context, 9) intellectual level, 10) prior treatment and response, and 11) idiosyncratic responses. Several different measurements for effect are suggested including global ratings, self-report, observations, and laboratory procedures. A large number of variables are suggested for possible inclusion to monitor safety: 1) intellectual, 2) social, 3) behavioral and emotional, 4) growth, 5) sexual maturation, 6) skeletal maturation, 7) standard physical and neurological examination, 8) cardiovascular, 9) hematological, 10) renal and metabolic, 11) hepatic, 12) endocrine, 13) electroencephalography, and 14) electromyography. Recommendations are given about the schedule and frequency of the measurements (which are discussed in detail in Chapter 2).

Under Phase II it is emphasized that change in target symptoms alone is not sufficient, "*but also the development of side effects if any, and the degree of change in non-target characteristics selected to monitor the child's general status.*" This point is important because far too often drugs have been evaluated only on the criterion of symptom suppression without concern for or investigation of other, sometimes detrimental, effects (Marholin & Phillips, 1976). The importance of follow-up for long durations is emphasized, "*This is particularly important in pediatric psychopharmacology because long term drug effects on growth, development, learning, and maturation are equally important to establish as drug efficacy itself.*" (See also Chapters 2, 3 and 6.)

Phase III recommendations stress patient selection ". . . *should reflect the spectrum of patients and symptom patterns encountered in the type of clinical practice in which the drug will be used.*" Other treatments, especially non-pharmacological procedures, are to be closely monitored. In this Phase, ". . . *studies should consist of double-blind, placebo-controlled studies with random assignment to experimental and control conditions and strict adherence to principles of sound experimental design and protocol. Where an existing drug is available for comparison, some studies at this stage should include comparison of the new agent with the standard.*"

If the impression has been obtained by reading this summary of only the highlights of the guidelines that they are comprehensive and tough, the impression is correct. Every member of the Subcommittee was concerned about the health and welfare of the children of the nation who are potential users of new psychotropic drugs, and the Subcommittee was cautious and conservative, although hopefully not so restrictive as to block the introduction of needed new medications.

Design of Clinical Trials

Purposes and Problems

The clinical trial is the method by which the indications for, and efficacy and safety of a drug are now ordinarily established. The design of such trials may be informal or highly formalized. Informal (uncontrolled) trials based on simple clinical observation have a respectable place in the history of medicine. However, for every discovery of a *potent drug* such as quinine for malaria or the usefulness of the amphetamines in behaviorally disturbed children by Bradley in 1937 (see Chapter 6), or the detection of serious *side effects* such as tardive dyskinesias with antipsychotic drugs (see Chapter 8), this method has spawned probably hundreds of falsely optimistic reports about the value or safety of drugs. For example, an analysis of all the studies in pediatric psychopharmacology carried out up to 1971 (756 in all) by Sulzbacher (1973) showed that informal studies were overwhelmingly indicative of drug potency while formal studies were much less enthusiastic in their findings.

Most readers are also probably aware of the way in the past that drug companies often field-tested their products, namely by using medical practitioners without training in clinical pharmacology, and often in unsupervised private practice. There were even accusations that some of the data had been fabricated in some instances. One need only reflect on the uncritical enthusiasm with which the dietary treatment of hyperkinesis was promulgated and accepted only to be reduced to size by subsequent formal studies (see Chapter 10) to realize that there seems to be some fundamental vulnerability in our society to the promulgation of false cures. Why is this? Only in a few instances are the promoters dishonest. The rather more usual circumstance is the one in which the doctor is misled by the *data* which do not or cannot show what he thought they did, or because he did not *control for error*, so that changes in the data which he attributed to the treatment are, in fact, attributable to other factors.

The interpretation of data is primarily a question of *measurement* (reliability and validity) discussed in detail in Chapter 2, and of *statistical and numerical analysis* which is also discussed there and in sections below. The control for error is aimed at four principal sources: The first is the well-known *placebo effect* which results from doctor and patient expectancies that benefit will result, and is ordinarily controlled by the use of double-blind, placebo-controlled procedures, too familiar to need further discussion. The second is *spontaneous improvement*—there is far too inadequate recognition of the fact that most medical conditions, including child psychiatric disorders, have a strong tendency toward improvement as a function of time alone (see review by Robins, in press b). Both these factors, but especially the latter, have kept and still keep doctors (and quacks) in business despite all the impressive bric-a-brac of modern medical practice. The third important source of error is *biased sampling* in which findings are typical only of a most unlikely group of patients, comparative groups are not equivalent, or unfavorable cases (such as treatment dropouts) are discarded, greatly exaggerating any treatment effects.

Other sources of error, which tend to have the opposite effect in that they miss drug effects, relate to *pharmacological* errors such as testing before or after a drug has acted, inadequate or excessive dosage, and *failure to take the medication* as prescribed (see Chapter 1 for discussion of these factors).

For all these reasons, control for error and proper attention to measurement issues and interpretation of results has made the technology of drug trials, especially in pediatric psychopharmacology where treatment effects are often quite small, measurement difficult and placebo effects and spontaneous improvement quite strong, exceedingly complex. While practitioners can and should contribute to the detection of novel therapeutic actions of established drugs (such as the anti-enuretic action of the antidepressants—see Chapter 7) and of unexpected treatment emergent effects such as the tardive dyskinesias with antipsychotic drugs (see Chapter 8), *the day of the amateur in clinical trials is very definitely over and to be actively discouraged.* The FDA pediatric guidelines are likely to hasten an end to this amateurism which is now no more appropriate than the Victorian Engilsh gentleman anthropologist and his retinue in Egypt or Africa.

In Table 1 is set out a useful checklist of points by which to evaluate any clinical trial which covers most of the common error points. More detail can be found in various texts (e.g., Hamilton, 1974) and reviews (Sprague & Werry, 1971; Werry & Sprague, 1972) and in the citations which follow in the sections below. However, two topics, experimental designs and statistics, require further discussion since they are not covered elsewhere in this volume.

Experimental Designs

There are basically four kinds of experimental designs which have been used effectively in studying psychotropic drugs.

TABLE 1

Check List for Assessing a Therapeutic Trial Report

Author and Journal reference   Encircle   Y = Yes
                                      as   N = No, or not clear
                                Appropriate   D = Doubtful
Title   n/a = not applicable
AIM: specific ...., or not clear ...., single ...., or multiple....

2-4. DESCRIPTION OF SUBJECTS, DRUG ADMINISTRATION, ETC.
ARE THE FOLLOWING SPECIFIED?
- 2.1 Healthy subjects or patients?   Y N
- 2.2 Volunteers or not?   Y N
- 2.3 Age   Y N
- 2.4 Sex   Y N
- 2.5 Race   Y N
- 2.6 Criteria of selection   Y N
- 2.7 Contraindications   Y N
- 2.8 Presence of disease other than that treated   Y N
- 2.9 Whether additional treatments were given   Y N
  If they were, are they described   Y N
- 3.1 Daily dose   Y N n/a
- 3.2 Frequency of administration   Y N n/a
- 3.3 Hour(s) o'clock when given   Y N n/a
- 3.4 Route of administration   Y N n/a
- 3.5 Source of drug (e.g., name of manufacturer)   Y N n/a
- 3.6 Presentation (e.g., tablet syrup, etc.)   Y N n/a
- 3.7 Timing of drug administration in relation to factors affecting absorption (e.g., meals)   Y N n/a
- 3.8 Checks that drug was taken   Y N n/a
- 3.9 Other therapeutic measures (if drug was not used)   Y N n/a
  If yes, are they described?   Y N n/a
- 3.10 Total duration of treatment   Y N n/a
- 4.1 Persons who made the observations   Y N n/a
- 4.2 Inpatient/outpatient   Y N n/a
- 4.3 Setting (e.g., one or several hospitals/clinics/wards)   Y N
- 4.4 Dates when trial began and was completed   Y N

5. METHODS AND DESIGN
   - 5.1 Are the methods of assessing therapeutic effects clearly described?   Y N
   - 5.2 Were these standardized methods?   Y N
   - 5.3 Were control measures used to reduce variation that might influence the results?   Y N
     If *yes*, specify:
     concurrent controls ....   patient his own control ....
     stratification or matched subgroups ....   identical ancillary treatment ....
     run-in period ....   other ....
   - 5.4 Were controls used to reduce bias?   Y N
     If *yes*, specify:
     "blind" observers ....   random allocation ....
     matching dummies ....   "blind" patients ....

TABLE 1 *(continued)*

6. ASSESSMENT OF THE TRIAL
   6.1 Were the subjects suitably selected in relation to aims
       (See sections 1 and 2)?   Y N
   6.2 Were the methods of measurement valid in relation to the aim?   Y N
   6.3 Were they adequately standardized?   Y N
   6.4 Were they sufficiently sensitive?   Y N
   6.5 Was the design appropriate?   Y N
   6.6 Were enough subjects used?   Y N
   6.7 Was the dosage appropriate?   Y N
   6.8 Was the duration of treatment adequate?   Y N
   6.9 Were carry-over effects avoided or allowed for?   Y N n/a
   6.10 (a) If no controls were used, were they unnecessary?   Y N
        (b) If controls were used, were they adequate?   Y N
   6.11 Was comparability of treatment groups examined?   Y N n/a
   6.12 Are the data adequate for assessment?   Y N
   6.13 (a) If statistical tests were not done, were they unnecessary?
        (b) If statistical tests are reported
            (i) Is it clear how they were done?   Y N
            (ii) Were they appropriately used?   Y N D

7. OTHER ASPECTS OF THE REPORT
   7.1 Are unwanted effects, or their absence, mentioned?   Y N
   7.2 Are the conclusions justified from the data presented?
       completely ....   partially ....   no ....
   7.3 Is the summary completely accurate?   Y N n/a

8. COMMENTS

9. IS THE TRIAL ACCEPTABLE?
   Definitely yes ....   Probably yes ....   No ....

Source: N. Lionel and A. Herxheimer, Assessing reports of therapeutic trials. Brit. Med. J. 3:637, 1970. Reproduced with permission of Drs. Lionel and Herxheimer and the editor of the *British Medical Journal*.

INFORMAL OBSERVATIONS

One of these is the *quasi-experimental* or informal design which capitalizes on the availability of natural, intact groups which often are unattainable in a planned, controlled experiment and which relies heavily on astute clinical observations. The experimenter does not establish the conditions or groups artifically but takes advantages of what nature or a clinical situation has provided and simply uses the resources available in a creative way. There are examples of the use of this design in pediatric psychopharmacology. Safer et al. (1972) first observed that children who happen to be placed on stimulants for a year or more seem to grow less when compared to classmates who were not on stimulant medication. This observation led to widespread concern about the possibility of growth suppression in children receiving stimulants and prompted controlled experimental designs (Greenhill et al., 1977; McNutt et al., 1977). As noted above, this method is particularly suited to detecting extensions of activity of a drug and unexpected side effects.

COMPARATIVE GROUPS

Probably the most common experimental design is the *between subjects* or groups design in which the experimenter arbitrarily (randomly) assigns one group of children to the placebo condition, and other groups to the experimental drug under investigation. Elemental to such a study of course is proper matching of groups, which is not always obvious or easily achieved. This design is becoming more difficult to conduct, largely due to the ethical problem of denying arbitrarily to one group of children the benefits of a needed treatment simply for methodological reasons (Sprague & Werry, 1971). But in many cases, this is the only design that is satisfactory, especially when one is dealing with a treatment that produces irreversible long-term effects or produces a sequential effect, i.e., an effect which occurs only in a certain order of administration.

CROSSOVER DESIGN

Possibly the most common design for use with children currently, primarily due to ethical considerations, is the *within subjects* or crossover design. In this design each child receives each condition, for example, placebo and drug, with the order of the presentation of the conditions randomized over time, i.e., placebo then drug as well as drug then placebo. Since each child receives a trial of each condition, there are fewer ethical problems because the child is not denied a needed treatment, other than for a brief, defensible period of time. The case certainly can be made that *a priori* very few treatments, particularly psychotropic drug treatments, can be determined to be beneficial for a particular child without a mini-trial. Such a trial would of necessity require a condition in which the child was observed without drug. There are several other advantages of this type of design including, usually, a greater sensitivity to drug effect (Sprague & Werry, 1971; Sulzbacher, 1973), which may stem, in part at least, from better control over a whole series of background, physical and other variables which, short of cataclysmic personal upheaval, are constant for each subject as he rotates through each condition, or acts as his own control. An added advantage is fewer children are needed than in between subject designs since each child forms a part of each treatment "group." However, as a consequence, each child has to undergo much more testing and make more visits to the evaluation center, which may present a real problem logistically and in acceptability. The crossover design is also dependent on reversibility of drug effects between phases and it is theoretically possible, for example, in the case of a drug that allowed learning to read to occur, that withdrawing the drug would not reverse the effect.

SINGLE SUBJECT DESIGNS

The last and newest design to be discussed is the *single subject* procedure. As the name implies, only a single subject or patient is used to test the various treatment conditions. Such a procedure has been used for years by researchers in behavior modification. The problem with this design is that it has been difficult to assess the *statistical* significance of any differences between baseline and treatment conditions. Recently, there has been a serious attempt to develop statistical techniques suitable to testing the significance of changes occurring in a single subject (Shine & Bower, 1971). Also indicative of the interest in the use of this design has been the appearance of 2 books in the last 7 years (Davidson & Costello, 1969; Hersen & Barlow, 1976). The advantages of this technique are its suitability for individual patients in unique situations, a common enough occurrence in child psychiatry, and for well-defined but infrequent conditions like classical infantile autism which need multi-center trials.

Statistics

Dependent on whether one is clinician or investigator, this word may evoke vilification or exaltation. In point of fact, statistics are no more than mathematical devices for *adjudicating* on results as to whether they could or could not have occurred simply by chance and for *manipulating* and *fitting* data into meaningful patterns and relationships according to their numerical properties. The latter process is somewhat akin to the crude so-called eye-balling of data or drawing of informal graphs, but is considerably more accurate. Few doctors understand statistics and it is important, therefore, that in doing research and clinical trials in pediatric psychopharmacology, they should have access to and consult with someone who has the requisite theoretical knowledge. They will, however, find this less disagreeable and confusing if they find someone who also has some practical clinical experience since this tempers the ideal with the possible, softens obfuscation, and results in rather more tolerance for the difficulties of conducting clinical research. This combination is most likely to be found in a clinical psychologist with a Ph.D. from a good university.

A few remarks about statistics are germane before describing some of the main methods. All statistical methods are subject to limitations based on assumptions about the data to which the methods are to be applied. For example, the commonly used product moment correlation coefficient (r) assumes that any relationship between variables will be linear. Such relationships are rare in nature and a zero or near zero r may, for example, miss a substantial dose/effect relationship the nature of which changes as the dose changes, especially if the relationship is actually an inverted U shape quite common biologically. The second point is that the *statistical significance* may have little to do with the *clinical significance* of the findings which may be quite trivial. For example, a recent study of two hypnotic (sleeping) drugs showed that they were statistically highly significantly ($p = .001$) superior to placebo in increasing sleep time but, inasmuch as this was only some half hour in amount, this effect was clinically insignificant.

Statistics, then, are tools, certainly useful and highly desirable but neither idols nor devils. They are there primarily to assist processing of data and the prevention of self-deception, but they are no substitute for thinking.

There are 3 main classes of statistical techniques which will be briefly discussed in this section.

NON-PARAMETRIC

Non-parametric statistics are essentially based on head *count or rank* (see Chapter 2) rather than measurement of the quantity of a variable, e.g., activity level or learning. There are many situations, particularly with between subjects designs, when the only information a researcher can obtain is the number of children who displayed a particular symptom versus those who did not. In such a situation the non-parametric statistic is the appropriate technique. Although numerous articles have appeared about these techniques, a book written by Siegal (1956) is still an excellent source of information. The commonest non-parametric technique by far is of course, Chi^2 (X^2), but other useful techniques are the sign test, the Wilcoxin Sign-Rank Test and Friedman Analysis of Variance. Correlation techniques include Spearman's rho and Kendall's tau.

PARAMETRIC

These refer to a wide range of techniques which assess the probability or likelihood of obtaining a difference as large as the one observed by chance on some *quantifiable* variable (see Chapter 2). Hundreds of articles and dozens of books have been written on this topic but the most used techniques are few—t test, analysis of variance, analysis of covariance and the product moment correlation coefficient. Analysis of covariance (ANCOVA) has been particularly popular in pediatric psychopharmacological studies because it permits initial differences between groups of children, for example on age or IQ, to be factored out insofar as they influence the effects of the treatments under consideration. In this way an assessment of the efficacy of the drug in general may be obtained. Like all statistical techniques ANCOVA is subject to certain assumptions which must be met and the technique has been misused to some extent. The proper use of this technique has recently been reviewed (Overall & Woodward, in press). However, as pediatric psychopharmacological studies move increasingly toward multi-assessment procedures, it becomes highly desirable, or necessary, to utilize multivariate analyses (Tatsuoka, 1971) rather than univariate or single variable analyses which have been so popular for the past 25 years. Examples of such techniques are multiple regression, multivariate analysis of variance, multiple discriminant analysis, and factor analysis. Such techniques offer an opportunity to *integrate* data from different sources such as doctor, laboratory, parent and school (see also Chapter 2).

TIME SERIES ANALYSIS

An analytic procedure new to behavioral sciences but used in other sciences, such as engineering, has recently gained attention as a technique for analyzing data in which there are cyclic patterns over time—much of human behavior measured over time displays such patterns. This technique is *time-series analysis* which measures patterns that are present but difficult to detect in data (Glass et al., 1974; Gottman et al., 1969). Time-series analyses offer a particular promise for single subjects designs. For those interested in this kind of analysis, a recent chapter by Kazdin (1976) is an excellent source of information and references.

Summary

The design, execution and interpretation of clinical trials in pediatric psychopharmacology are complex technological matters which require a sound knowledge of pharmacology, behavioral science and clinical child psychiatry or behavioral pediatrics. No one person or profession is likely to have all the requisite knowledge and a team of peers is necessary.*

---

* In case anyone thinks Dr. Sprague is grinding a psychologist's axe, it should be noted that this summary was inserted by the editor; see also Chapter 2.—(Ed.)

Recent Litigation and Legislation

Legislation

Legislative interest into the issue of psychotropic drug treatment of children can be traced to the previously described congressional hearings convened by Representative Gallagher. Although a number of legislatures in several states established committees to investigate the usage of stimulant medications in children following the Gallagher hearings (Robin & Bosco, 1976), none of these investigations resulted in legislation until Massachusetts passed a law which "bans" (Brown & Bing, 1976) research on pediatric psychopharmacology. The legislation was proposed as a reaction to a pediatric psychopharmacology project funded by NIMH, scheduled to be conducted in Boston with the cooperation of the public schools. A local community group comprised primarily of minority citizens pressured the Institutional Review Board of the Massachusetts Department of Mental Health until that Board withdrew its previous approval of the project. The participants in this controversy, including the researcher, the community advocates, the state representative who introduced the bill, and national leaders, met in a two-day "confrontation" session in 1976 which has been summarized by the Hastings Center (MBD, 1976).

The most unfortunate aspect of the entire incident, in this reviewer's opinion, is that a law was passed that *banned only research in cooperation with the schools and not the clinical use of the drugs in any way!* The proscribing of such research has been praised by one of the community advocates, thus: "The same year, partially as a consequence of the above experiment, Massachusetts adopted a *model psychotropic drug law. The statute bans the use of such drugs* on school children for the purposes of *clinical research* (italics added)" (Brown & Bing, 1976). Thus, the issue was resolved in Boston not by banning drug use, not by requiring more rigorous monitoring of drug effects under treatment conditions, *but by prohibiting further investigations to obtain needed information about the claims and counter claims in the controversy*. This is particularly a sad commentary because it occurred in the city of some of the greatest universities and research centers in the United States.

In a thesis primarily concerned with the issue of stimulant medication with hyperactive children, Appleman (1974) surveyed the Offices of Education in the 50 states and received responses to 42 (84%) of his questionnaires. At that time, three states had laws regarding the use of stimulant medication: Massachusetts, as previously discussed, prohibited clinical research with public school children; New Hampshire had a law recommending that medication should only be used when clearly appropriate and that careful monitoring and observation of the child by the physician, school personnel, and parents be done; New Jersey prohibited the administration of any drug for experimental purposes unless on the written consent of the parent or guardian *and* the family physician. Four other states have issued administrative regulations under broader preexisting legislation: Connecticut, Hawaii, Indiana, and Oregon, while 6 states also issued guidelines for the use of stimulant medication: Connecticut, Delaware, Iowa, Minnesota, New Hampshire, and New York.

Regulatory Changes

In addition to the state offices of education which have taken action as described above, state departments of mental health have taken regulatory action in regard to the general issue of psychotropic drugs including use with children, the best example of which was issued by the Michigan Department of Mental Health in 1976 (available upon request). The regulations contained 18 standards for the use of psychotropic drugs, and these will be summarized and quoted in part. The most important standard, in my opinion, is the second standard which states, "*The target symptoms and behaviors to be treated should be recorded in the clinical record. These signs and symptoms constitute a baseline against which the patient's clinical condition is evaluated and also permit an evaluation of the efficiency of the treatment interventions.*" Monitoring is properly emphasized in standard three, "*Effects of medication on the target symptoms and the patient behavior should be recorded weekly in the patient's progress notes.*" Appropriate dosages are discussed in standards five and seven, "*Dosage should be reduced to minimum maintenance dose after the desired clinical result is obtained and the patient's condition has stabilized. . . . A single daily dose should be used after the patient is stabilized on a maintenance dose whenever this is possible.*" Polypharmacy or the prescription of several drugs at one time, is discouraged in standard 12, "*Only one psychotropic drug shall be prescribed at one time.*" Finally, the regulations acknowledge the continuing need for information and training in standard 17, "*Each institution . . . should develop in-house training—retaining seminars at which consultants in the use of anti-psychotic and other behavioral drugs can discuss chemotherapy with the hospital or center medical staff, including those responsible for outpatient care.*"

Soon after establishment by the FDA of the Pediatric Subcommittee, a petition was presented to the FDA by the Washington law firm of Hogan and Hartson regarding alleged misuse of psychotropic drugs in institutions for the mentally retarded in the United States. Considerable time and effort was devoted to the study of this problem including a special workshop at the convention of the American Association on Mental Deficiency, the professional group which is most concerned with the mentally retarded. Lehr and Tatel (1975) of the law firm concerned also presented their case to the AAMD then, citing considerable material in newspaper reports. The role of the FDA in this matter was outlined by Hayes (1975). The result of this presentation and deliberations by the Subcommittee has been summarized (Sprague, 1977b). The petitioners asked for seven specific actions to be taken by the FDA, several of which were approved by FDA Commissioner Schmidt: revised labeling of some of the phenothiazines, revised labeling of some drugs to clarify specific behavior problems for which they should be administered, labeling to include cautions about monitoring effects with the retarded who have difficulty in verbal communication, and a promise that warnings and precautions about the use of psychotropic drugs would be issued from time to time when necessary.

In response to serious questions raised about growth suppression with stimulants (Safer et al., 1972; see also Chapter 6), the Pediatric Subcommittee has addressed the issue of how to study possible drug effects on the growth and development of children. Longitudinal studies are extremely difficult due to numerous complexities and sources of confounding in trying to ascertain the possible effects of medication separated from environment, diagnostic condition, and time (see also Chapter 2). The Subcommittee held a workshop with experts in physical growth, methodology and statistics, and developmental endocrinology in an attempt to establish possible models for such studies, which will help in the formulation of guidelines in this area.

Litigation

Foreigners are inclined to regard the U.S. as a litigious society and, certainly in the 1970's, there has been a marked trend there to turn to the courts, especially the Federal courts, to seek a whole series of rights of various individuals, groups, and classes of people. There is no better example of this trend than a series of lawsuits regarding the rights of children, especially the *right to treatment* and the *right to education*. Most, but not all, of this litigation has involved mentally retarded residents in state institutions. Because of their indications of social concern and deficiencies in professional knowledge and practice in pediatric psychopharmacology, a brief survey in chronological order of this litigation will be given, outlining the major points of the lawsuits.

The landmark case is *Wyatt v Stickney* in which Judge Frank M. Johnson forcefully detailed the specific meaning of the constitutional right to treatment. He dictated that the right to treatment involves appropriate treatment for the condition of the retarded resident for "habilitation" which he defined as *"the process by which the staff of the institution assists the resident to acquire and maintain those life skills which enable him to cope more effectively with the demands of his own person and of his environment and to raise the level of his physical, mental, and social efficiency"* (*Wyatt* v *Stickney*, 1972, p. 395). The governor of Alabama and the commissioner of mental health appealed this decision to the Court of Appeals which, however, upheld Judge Johnson (*Wyatt* v *Aderholt*, 1974).

In *Wyatt* the court developed a 12-page "Minimum Constitutional Standards for Adequate Habilitation of the Mentally Retarded." Numerous clauses and phrases in these minimum standards have become almost household words, at least among professionals. Some examples of the requirements which are now commonly accepted are: *"Residents shall have a right to habilitation, including medical treatment, education and care, suited to their needs, regardless of age, degree of retardation or handicapped condition. . . . Residents shall have the right to the least restrictive conditions necessary to achieve the purposes of habilitation"* (p. 396). Standard 22 refers to medication. The most important concept in this standard is, *"Residents shall have a right to be free from unnecessary or excessive medication. The resident's records shall state the effects of psychoactive medication on the resident. When dosages of such are changed or other psychoactive medications are prescribed, a notation shall be made in the resident's record concerning the effect of the new medication or new dosages and the behavior changes, if any, which occur"* (p. 400). Embodied in this statement are several important concepts including the right to be unhampered by excessive medication, the necessity of adequately monitoring and recording behavioral change, and the importance of dosage in regard to monitoring and recording. The concept of monitoring is further supported in section b, *"Notation of each individual's medication shall be kept in his medical records. . . . At least weekly the attending physician shall review the drug regimen of each resident under his care. All prescriptions shall be written with termination date, which shall not exceed 30 days."* Another section deals with the tendency, at least in institutions, to use psychotropic drugs as a means of suppressing undesirable behavior in the absence of active treatment programs to bring about behavioral changes in the residents: *"Medication shall not be used as punishment, for the convenience of staff, as a substitute for a habilitative program, or in quantities that interfere with the resident's habilitation program."*

Other parts of the 7-part Standard 22 deal with more mundane items, rather than setting constitutional precedents, such as the order that medication should not be administered without a written order of a physician and that adequate pharmacy services must be provided.

Another major case was settled by consent decree, i.e., both plaintiff and defendants agreed on terms of the settlement (*New York State ARC v Rockefeller*, 1975). In that decree there were 23 sets of standards imposed ranging from community placement to medication to speech and audiology services. Appendix Q, Medication, includes the orders issued in *Wyatt* plus new orders: *"Only appropriately trained staff shall be allowed to administer drugs. . . . Written policies and procedures that govern the safe administration and handling of all drugs shall be developed . . ., and medication errors and drug reactions shall be recorded and reported immediately to the practitioner who ordered the drug."*

The above cases involved governmental units, namely state facilities for the mentally retarded. A loophole existed in this series of litigations in the sense that the federal government through various aid programs supports tens of thousands of children in private facilities in the United States. In fact, some states with lax regulations for private, profit-making facilities have attracted a number of entrepreneurs who have developed and built facilities for children (Velie, 1976). Another case (*Gary W. v State of Louisiana*, 1976) has been decided which will probably also become an influential case. An attorney filed suit against Louisiana on behalf of a Louisiana adolescent who was placed by Louisiana officials in a privately owned Texas facility. The attorney was joined by consumer legal groups and by the Office of Special Litigation of the U.S. Department of Justice. The author made site visits to many of the private facilities for the Office of Special Litigation and found intolerable conditions for many of the children. In one facility for severely retarded children, the average stay for residents was 7.8 years with 66% of the residents receiving regular antiepileptic medication (see Chapter 9). The monitoring of this medication was almost nonexistent in that the physician supervising these patients only ordered a laboratory test to check the physical effects of the medication once in 184.3 patient-years (a patient-year is one patient in the facility for one year). Judge Alvin B. Rubin in his decision has ordered standards similar to those previously discussed.

In another lawsuit which has attracted widespread attention in the media even though it has not been decided (Bell, 1977; Bruck, 1976), 17 parents of children in the public schools of Taft City, California filed suit against the school district and administrators claiming (among other things) that the school officials coerced them into accepting stimulant medication for their children, that the physician and school personnel did not adequately monitor the effects of the medication, that the children were improperly placed in special education classes, and that proper informed consent was not obtained (*Benskin* v *Taft City School District*, 1975). Because of the national publicity which the *Benskin* case has received, it has had an impact even before a decision has been rendered. It has made clinicians more cautious and presumably more careful in their monitoring effects of stimulant medication.

Future Trends

It should be clear from the previous discussion of litigation that much tighter controls on research on children are rapidly approaching in the United States, and the real possibility exists that, at least from a practical standpoint, pediatric psychopharmacological research may be slowed to a standstill. Such research will probably not be severely limited nationwide as it was in Massachusetts, but the regulations are becoming so onerous and the paper work so overwhelming that for all practical purposes researchers may not be able to function.

Besides the committees at the federal level making rules and guidelines, the courts are becoming involved with experimentation, particularly research that involves children. In the *New York ARC* v *Rockefeller* (1975), the court ordered that certain types of research not be done: "... *no physically intrusive, chemical, or bio-medical research or experimentation shall be performed at Willowbrook or upon members of the plaintiff class*" (Appendix P, item 4). Such a ruling is likely to be interpreted that *any research* that poses some risk regardless of its need or benefits to the residents will not be permitted.

It is questionable that it is the general public in the United States which is demanding such strict controls or outright prohibitions against research with children. What is clear is that these rules and regulations and court decisions have been supported by activist groups, usually legal advocates, who like antivivisectionists have a viewpoint that all experimentation is dangerous and inhumane. In a sitting of the National Commission for the Protection of Subjects of Biomedical and Behavioral Research a legal advocate group compared researchers to Roman emperors and Nazi storm troopers.* It is possible that these groups may prevail and obtain either regulations and/or laws which prevent needed research in this area. This outcome is especially likely if parent groups, which have a profound interest in obtaining new treatments for certain disorders, do not unite with concerned researchers before state laws or restrictive court orders are made. It is obvious that researchers in various professions should organize for this kind of lobby effort, but typically they have been notoriously disorganized and, in the words of a state legislator (Delahunt, 1976), "overwhelmingly . . . ignorant" of the political process.

It is equally apparent, on the other hand, that the public is demanding research information relevant to many pressing practical problems. For example, in response to the public clamor over the Feingold diet and the possible harmfulness of good additives, the federal government appointed 28 scientists and administrators to a group known as the Interagency Collaborative Group on Hyperkinesis to study the problem, to make recommendations for experimentation in this area, and to support research into the claim that the diet significantly reduced the symptoms of hyperactivity (Kolbye, 1976) (see also Chapter 10).

Opposing and incompatible trends concerning the treatment of children with medication for behavioral problems are present in our modern society. On the one hand, society is rapidly tightening and vigorously controlling the patient and systematic search for information about the effects of a wide range of medications with children. Yet, on the other, surveys regarding prevalence of usage certainly show that the use of psychotropic medication has not declined, but in fact *increased,* despite the general agreement among writers and researchers that there are still many unknowns and much ignorance about the effects of these medications. What will be the final outcome of these two contradictory trends? One can only hope that the swing of the pendulum toward tighter control or prohibition encounters some counterforce espousing the need for continuing information for and development of pediatric psychopharmacology. Persons in other countries may view with disdain or unconcern these American antics but what goes on in America has a habit of spreading well beyond its borders!

---

*The U.S. has always been subject to recurring cycles of anti-intellectualism which result in "pogroms" such as Palmerism or McCarthyism but the chilling aspect of the current one is that it is led by University educated persons of no mean intellect who have a conspiracy theory of and a contempt for Science.—(Ed.)

5

DIAGNOSTIC CLASSIFICATIONS AND PSYCHOPHARMACOLOGICAL INDICATIONS

RACHEL GITTELMAN-KLEIN, Ph.D.,
ROBERT L. SPITZER, M.D. and
DENNIS CANTWELL, M.D.

INTRODUCTION

Why Diagnose?

Anyone wishing to study phenomena, whether they be geological, biological, or social, must identify them, group them, and probably label them, or, in short, develop a taxonomy. In medicine, the concepts underlying classification have come to be known as the *medical or disease model*. The essence of this model is that it groups clinical and pathological phenomena into a single abnormal diagnostic entity which is, or is assumed to be, of some discrete underlying etiology, and of predictable outcome.

This model has served medicine well and it is not surprising that psychiatrists have tried to apply it to psychological and behavioral clinical phenomena. Much of the negative feeling which the concept of diagnosis has generated in psychiatry is due to a misinterpretation of the etiological implications of a psychiatric nomenclature. It is often erroneously assumed that psychiatric nosology automatically presumes the presence of *ubi-*

This paper was supported in part by USPHS grant #MH18579

The Advisory Committee on Childhood and Adolescence Disorders to the American Psychiatric Association Task Force on Nomenclature consisted of: Robert Arnstein, M.D., Dennis Cantwell, M.D., Stella Chess, M.D., Everett Dulit, M.D., Rachel Gittelman, Ph.D., Richard Jenkins, M.D., J. Gary May, M.D., Judith Rapoport, M.D., Robert L. Spitzer, M.D., Richard Ward, M.D., Paul Wender, M.D.

quitous underlying organic causes. This assumption is wrong and unwarranted—all that a psychiatric diagnostic classification suggests is that the *various categories may represent relatively discrete sets of behavioral phenomena,* or in behavioral parlance, response classes. Some might be caused by various psychopathological family influences, others by unresolved intrapsychic conflicts, yet others by biological or social factors, or by varying combinations of these. Even within each of these broad categories of causality, attempts could be made to derive a taxonomy or classification system, for instance, by describing types of personal adjustments associated with contrasting family milieus.

The arguments against psychiatric classification are fueled by strong reactions against yet another, more accurately perceived consequence of the psychiatric nomenclature. A psychiatric diagnosis defines a person as *sick,* with possible consequent social stigma. There is little doubt that, in some ways, sick people are at a disadvantage in our society. However, this is probably so whether their "sickness" is diagnosed or not. So far, it has not been demonstrated that any prejudice befalling those whose behavior deviates from the accepted social norms is the result of any label attached to the behavior rather than the result of the deviance itself. On the other hand, in some instances, being considered "ill" may be an advantage since the sick role excuses the person from many ordinary societal demands and expectations (though while invoking others such as the seeking and accepting of treatment). Therefore, the consequences of a psychiatric diagnosis need not all be handicapping.

Yet, if it is true that psychiatric diagnosis may put a child at a disadvantage (as it may), it might well be asked whether there is any value or, indeed, any justification in pursuing it? For the individual child the cost/benefit ratio of having a diagnosed psychiatric disorder varies, but the same dilemma occurs in other branches of medicine where certain diagnoses have negative social implications, for example epilepsy. As discussed in Chapter 9, it is clear that, since the advent of modern antiepileptic drugs, the epileptic child when properly diagnosed and treated is at a marked advantage by having the disorder diagnosed. In child psychiatry, there are some instances where it can be argued that a similar (though not identical) situation exists. That is, with current diagnostic classification, the child stands a better chance of finding relief from social difficulties and psychological pain. Even when such advantage is not incurred, the process of classification in child psychiatry must still continue at an investigative level since to forego it is to adopt a nihilistic, anti-scientific stand which essentially abandons all hopes of identifying other clinical syndromes, their causes, their treatment, and eventually their prevention.

Qualities of an Ideal Diagnosis

The minimum information a diagnosis can communicate is the *phenomenology* of the disorder or the constellation of clinical symptoms grouped under the common label. Doing so provides a consensus which enhances the communicative value of diagnostic terms. This grouping process can be arbitrary simply as a starting point, or based on careful, objective clinical evaluation characteristic of Hippocratic medicine, or derived from a variety of statistical techniques such as factor, cluster, or multiple regression analysis, which estimate the relationships of observed clinical phenomena mathematically (Klein & Davis, 1969). However, if all a diagnosis can do is to indicate a clinical picture and no more, it has limited value indeed.

In the ideal, a diagnosis has several characteristics. It should provide a good estimate of the *natural history* of the disorder (outcome or prognosis without treatment), its outcome given current *treatment*, its *etiologies*, the *pathophysiology* of the disorder if there is a specific biological cause, and, if there is a psychosocial cause, the *psychological mechanisms* underlying the disorder. These prognostic and etiological data are those necessary in the end to validate the syndrome and show that it is more than an arbitrary concatenation of signs and symptoms. When all these factors are known, the ground is laid not only for curing the disorders, but, better yet, for preventing it. Of course, the process of discovery need not always proceed in this orderly fashion and the establishment of specific treatments may help to define clinical syndromes (Klein, 1970, 1973) such as may well prove to be the case with depression or hyperkinetic disorder (Wender, 1971).

Unfortunately, very few psychiatric disorders of children have been investigated sufficiently so that it may be stated with confidence that they have the associated etiological, prognostic, therapeutic and preventive validating factors discussed above. Though this uncertainty is unfortunate, it should act to stimulate systematic research in diagnosis in child psychiatry rather than lead to a defeatist attitude.

Diagnosis and Pediatric Psychopharmacology

Interest in and attention to diagnosis are especially characteristic of psychopharmacology, since ideally a particular drug should be indicated in a *specific* disorder, rather than for a symptom which may be present as part of the clinical picture of several syndromes. A case in point is the treatment of hyperactivity with stimulants (see Chapter 6). Stimulants are not antiactivity drugs, since they normalize motor activity in children hitherto referred to as having the Hyperkinetic Reaction (Diagnostic and Statistical Manual, 1968), but apparently not in other conditions such as severe pervasive conditions hitherto known as childhood psychoses where overactivity may be prominent too. Therefore, it can be claimed that the use of stimulants for hyperactivity should be restricted to this specific diagnostic group, and not used promiscuously to modify hyperactivity regardless of its context. Further, this empirical clinical fact suggests that the Hyperkinetic syndrome may represent a discrete, unique array of physiological dysfunctions. This specific indication is ideal for the clinician and the patient since now there is "The right drug for the right patient."

However, such a close relationship between drug and diagnosis is all too uncommon in pediatric psychopharmacology. For example, as may be seen in Chapter 8, in contrast to the stimulants, the antipsychotics such as the phenothiazines are not effective as specific antipsychotics in children, but are used symptomatically to reduce motor activity in overactive children, regardless of any other diagnostic considerations. In this instance, the efficacy of the phenothiazines in reducing children's activity is of no diagnostic significance and cannot be used as a validating criterion for the category of Hyperkinetic Reaction as separate from other conditions in which hyperactivity occurs.

Improving Diagnosis

The degree to which the desideratum of the "right drug for the right patient" can be met is, in part, a function of how reliably we can measure the child's behavioral signs and symptoms, on which, at the moment, diagnosis in child psychiatry largely rests. This is discussed in Chapter 2 where it can be seen that there is room for significant improvement in current diagnostic practice. But the utility of diagnoses also rests on the ability of the symptoms to reflect discrete clinical categories meaningful for pharmacotherapy or other interventions. Is this claiming that there is indeed still a better chance of finding the *right drug* after having identified the *right diagnosis* through an improved taxonomy? An obvious example of the value of a good taxonomy for pharmacological discovery is the use of lithium in manic-depressive disorders (see Chapter 10). The syndrome was identified long before the use of the drug and thus facilitated the discovery of lithium treatment in those disorders. Is it expecting too much to hope that the improvements in the current diagnostic system for children (which most are agreed is unsatisfactory) may set the stage for the discovery of relationships between specific disorders and specific treatments (not necessarily all pharmacological)? The new American and

International classifications described below are an act of faith that this can be so, though the proof of the pudding will be in the eating!

However, the question is raised in Chapter 2 whether, despite improved precision in measurement and in diagnostic classifications, the remoteness of behavioral measures from the cellular actions of drugs may not limit the ability of behaviorally derived classifications to indicate a specific pharmacotherapy. Indeed, arguments have been advanced in favor of another approach to diagnostic classification whereby *drug response* would be used as the basis for identifying homogeneous patient groups (Klein, 1970, 1973; Wender, 1971). However, this strategy is not at variance with the phenomenological approach in diagnosis, and the two should complement each other. Another solution, again complementary, would be to round out behavioral with physiological measures. This is an active, though to date disappointing area in measurement in pediatric psychopharmacology (see Chapter 2).

Alternative Concepts in Diagnosis

Medical diagnoses, of which present psychiatric classifications are part, are basically qualitative and dichotomous—the attributes of conditions differ and the patient either has the condition or does not. In contrast, behavioral scientists often espouse a dimensional approach to diagnosis in which behavior is believed to consist of a number of dimensions rather like, say, height and weight, along which any individual's behavioral or personality profile may be plotted in N dimensional space. Abnormality then is simply an extreme position on one or more dimensions with the "syndrome" being defined by the *profile* rather than a simple yes/no categorization. This method has been used extensively with personality tests like the MMPI and in children's behavior rating scales (Quay, in press), some examples of which are described in Chapter 2. It is of interest that, when these are used as *classification devices*, a classification is usually achieved by truncating extreme scores into "profiles" or syndromes which have all the features and assumptions of the medical model. For example, Quay's "conduct problem" child seems much the same as the American DSM II's Unsocialized Aggressive Reaction.

Ordinarily, and probably more properly, these dimensions have been used in pediatric psychopharmacology as *predictors* or *measures* of drug effect rather than as diagnostic categories. The new American DSM III and International Classifications have some dimensional features but the heart of it is the typical medical model.

New American and International Systems

Historically, pediatric psychiatric diagnosis has received little systematic attention in the English speaking world apart from one previous attempt to provide a comprehensive diagnostic schema for children which, perhaps because of its lack of official origin, was not widely applied (GAP, 1966). Recently, both official American and international psychiatric bodies have given intensive consideration to children's diagnostic systems and have advanced relatively elaborate descriptive systems for implementation in the near future.

Because of their importance both will receive detailed discussion here. Since they are both relatively new efforts, it is expected that further extensive revisions will be in order as knowledge is accumulated.

The third edition of the American Psychiatric Association Diagnostic and Statistical Manual (DSM III) was initiated with the goal of preparing a classification system based on current knowledge and practice. The correspondence of the new classification to the Ninth Revision of the International Classification of Diseases (ICD-9) was an important, but not an overriding consideration (Spitzer & Sheehy, 1976). Consequently, though ICD-9 and DSM III may not cause problems for diagnosticians using either system exclusively, those seriously interested in diagnosis in child psychiatry must be interested in a comparison of the two classifications.

Table 1 presents the conditions listed in the section of DSM III reserved for *Disorders Usually Arising in Childhood or Adolescence* and their ICD-9 equivalents. These are disorders which usually originate during childhood and which, typically, are not known to have adult onsets. On the other hand, other disorders arise across a wide age span, from early childhood through adulthood; for example, obsessive-compulsive disorders may begin in childhood, but are also known to occur *de novo* in adulthood. Such disorders are not listed in the section of DSM III specific to childhood. Therefore, if a child presents with difficulties which coincide with those stipulated for any disorder outside the section for childhood disorders, the appropriate *adult* diagnosis is to be applied. *Consequently, it would be erroneous to assume that the list of conditions enumerated under Disorders Usually Arising in Childhood or Adolescence represents the universe of diagnoses applicable to children.* Children may receive diagnoses from the other major diagnostic rubrics included in DSM III: Organic Mental Disorders, Drug-use Disorders, Schizophrenic Disorders, Paranoid Disorders, Psychoses Not Elsewhere Classified, Affective Disorders, Anxiety Disorders, Factitious Disorders, Somatoform Disorders, Dissociative Disorders, Personality Disorders, Psychosexual Disorders,

Table 1

DSM III and ICD-9 Classifications for Childhood Disorders

Axis One—Clinical Disorder

DSM III Disorders Usually Arising in Childhood or Adolescence	ICD-9 Equivalent Categories
Mental Retardation	*Mental Retardation*
Mild	Mild
Moderate	Moderate
Severe	Severe
Profound	Profound
Unspecified	Unspecified
Pervasive Developmental Disorders	*Psychoses Specific to Childhood*
Infantile autism	Infantile autism
Atypical childhood psychosis	Other
Disintegrative psychosis	Disintegrative Psychosis
Unspecified	Unspecified
Pervasive developmental disorder, Residual state	No Equivalent
Attention Deficit Disorders	*Hyperkinetic Syndrome of Childhood*
With Hyperactivity	Simple disturbance of activity and attention
Without Hyperactivity	No Equivalent
No Equivalent, Mixed Diagnosis	Hyperkinesis with developmental delay
No Equivalent, Mixed Diagnosis	Hyperkinetic Conduct Disorder
Stereotyped Movement Disorders	*Special Symptoms or Syndromes Not Elsewhere Classified*
Transient Motor Tic Disorder	Tics
Chronic Motor Tic Disorder	Tics
Tourette's Disorder	Tics
Unspecified Tic Disorder	Tics
Other Stereotyped Movement Disorder	Stereotyped repetitive movements
Speech Disorders Not Elsewhere Classified	
Stuttering	Stammering and stuttering
Elective mutism	[Other adjustment reaction] *or* [Disturbance of emotions specific to childhood and adolescence with anxiety and fearfulness] *or* [with sensitivity, shyness and social withdrawal]*
Conduct Disorders	*Disturbance of Conduct Not Elsewhere Classified*
Undersocialized Conduct Disorder, Aggressive Type	Unsocialized Conduct Disorder

TABLE 1 (*continued*)

DSM III	ICD-9
Undersocialized Conduct Disorder, Unaggressive Type	[Unsocialized Conduct Disorder]*
Socialized Conduct Disorder	Socialized Conduct Disorder
Eating Disorders	*Special Symptoms or Syndromes*
Anorexia nervosa	Anorexia nervosa
Bulimia	Other Disorders of Eating
Pica	Other Disorders of Eating
Rumination	Other Disorders of Eating
Other or unspecified	Other Disorders of Eating
Anxiety Disorders	
Overanxious Disorder	Disturbance of emotions specific to childhood and adolescence with anxiety and fearfulness *or* Neurotic Disorder, Anxiety State
Shyness Disorder	Disturbance of Emotions with sensitivity, shyness and social withdrawal
Separation Anxiety Disorder	[Adjustment Reaction with predominant disturbance of other emotions]* *or* [Neurosis, phobic state]*
Other Disorders	
Asocial Disorder	Disturbance of Emotions with Sensitivity, Shyness and Social Withdrawal
Oppositional disorder	[Relationship problems]*
Academic underachievement disorder	No Equivalent

Axis Two—Specific Developmental Disorders

Specific Developmental Disorders	*Special Delays in Development*
Specific reading disorder	Specific reading retardation
Specific arithmetical disorder	Specific arithmetical retardation
Developmental language disorder	Developmental speech/language disorder
Developmental articulation disorder	Developmental speech/language disorder
Coordination disorder	Specific motor retardation
Enuresis	Enuresis (On Axis I in ICD-9)
Encopresis	Encopresis (On Axis I in ICD-9)
Mixed	Mixed
Unspecified	No Equivalent coding
Other	Other specific learning difficulties

* The disorders in brackets represent possible ICD-9 equivalent disorders, not identical categories.

Reactive Disorders Not Elsewhere Classified, and Disorders of Impulse Control Not Elsewhere Classified.

Several basic general principles were established to guide the work of the task force responsible for the formulation of the third edition of the American Psychiatric Association Diagnostic and Statistical Manual (DSM III) (Spitzer & Sheehy, 1976). These have led to differences between ICD-9 and DSM III which are conceptual and pertain to the entire classification, and which, by extension, inevitably affect the childhood codings. In addition, ICD-9 and DSM III differ in ways which are *specifically pertinent to children's psychiatric disorders*. For the sake of clarity, a discussion of the overall general discrepancies precedes that of the children's nomenclature.

General Differences between DSM III and ICD-9

The points raised below are not comprehensive in scope with regard to differences between the two classification schemas. Only the major points which affect the diagnosis of children's psychiatric disorders are summarized. Many other discrepancies exist, such as those among Organic Mental Disorders, but their relevance to the pediatric diagnostician is remote and therefore do not require attention here.

MAJOR CATEGORIES

Certain classificatory umbrellas have been abandoned in DSM III and consequently affect the way in which mental disorders for children are organized. The classical terms Psychosis and Neurosis are no longer grouping concepts for mental disorders.

1) *Psychosis.* The term *psychosis* connotes a multitude of clinical phenomena and is therefore confusing. It does not represent a homogenous group of conditions, but is a particular aspect of mental dysfunction which may occur across many types of disorders; for example, in organic mental disorders, it often refers to changes in *intellectual functions* such as memory and orientation; in schizophrenia it may connote the presence of *abnormal ideas or perceptions*, delusions and/or hallucinations; in affective disorders the concept of psychosis may be applied to patients with delusional ideation, or alternatively to those severely dysfunctional in mood but with no delusions; finally, it can be applied to individuals who, under the influence of psychotomimetic or other drugs, undergo marked changes in their experience of reality. Therefore, the notion of psychosis as a class of disorders is untenable. Further, in children, the term *psychosis* poses additional definitional problems. Adult psychotic individuals are

usually not mentally retarded; they are thought to have achieved a certain level of adjustment (with varying degrees of adequacy) and at some time to have undergone marked changes in personality. This picture does not apply to children with infantile autism which is the commonest psychosis of childhood (see Werry, in press c), since, typically, they have not experienced a period of social normalcy interrupted by psychosis, but are developmentally deviant from infancy on, and are frequently intellectually retarded. In addition, and of some importance, the therapeutic connotations which the term psychosis often carries in adults are misleading. The neuroleptics have come to be known as antipsychotic agents. Given their documented efficacy in adult schizophrenia, this practice may not be wholly unjustified. However, their action in so-called psychotic children cannot be inferred from adult "psychotics" since the medications do not normalize the behavior of the children in the same fashion as that of adults (see Chapter 8). Finally, the family histories and manifest clinical symptoms of most psychotic children and adults are markedly different (see Werry, in press c). Therefore, there seems to be little point to using the same diagnostic term in children and adults with different respective phenomenologies, different prognosis, different treatment indications and probably different etiologies.

2) *Neurosis* as a classificatory concept was abandoned for different reasons. Unlike psychosis, it carries etiological inferences—the assumption being that the overt neurotic symptoms represent superficial manifestations of unconscious, repressed intrapsychic conflicts, the exact nature of these conflicts varying with the psychopathological theory of the diagnostician's predilection. Since it was agreed upon that *etiological speculations* would not be part of the new objective descriptive diagnostic schema, retaining the concept of neurosis was unjustified. The usual reaction to learning that the term neurosis does not appear in DSM III is usually one of shock and disbelief. However, recovery is usually prompt when it is realized that only the *designation* is omitted and all the disorders it formerly encompassed have been retained. Therefore, substantively, the change is of no import except for those with strong logophilia for the term.

3) *Hysteria*. The term Hysteria, a subset of the neuroses in prior classifications, has also been removed from the nomenclature in DSM III. As neurosis, it too implies causal factors which remain unproved and has acquired confusing and often pejorative connotations. In its place, more descriptive labels and more specific disorders formerly grouped within "hysteria" have been included under the rubrics of Factitious disorders,

Somatoform disorders, and Dissociative disorders. It is hoped that these labels are novel enough to have some chance of exact meaning.

4) *Adolescent Disorders.* Adolescent psychiatry, as a subspecialty, is developing in the United States. Reflecting this trend, three disorders specific to late adolescence are included in DSM III: Emancipation Disorder, Identity Disorder, and Specific Academic or Work Inhibition Disorder. ICD-9 does not contain disorders special to adolescence. Though the above three conditions reflect the clinical experience of some who specialize in the treatment of young adults, especially university students, it must be conceded that they derive only from clinical experience and not from empirical investigations. The task remains to establish that late adolescence is an age period associated with mental disorders distinct from those of childhood or adulthood. Unless it can be demonstrated that this is the case, the provision for conditions exclusive to late adolescence will be an instance where the splitting has gone too far.

DIAGNOSTIC DESCRIPTORS

The content of all of DSM III diagnostic descriptions will include a summary of the following descriptors: 1) *primary clinical features;* 2) frequently but inconsistently associated *secondary symptoms;* 3) *age* at onset; 4) *course* of the disorder; 5) *complications;* 6) *predisposing* factors; 7) *familial* pattern; 8) *prevalence;* 9) *sex* ratio; 10) *differential* diagnosis; and as discussed below in more detail, 11) *operational criteria* for making the diagnosis. No such comprehensive attempt has been made for ICD-9.

This schema will also allow a very quick perusal of the state of knowledge for each condition, and will provide a wealth of information to the clinician. At the same time, it will present a sobering exposé of lacunae in the knowledge about basic characteristics of many mental disorders and a pointer to much needed research areas. A typical write-up of a childhood condition of particular interest in pediatric psychopharmacology is presented in Table 2.

TABLE 2

DSM III Description of Attention Deficit Disorder
with Hyperactivity

Essential features. This category is for children who display excessive motor activity for their age as well as attentional difficulties and impulsivity. Children with this disorder are described in school as having a short attention span, as being impulsive and distractible, as failing to follow through on instructions and complete work, and

TABLE 2 (continued)

as being disorganized and inattentive. In addition, the children are reported to be fidgety, restless, overactive, over-demanding of the teacher's attention, and disruptive of others at play and at work.

At home, attentional problems are characterized by a failure to follow through on parental requests and instructions, or by the inability to engage in activities, including play, for periods of time appropriate for age. The child is often described as being on the go, "running like motor," and having difficulty sitting still.

In young children hyperactivity is manifested by excessive gross motor activity such as running or climbing. In older children and adolescents, hyperactivity may be indicated by restlessness and fidgeting. Often, the impression obtained is that the quality of the motor behavior is what distinguishes this disorder from ordinary overactivity. The activity tends to be haphazard, poorly organized, lacking in clear goal orientation. In situations where high levels of motor activity are expected and appropriate, such as the playground, children with this disorder do not obviously display more activity than others.

The behavior of children with Attention Deficit Disorder with Hyperactivity is extremely variable. Typically, symptoms fluctuate across situations as well as within situations, and inconsistent functioning is a very common characteristic of the disorder. A child's behavior may be well organized and appropriate on a one to one basis, but become dysregulated in a group situation or the classroom; or home adjustment may be satisfactory and difficulties may emerge only in school. In addition, the child's level of motor activity may vary considerably within any situation. The usual pattern is an inconsistent one. It is the rare child who displays uniform, constant symptoms of hyperactivity either within or across settings.

Associated features. Associated clinical features change as a function of age. Some of the concurrent difficulties include alteration of interpersonal relationships with obstinacy, stubbornness, negativism, bossiness, or bullying; altered emotionality, for example, increased lability, low frustration tolerance or temper outbursts; low self-esteem; lack of response to discipline; and antisocial behavior especially in adolescence.

Specific Developmental Disorders are common and should be noted on Axis II. Impaired academic performance is common.

Non-localized "soft" neurological signs, learning disabilities, motor-perceptual dysfunctions, and EEG abnormalities may or may not be present. Negative findings with regard to the presence of central nervous system dysfunction do not preclude the diagnosis of Attention Deficit Disorders with Hyperactivity.

In the vast majority of these children there is no known neurological disorder, but in about 5%, the disorders are associated with diagnosable brain disease. In such cases, the organic factors should be coded on Axis III.

When this disorder is an expression of an Organic Personality Syndrome, the diagnosis of Attention Deficit Disorder with Hyperactivity should be used.

Age at onset. Onset is typically early in childhood (around the ages of 2 or 3 and even in infancy), although the condition frequently does not come to professional attention until the child enters school.

Course. The course of the disorder is not fully known. Current information suggests that in some children the symptoms may disappear in puberty, but a significant proportion retain attentional difficulties well into adult life. In addition, both social and academic difficulties may persist through adolescence.

TABLE 2 (*continued*)

Impairment. The severity of impairment ranges widely. The difficulties may be limited to the school situation alone but are often experienced in all environments. Infrequently children with this disorder require residential treatment.

Complications. Complications include school failure, placement in special classes, interpersonal difficulties with peers and authority figures, and the development of Conduct Disorders of varying severity.

Predisposing factors. The factors predisposing to the disorder include Mental Retardation, epilepsy, some forms of cerebral palsy, and probably other neurological disorders.

Prevalence. The disorder is common. In the United States, it may occur in as many as 3% of the prepuberty children.

Sex ratio. The disorder is much more common in boys than girls. The sex ratio is about 10 to 1.

Familiar pattern. Among affected children, there seems to be an increased frequency of the disorder in siblings and, by history, in the parents when they were children, especially among fathers.

Differential diagnosis. Diagnostic difficulties may occur when there are inconsistent reports regarding the presence of the symptoms. In such cases, primary consideration should be given to the child's current and past functioning in school over his reported behavior at home.

The disorder must be distinguished from Attention Deficit Disorder without Hyperactivity which does not present with excessive motor activity for age. Further, the disorder must be distinguished from the Conduct Disorders in which antisocial behavior predominates. However, Conduct Disorders may coexist with an Attentional Deficit Disorder with Hyperactivity, and in such cases both should be coded.

It is important to note that the diagnostic significance of the signs and symptoms of this disorder may be difficult to interpret when they are found in children in an inadequate, disorganized, or chaotic environment.

DIAGNOSTIC CRITERIA FOR ATTENTION DEFICIT DISORDER WITH HYPERACTIVITY

A. Excessive general hyperactivity or motor restlessness for age is a prominent feature of the current clinical picture. In preschool and early school years, there may be haphazard, impulsive running, climbing, or crawling. During middle childhood or adolescence, inability to sit still, up and down activity, and fidgeting are characteristic. The activity differs from the norm for age both in quality and quantity.

B. Difficulty sustaining attention such as an inability to complete tasks initiated, a disorganized approach to tasks. Frequent "forgetting" of demands made, or tasks assigned, a worsening of attentional processes in unstructured situations or when demands are made for independent, unsupervised performance.

C. Impulsive behavior as manifested by at least two of the following:

   (1) Sloppy work in spite of reasonable efforts to perform adequately.
   (2) Frequent calling out of turn or making inappropriate sounds in class.

(3) Frequent interruption of, or intrusion into, other children's activities or conversations.
(4) Difficulty waiting for one's turn in games, or in group situations.
(5) Poor frustration tolerance.
(6) Fighting with children in a fashion indicating low frustration tolerance rather than sadistic or mean calculated intention.

D. Duration of at least one year.

Criteria for Diagnosis

A critical step forward has been taken by DSM III by providing diagnostic criteria for each disorder so that the clinician will have guidelines to apply in the diagnostic decision process. An obvious question is how can these criteria be formulated in the present absence of objective empirical data which define the limits of each disorder? There is no wholly satisfactory answer; yet, there has to be a point of beginning somewhere. Therefore, those clinicians involved with the development of DSM III formulated a set of arbitrary but, it is hoped, sensible rules based on current knowledge and experience. As a result, the *objectivity* of the diagnostic criteria is very variable. In cases where considerable information regarding a condition has been accumulated, the job of formulating criteria was both easier and more rational. In contrast, where disorders have been included because of a consensus that the category exists, but no systematic studies have been conducted, the criteria are arbitrary. In practice, it will be difficult at times to be certain whether the criteria for a particular diagnosis are met by some patients. Thus, a patient might fit some, but not all the criteria of a particular diagnosis. In such instances the diagnosis should be used if it appears clinically to be the *best diagnostic fit* possible.

Operational diagnostic criteria improve diagnostic reliability (Spitzer et al., 1975) and therefore make a major contribution to the progress of psychodiagnosis. Understandably, hitherto the importance of psychiatric diagnosis often has been denigrated within and without the psychiatric profession because of lack of documented adequate reliability. The adoption of operational criteria should help to meet these criticisms. Further, and as importantly, the criteria will render investigations of the validity and the epidemiology of mental disorders much more feasible.

Finally, the criteria will probably enable individuals without extensive training in psychodiagnosis to use the manual with less confusion and ambiguity, thereby making it more useful to pediatricians and other non-mental health professionals involved in the care of children.

Field Trials Prior to Publication

For the first time in the history of psychiatric nomenclature, the proposed content is being subjected to clinical trials in clinical settings *before* finalizing its contents. Doing so will identify the disorders which, though proposed, are not readily applicable to patients; it will identify some of the ambiguities of the descriptive content and the diagnostic criteria; it will point to omissions by identifying patients who cannot be diagnosed by DSM III; it will indicate recording and data processing difficulties, if any, and will elucidate to what extent DSM III and ICD-9 diagnoses are incompatible, if at all. Therefore, there will be an opportunity to revise the manual prior to publication so that any difficulties identified can be removed and need not wait a decade to be incorporated in the next manual. This may create a sense of uncertainty and frustration in readers, but the authors feel that the system is so different and so well advanced that it is more reasonable to describe the DSM III as it is now than to perpetuate an archaic system.

The ICD-8 childhood disorders have also been field tested (e.g., Rutter et al., 1973) which has led already to substantial revisions in the childhood disorders section of ICD-9.

Differences Specific to Children Between ICD-9 and DSM III

In addition to the considerations discussed above which have a pervasive impact on the whole of DSM III and lead to divergencies from ICD-9, there are variations in the two classifications which are specific to the psychodiagnosis of children. A summary of the major substantive points is presented.

Multiaxial Classification System

The Multiaxial diagnostic approach proposed by some of those involved in ICD-9 under the aegis of WHO (Rutter et al., 1973, 1976) has been adopted for DSM III but with some modifications. A major difference is that, whereas the multiaxial approach proposed in ICD-9 is *optional and limited to children,* in DSM III it will be applied to adults as well as children and be an integral part of the diagnostic coding.

ADVANTAGES OF MULTIAXIAL CLASSIFICATIONS

It should be made clear that a multiaxial classification in no way precludes the use of *several* clinical diagnoses, so that a child with an Attention Deficit Disorder and a Conduct Disorder would receive two codings to reflect the presenting psychiatric symptomatology. *The multiaxial approach simply insures that certain specified domains of function are regularly assessed in all cases* and thus should improve diagnosis in child psychiatry.

Besides the research advantages of providing a large pool of cases evaluated along similar dimensions, commonly assessed at present, but obscured in current systems, the multiaxial coding maximized diagnostic reliability. For example, Rutter et al. (1973) demonstrated that when children presented with mixed clinical pictures such as a concatenation of severe behavior disorder, epilepsy, and mental deficiency, categorization was inconsistent since primary consideration and weight was given to different aspects of the children's conditions by different diagnosticians. Regardless of which of the three classes of dysfunctions was chosen as the clinical diagnosis (epilepsy, psychosis or mental retardation), a correct decision was actually made, but in each instance, being uniaxial in nature, was incomplete and *seemingly* in complete disagreement with any of the other diagnoses. However, given multiaxial ratings, no such diagnostic confusion should occur. Therefore, the system should enhance the validity of the diagnostic decisions, always assuming, of course, that the axes selected reflect attributes which are relevant either to the origin, course, or treatment response of the disorder. Even if this ambitious clinical goal is not met with the use of multiple axes, the latter will still be useful by enhancing the scope and accuracy of descriptive content communicated by the diagnosis formulated—a small advance, but a real one nonetheless.

TABLE 3

Multiaxial Classifications of ICD-9 and DSM III for Children

DSM III		ICD-9 (Proposed)
Clinical Psychiatric Syndrome(s)	Axis I	Clinical Psychiatric Syndrome
Specific Developmental Disorders*	Axis II	Special Delays in Development
Non-Mental Medical Disorders	Axis III	Intellectual Level
Severity of Psychosocial Stressors	Axis IV	Medical Conditions
Highest Level of Adaptive Functioning During Past Year	Axis V	Psychosocial Stressors

* In adults, Axis II is used for coding Personality Disorders, when appropriate.

ICD-9 AND DSM III COMPARED

The content of the axes of DSM III and ICD-9 are compared in Table 3. It will be seen that Axes I and II of both systems are identical. Axis I reflects the *clinical disorder*, and, as noted, multiple diagnoses may be used. Axis II is for ratings of specific *developmental disorders* (see Table 1). These are deficiencies in development which cannot be attributed solely to mental deficiency or gross deprivation (such as absence of schooling) and encompass such problems as specific learning disabilities, motor incoordination and delays in bowel and bladder control.

Somewhat confusingly Axis III in DSM III corresponds to Axis IV of ICD-9. In DSM III, Axis III provides the opportunity to note the concurrence of *physical* or biological disorders which are felt to be, in some way, pertinent to the clinical psychiatric condition *by affecting its course, severity or management*. This association need not be clearly established for the former to be recorded. For instance, the presence of epilepsy,* diabetes, or asthma would be coded even when no obvious link existed between them and the psychiatric syndromes, since their association with psychiatric disorders is not infrequent. However, clearly *transient, acute medical disorders* would not be noted except under extraordinary circumstances. In both ICD-9 and DSM III more than one rating may be recorded on this axis. However, the principles of ICD-9 and DSM III underlying this axis are different. The ICD-9 proposal, in contrast to DSM III, requires codings of medical conditions *regardless of any putative relationship* between the psychiatric syndrome and the physical condition. However, the examples given by the authors of the ICD-9 multiaxial system clearly indicate that in spite of this, they are actually concerned with physical disorders which might have a relationship to behavior problems.

The automatic evaluation of possible biological factors may help elucidate some antecedents or complications which would otherwise be ignored or overlooked by the clinician. From a research viewpoint, ultimately, the systematic accumulation of clinical diagnoses coupled with their associated physical conditions may lead serendipitously to the discovery of unexpected relationships and provide new knowledge.

The coding of intellectual levels which appears on Axis III of ICD-9 does not appear in DSM III. The reason for this discrepancy is explained below in the discussion of Mental Retardation.

On Axis IV of DSM III, the diagnostician notes whether a significant psychosocial stress appears to have contributed to the clinical disorder and if so, the severity of the stressor from minimal to catastrophic. In contrast to Axis III, an etiological relationship between the presence or

---

* Because of its particular effects on behavior, its association with brain dysfunction and the psychotropic effects of antiepileptic medication, epilepsy is the subject of a detailed discussion in Chapter 9.—(Ed.)

Table 4

ICD-9 Disorders Likely to be Used With Children and Their DSM III Equivalents

ICD-9 Disorders	DSM III Disorders
Neurotic Disorders	
Anxiety States	Panic Disorder
	Generalized Anxiety Disorder
	Atypical Anxiety Disorder
Hysteria	Factitious illness with psychological symptoms
	Chronic "factitious" illness with physical symptoms
	Other "factitious" illness with physical symptoms
	Somatization Disorder
	Conversion disorder
	Psychogenic Amnesia
	Psychogenic Fugue
	Multiple personality
	Other or unspecified
Phobic State	Agoraphobia with panic attacks
	Agoraphobia without panic attacks
	Social phobia
	Simple phobia
	Unspecified phobia
Obsessive Compulsive Disorder	Obsessive Compulsive Disorder
Neurotic Depression	No Direct Equivalent
Neurasthenia	No Equivalent
Depersonalization syndrome	Depersonalization Disorder
Hypochondriasis	Atypical somatoform disorder

severity of the psychiatric disorder and the stress is inferred. This rating has not been included in ICD-9.

Axis V of DSM III indicates the highest level of the patient's psychosocial functioning during the year preceding the evaluation. This aspect of adjustment is felt to be often important in planning treatment. The behavior rated on Axis V is independent of other clinical considerations such as overt symptoms, or subjective distress, and reflects exclusively the patient's level of adaptive functioning, rated on a scale from an optimum or "superior" to a minimum of "grossly impaired."

DIFFERENCES IN DIAGNOSTIC CATEGORIES

In addition to the DSM III categories presented in Table 1, over 100 additional diagnoses not listed as specifically arising in childhood also may be used for children. Table 4 lists the ICD-9 disorders, not specific to childhood, highlighted as likely to be used commonly in child psychiatry (Rutter et al., 1976) and their DSM III equivalents.

It is apparent that, on the whole, the sheer number of discrete diagnostic categories is greater in DSM III than ICD-9, so that one ICD-9 coding may correspond to several DSM III codings. The reason for this discrepancy stems from the philosophy which guided DSM III codings—*any distinct, internally consistent phenomenological symptom pattern merited its own code,* so that more knowledge could be accumulated for the disorder. Diagnostic refinement was felt to be unlikely to lead to loss of information, whereas lumping discrete conditions on purely traditional grounds might obscure important clinical differences among the combined disorders. This situation is well illustrated by the differences among the *phobic* disorders in the two classifications. In ICD-9 it is a single category, Phobic State, whereas it has become a six-category grouping in DSM III. This change reflects growing belief that there are subsets of disorders among phobias, with different ages of onset and different treatment responses (Klein, 1964; Marks & Gelder, 1966). It is unlikely that progress in clinical refinement can be obtained unless efforts are made to isolate groups with discrete syndromes.

The danger in this splitting process is that it can go too far. There is an awareness of, and no wish to revert back to, the chaos of the pre-Kraepelinian European psychiatry, with a myriad of disorders all lacking in validation. Fortunately, in contrast to then, there are now investigational tools available to enable rapid and sophisticated documentation of the validity of a category—for example: the research technology of epidemiology, drug responsivity, outcome, genetics, and inferential statistics, to say nothing of electronic data processing and a vastly increased body of psychiatrists and knowledge. We are therefore at a marked advantage over our B.K. (before Kraepelin) 19th century colleagues, and it is unlikely that we run the danger of creating the same monster they did!

In a few cases there is no DSM III equivalent for an ICD-9 category (see Table 1); this is usually the case when the ICD-9 coding reflects a composite clinical picture consisting of more than a single syndrome, viz. Hyperkinetic Conduct Disorder. For DSM III, it was opted to avoid mixed diagnoses, but to recommend that the several clinical disorders which make up the composite clinical picture be coded separately on Axis I.

Ratings of Severity

For each disorder, ICD-9 provides a four digit code, DSM III a five

TABLE 5
Childhood Diagnoses and Their Pharmacotherapy

DSM III Category	Specific	Symptomatic
Pervasive Developmental Disorders	None	Antipsychotics
Attention Deficit Disorders		
with Hyperactivity	Stimulants	Antipsychotics
	?Antidepressants?	Antidepressants
Stereotyped Movement Disorders		
1. Transient Motor Tic Disorder	None	?Antipsychotics?
2. Chronic Motor Tic Disorder	None	?Antipsychotics?
3. Tourette's Disorder	?Antipsychotics?	Antipsychotics
Conduct Disorders		
Undersocialized, aggressive	None	?Stimulants?
		?Antimanics?
Eating Disorders		
Anorexia Nervosa	None	?Antipsychotics?
Anxiety Disorders		
1. Overanxious Disorder	None	?Anxiolytics?
2. Separation Anxiety Disorder	?Antidepressants?	Antidepressants
Developmental Disorders		
Enuresis	None	Antidepressants

Note: For details see Chapters 5-10. Diagnoses omitted have no indications currently.

digit code. Because of the additional rating in DSM III, the diagnostician will be able to rate the severity of two classes of childhood disorders, the Attentional Deficit Disorders and the Conduct Disorders, and will be able to indicate whether the disorders of Enuresis and Encopresis are primary or secondary disturbances. The information regarding severity may prove useful since it is possible that the long-term outcome of childhood conditions may be related to their initial status. There are already some data indicating that this is so for conduct disorders, the more seriously affected youngsters showing greater difficulty in later life than the milder cases.

CHILDHOOD DISORDERS AND THEIR PHARMACOTHERAPY

The disorders discussed below follow the DSM III classification. For the ICD-9 equivalents, the reader should refer to Table 1. The brief notes and the summary in Table 5 regarding the pharmacological management of the respective DSM III categories are not intended to provide a comprehensive view of the field which is covered in other chapters (Section II). Rather, it is mentioned only to point out *existing* relationships between pediatric psychopharmacology and the proposed new systems. Obviously much more work will need to be done to cover new and/or pharmacologically untested diagnostic categories and subcategories. Cross references to other chapters are stressed.

Mental Retardation

DIAGNOSIS

Criteria for mental retardation differ considerably between ICD-9 and DSM III. In ICD-9 mental retardation requires an IQ score two standard deviations below the test mean, with provisions made for recording the severity of the intellectual deficit, from mild to profound. ICD-9 diagnosticians are informed that these IQ levels are not to be used rigidly; unfortunately, there is no specification of the factors to be taken into consideration for a flexibility of judgment. The DSM III diagnosis of mental retardation requires a similarly subnormal IQ, but, in addition, *a concurrent deficit in the capacity for adaptive behavior.* Given this bivariate definition of the mental retardation, a child with an IQ below 70 who was managing well in meeting the usual role expectations for his age, such as going to school (though in a special class), self-care, and so on, would not be considered to have mental retardation in DSM III, whereas in ICD-9 he might. These DSM III criteria were adopted so as to be consistent with those of American Association for Mental Retardation (Grossman et al., 1973). However, the *severity* ratings for Mental Retardation in DSM III are identical to those in ICD-9—they are strictly dependent on level of quantified IQ, and not affected by other considerations. There is some inconsistency, therefore, within the DSM III schema *since the diagnostic criterion for the disorder rests on the presence of two sets of dysfunctions, but its severity only on one.* This lack of internal consistency is due to the fact that ratings of adequacy of adaptive behavior are relatively subjective and therefore more unreliable than IQ measures, and including an evaluation of psychosocial adaptation in the severity codings of mental retardation would have affected the reliability of the diagnosis negatively. Further, eliminating considerations of level of general functioning from the severity ratings will make DSM III diagnoses of mental retardation more congruent with ICD-9. However, the ICD-9 diagnosis seems more inclusive—not all children considered as having mental retardation according to ICD-9 would qualify for the diagnosis of DSM III, whereas all children classified as such by DSM III would be included in the ICD-9 category.

It is difficult to evaluate the relative merits of the respective classifications of Mental Retardation. Emphasis on level of adaptive function in the diagnosis stems from the fact that, particularly in inner-city areas in the U.S., children do not come to the attention of professionals because they have low IQ's, but because they are unable to cope satisfactorily with the usual demands placed on youngsters of their age from similar backgrounds. Consequently, therapeutic efforts are focused regularly upon developing greater adaptive skills, rather than raising IQ *per se*. If specific means were developed for improving IQ level among individuals with intellectual retardation with concomitant enhancement of coping skills, the definitional content of Mental Retardation as conceptualized in DSM III would require revision. Thus at this time, in the American view, Mental Retardation is a complex set of interacting disabilities, social and intellectual. Given the different preoccupations and, possibly, problems of the two societies, the reasons for this socio-political view compared with the purist European view are understandable.

PSYCHOPHARMACOLOGICAL TREATMENT

There is no specific pharmacological treatment for Mental Retardation. However, children with the disorder often have behavior problems, not infrequently severe. Symptoms of hyperactivity, aggression, destructiveness, self-damage (such as hitting, biting, banging oneself) occur. As discussed in more detail in Chapter 8, the neuroleptics have been found to ameliorate these secondary clinical complications, but do not affect the primary intellectual deficit, in fact may depress cognitive function (see Chapter 3 also). Stimulants, despite their facilitative role on cognitive function in the laboratory, have yet to be shown to influence academic skills in general (see Chapters 3 and 6).

Pervasive Developmental Disorders

DIAGNOSIS

There is large overlap between the two classifications with regard to this class of childhood disorders; differences are minor and more apparent than real. Infantile Autism refers to severe deviance in the development of social responsiveness, occurring very early in life as originally described by Kanner (1943). The disorder has three key features: onset during the first three years of life, lack of social responsiveness, and deficits in language development.

The disorder of Atypical Childhood Psychosis is a less distinct grouping which will need refinement. Its clinical picture is more varied than that of Infantile Autism. It is partially defined by exclusion, in that children with Infantile Autism, Disintegrative Psychosis, or Schizophrenia are not included in this category. The disorder is for children who, after the age of three years, develop gross social and emotional impairment often accompanied by bizarre beliefs or preoccupations. The clinical picture does not meet the criteria for a diagnosis of schizophrenia in that the essential clinical features of schizophrenia, consisting of certain types of delusions, such as delusions of passivity, hallucinations, or formal thought disorder, are not present. The disorder includes the ICD-9 Childhood Psychosis, Other.

Disintegrative Psychosis of DSM III and ICD-9 is an extremely rare organic disorder. It includes children who develop brain disease with concomitant loss of speech and behavior deterioration. The disorder usually has a degenerative course. A number of organic disorders may be responsible for this clinical picture; one of them is known as Heller's disease, a disorder of lipid metabolism. The term psychosis as a description for the category of Atypical Childhood Psychosis and Disintegrative Psychosis has been retained since, by definition, the children display marked changes in object relationships.

To recapitulate, Pervasive Developmental Disorders whose onset is within the first three years are considered Infantile Autism; those with onset after three and no specific organic disease, Atypical Childhood Psychosis; those with a definite organic etiology, Distintegrative Psychosis.

PHARMACOLOGICAL TREATMENT

The antipsychotics have been demonstrated to have some beneficial effect on the secondary signs and symptoms of this group of childhood disorders (see Chapter 8). However, the drugs do not have a normalizing or true antipsychotic action as in adults, nor do they eliminate or reduce significantly much of the children's bizarre interests and inappropriate social interactions, but they may have dramatic beneficial effects on certain disturbing symptoms such as severe hyperactivity and mood lability. Troublesome side effects, such as dyskinesias, have been reported and the cost-benefit ratio of using high levels of neuroleptics over extended periods of time must be weighed for each child (see Chapter 8).

Attention Deficit Disorders

DIAGNOSIS

This category is for disorders often referred to as Minimal Brain Dysfunction, or Hyperkinetic Reaction of Childhood, the hallmark of these disorders being now considered (though by no means unanimously) to be marked impairment in sustained attention processes. (Attention and its measurement are discussed in detail in Chapter 3).

DSM III distinguishes between two categories, Attention Deficit Disorder *with* Hyperactivity, and Attention Deficit Disorder *without* Hyperactivity. The latter disorder is not present in ICD-9; it refers to children with *pure attention deficit disorders without motor hyperactivity*. It is a controversial category, based on clinical reports that some children exhibit difficulty in sustaining attention and applying themselves, without any dysregulation of patterns of motor activity. The existence of the syndrome itself has not been documented. It is hoped that its inclusion in DSM III will lead to attempts at providing objective evidence for the disorder, or lack thereof. The DSM III Attention Deficit Disorder *with* Hyperactivity is equivalent to the ICD-9 Simple Disturbance of Activity and Attention.

DSM III does not provide for mixed classification of Hyperkinesis with Developmental Delay or with Conduct Disorder as does ICD-9. In such cases, multpile clinical diagnoses would be used in DSM III. The reason for avoiding a mixed diagnosis in DSM III is due to the difficulties in establishing a primary and secondary diagnosis in a child who presents with several patterns of dysfunction. In ICD-9, if a child has both a hyperkinetic and conduct disorder, in keeping with European opinion that hyperkinesis is rare and overdiagnosed in the U.S., precedence, or emphasis, is given to the latter in the diagnosis of Hyperkinetic Conduct Disorder rather than Conduct Disorder with Hyperactivity. It was felt by the DSM III consultants that assumptions regarding which disorder should be emphasized were premature, and it was opted to give multiple clinical codings in such cases rather than provide comibnation diagnoses.

PHARMACOLOGICAL TREATMENT

Of all the childhood disorders, the Attention Deficit Disorder with Hyperactivity is the one for which drug treatment is best documented. The stimulants have been shown repeatedly to improve dramatically the clinical symptoms of the disorder (see Chapter 6). Some antipsychotics such as certain phenothiazines (see Chapter 8) can also ameliorate motor hyperactivity, but they do not have the broad normalizing therapeutic effect of the stimulants. It is unknown whether stimulants are also useful in the treatment of children with Attention Deficit Disorder without Hyperactivity. The clinical impression is that they probably are (see Chapter 6). Tricyclic antidepressants (see Chapter 7) are also useful though less so than stimulants and they may be more toxic. Also, it is still unclear whether they normalize behavior or act symptomatically.

Stereotyped Movement Disorders

The corresponding ICD-9 categories of the DSM III Stereotyped Movement Disorders are grouped under the ICD-9 heading of *Special Symptoms or Syndromes*. The Gilles de la Tourette's syndrome (renamed Motor-Verbal Tic Disorder in order to avoid eponyms), has been split from pure motor tics in DSM III, but not in ICD-9. It is not clear whether the distinction is warranted. Part of the reason for distinguishing individuals who, in addition to motor tics, also have involuntary verbal outbursts is due to the efficacy of a butyrophenone (haloperidol) (see Chapter 8) in the treatment of the Motor-Verbal Tic Disorder. The indications are that pure motor tics probably respond similarly, but this has not been well demonstrated (see Chapter 8). Further, the social and functional implications for both sets of symptoms are so different, the Tourette's Disorder portending a more serious outlook for the affected individuals, that the distinction seemed warranted on this basis alone.

In addition, DSM III distinguishes between motor tics which very commonly remit within a period of a few months or less (Transient Motor Tic Disorder) and the rarer cases of motor tics which extend for long periods of time, at times up to adulthood (Chronic Motor Tic Disorder). This distinction does not appear in ICD-9.

The DSM III "Other stereotyped movement disorder" category corresponds to the Stereotyped Repetitive Movements of ICD-9.

PHARMACOLOGICAL TREATMENT

The only condition of the Stereotyped movement disorders for which drug treatment is documented is the Motor-Verbal Tic Disorder, haloperidol being the treatment of choice (see Chapter 8). The less pervasive and less severe motor tic disorders and the Other Stereotyped Movement disorders have no established drug treatment. As noted, haloperidol may be effective in them too, though the risk of tardive dyskinesia begets a certain reluctance to use it in the high doses required.

Speech Disorders Not Elsewhere Classified

The awkward modifier *not elsewhere classified* is necessitated by the fact that some speech and language disorders are listed under Specific Developmental Disorders. There are two disorders included here, Stuttering and Elective Mutism. Stuttering has a direct ICD equivalent. Elective Mutism does not receive a separate coding but is mentioned in ICD-9 as possibly occurring among children diagnosed as having an emotional disorder *with sensitivity, shyness and social withdrawal*, or among those *with anxiety and fearfulness*, or as part of an Adjustment Reaction. At this time, knowledge regarding the status of the disorder is limited. It is not clear whether Elective Mutism is a syndrome in and of itself, or a symptom occurring in a variety of clinical contexts. It was felt that the condition had sufficient distinctiveness to warrant its inclusion as a category. It is possible that research may not bear out this judgment.

PSYCHOPHARMACOLOGICAL TREATMENT

This class of disorders has no known appropriate pharmacological treatment.

Conduct Disorders

This category is for children who display antisocial behavior and a lack of concern for social norms.

DIAGNOSIS

Two broad classes are usually observed. One consists of children who have established social bonds and social involvements indicating a sense of sharing and reciprocity and whose antisocial behavior is often performed as part of a delinquent peer group activity (Socialized Conduct Disorder). The other includes children who have no or inadequate social relationships and whose antisocial behavior does not occur in conjunction with a peer group (Undersocialized Conduct Disorders). The term *undersocialized* has been preferred in DSM III over the traditional epithet *unsocialized* used in ICD-9 since the latter implies a total absence of socialization which was felt to be overly categorical.

The major difference between the DSM III and ICD-9 classifications of the conduct disorders is the differentiation in the former between the aggressive and nonaggressive forms of the undersocialized forms of the disorder. It was felt that a diagnostic distinction should be provided between children with conduct disorders who are aggressive, and those who show no overt aggression. The presence of violent behavior may have distinct implications for the long-term outcome of children with conduct disorders as well as for their pharmocotherapy (see Chapter 10).

The clinical criteria for the Socialized Conduct Disorder of DSM III and ICD-9 are dissimilar. Whereas ICD-9 defines the disorder as delinquency (though gang membership alone is insufficient), the DSM III criteria stipulate that deviating from social norms, or delinquency is insufficient. The DSM III diagnosis requires that, in adidtion to socially disapproved behavior with a peer group, youngsters must also display a variety of dysfunctions (such as relationship difficulties at home and school) to qualify for this coding. Therefore, delinquent behavior alone is not considered a mental disorder in DSM III but can be noted in a section called *Conditions Not Attributable to a Known Mental Disorder* as Childhood Antisocial Behavior.

In addition, in ICD-9 the distinction between the socialized and unsocialized conduct disorders rests upon the presence or absence of group delinquency *per se*. In contrast, in DSM III the development of age-appropriate social relationships is emphasized as the crucial differentiating clinical feature between the socialized and unsocialized conduct disorders.

PHARMACOLOGICAL TREATMENT

There is no established pharmacological intervention in the management of conduct disorders, though because of laxity in current diagnostic systems, the evidence is difficult to disentangle from that relating to the Hyperkinetic Reaction. There have been speculations that some adolescent conduct disorders represent later manifestations of Attention Deficit Disorders which, with time, have become complicated with antisocial behavior. In such adolescent cases, the use of stimulants has been reported to be therapeutic (see Chapter 6). However, this drug effect is far from substantiated as is that of lithium in the Aggressive Conduct Disorder (see Chapter 10). At this time, the most accurate statement concerning the usefulness of pharmacological treatment in *pure* conduct disorders uncomplicated by Disorders of Attention or, in former parlance, hyperactivity, is that no such treatment has been demonstrated to be clinically efficacious, though more study based on properly honed diagnosis is highly desirable since indications that some drugs such as stimulants may be useful need confirmation (see Chapter 6).

Eating Disorders

DIAGNOSIS

Anorexia nervosa is the only DSM III category of the Eating Disorders for which there is a direct ICD-9 equivalent. The DSM III diagnoses of Bulimia, Pica and Rumination are subsumed under Other Disorders of Eating in ICD-9.

PHARMACOLOGICAL TREATMENT

There is no demonstrated effective treatment for any of the eating disorders. A controlled investigation of cyproheptadine (Periactin) failed to find a significant advantage for the drug over placebo in women with anorexia nervosa. Interestingly, a history of birth difficulties, as well as severity of emaciation, was positively associated with improvement on the drug compared to that on placebo (Goldberg et al., 1977). Chlorpromazine is commonly used in anorexia nervosa (Dally, 1969), though its combination with bedrest, insulin, contingency management and/or psychotherapy makes elucidation of its therapeutic role difficult (Chapter 8). Recently, amitryptiline has been reported to have considerable ameliorative effect in a few children and adolescents with anorexia nervosa (Needleman & Weber, 1976).

Anxiety Disorders

DIAGNOSIS

Three anxiety disorders specific to childhood are included in DSM III: Overanxious Disorder, Separation Anxiety Disorder, and Shyness Disorder. The Overanxious Disorder corresponds to the ICD-9 category of Disturbance of Emotions Specific to Childhood and Adolescence with Anxiety and Fearfulness. However, there are some differences in the clinical content of the category. The ICD-9 coding includes in it "many cases of school refusal," whereas the DSM III would not. The DSM III diagnosis is for children *with excessive, pervasive worry and fearfulness not related to specific events or situations.*

The Separation Anxiety Disorder of DSM III has no specific ICD-9 equivalent. It represents a refinement of the overall phobic category. In ICD-9, children with abnormal separation reactions are included within the Adjustment Reactions with Predominant Disturbance of Other Emotions. Since culture shock is also part of this category, it is clearly a heterogeneous grouping.

The DSM III Shyness Disorder is for children who are reticent to initiate social contact and who feel anxious in new social situations, *but* who enjoy social interactions and function well once the contacts are established. The Shyness Disorder corresponds to two ICD-9 categories:

Neurotic Disorder, Anxiety State, and Disturbance of Emotions with sensitivity, shyness and social withdrawal. The above ICD-9 childhood condition is diagnostically less pure than the DSM III Shyness Disorder, since ICD-9 lumps shy children together with withdrawn, isolated children. Yet, clinically, they seem to represent distinct groups.

PSYCHOPHARMACOLOGICAL TREATMENT

The use of antianxiety agents such as the benzodiazepines has been reported in several clinical studies which claim that their findings support the clinical efficacy of antianxiety medication in children (see Chapter 10). However, the reports often defy a clear identification of the diagnostic characteristics of the children treated. For example, the samples are often described as *neurotic*, a term which does little to communicate clinical inclusion criteria. The studies which have advanced claims of efficacy for antianxiety agents suffer from so many shortcomings that it is not possible to draw any reliable information from them (Gittelman-Klein, 1978b, and Chapter 10).

The efficacy of drug treatment of a clinical subgroup of the childhood anxiety disorders consisting of children with pathological levels of separation anxiety has been studied and the antidepressant imipramine was found to be markedly superior to placebo, but unfortunately, only one study has been conducted so far (see Chapter 7). This work is in part responsible for delineating the syndrome as separate from other childhood anxiety disorders—an example of how progress in psychopharmacology may influence psychodiagnostic concepts.

Other Disorders of Childhood or Adolescence

DIAGNOSIS

The three disorders in this rubric do not fall logically into any of the above classes of conditions and do not represent a clinically homogeneous subgrouping.

The Introverted Disorder refers to children who are loners and who have introverted interests. They typically have no friends and lack social interest in general. These youngsters have been referred to, in the past, as having "shut-in" personalities. In the DSM II as well as ICD-9, these children have been lumped together with shy, anxious children who are reluctant to initiate social contact, but who enjoy peer interactions once these are established. Distinguishing the asocial, isolated child from the shy group will make it possible to determine whether the two diagnoses have different associated treatments and long-term outcome.

Oppositional Disorder includes children who are pervasively negativistic and oppositional in their interaction with authority figures, but who, unlike the Conduct Disorders, do not display marked antisocial behavior. Whether this type of behavior represents a distinct clinical entity, or whether the behavior occurs as part of a variety of disorders is unclear. The category has no direct ICD-9 equivalent, but one might consider the Oppositional Disorder as a form of the ICD-9 childhood diagnosis of Relationship Problems.

The last disorder of childhood, Academic Underachievement Disorder, does not have an ICD-9 equivalent. The category is for children of normal or above normal academic competence who, because of emotional conflict, fail to perform. They are children traditionally referred to as underachievers. It is questionable whether this category, as well as some others discussed, represents a discrete syndrome or whether the dysfunction is one clinical aspect of a variety of conditions. Its inclusion in DSM III stems from informal reports by clinicians that a pattern of underachievement in the absence of other psychopathology (particularly specific developmental disorders) is encountered among practitioners who treat middle class children, frequently the offspring of well-educated professional parents. It is conceivable that some of those children would fall in the ICD-9 diagnosis of Neurosis, Other.

PHARMACOLOGICAL TREATMENT

No definite statements can be made, not surprisingly in view of the uncertainty of these entities.

Specific Developmental Disorders

DIAGNOSIS

The Specific Developmental Disorders reflect conditions due to deviations from levels of function expected to occur in children, *given usual opportunities for growth and development.* These disorders are noted on Axis II in the two classifications. The functions selected are those which are felt to have a potentially disruptive effect on a child's general ability to cope with usual task demands, especially in school. These areas of development include reading and arithmetic skills, language, speech, motor coordination, and control of elimination. They are referred to as *specific* because they can occur in isolation without any other clinical concomitants, though children with a variety of psychiatric disorders are more likely to suffer from Specific Developmental Disorders. The failure to develop cognitive skills necessary for reading and arithmetic, and problems in motor coordination are noted in similar fashion in ICD-9 and DSM III. These disorders are discussed in detail in Chapter 3.

Enuresis and Encopresis are rated as clinical syndromes in ICD-9. In contrast, in DSM III they are considered simply deviations from normal childhood development and not necessarily part of other, more pervasive clinical disorders. They are therefore included among the Specific Developmental Disorders to be coded on Axis II. The clinical content of the disorders in ICD-9 and DSM III is somewhat dissimilar. DSM III makes a distinction, but ICD-9 does not, between the primary form in which the individual has never developed bladder or bowel control, and the secondary form in which, after a period of continence, loss of elimination control occurs. In both nomenclatures, the psychiatric rating is made only when there is no known organic abnormality causing the disorders.

A distinction is made in DSM III, but not ICD-9, between speech or articulation difficulties and language or communicative disorders. Most likely articulation and language difficulties are the result of different neurophysiological disorders; clinically they have very dissimilar consequences and call for different interventions. Therefore, distinguishing between them appears reasonable.

PHARMACOLOGICAL TREATMENT

Except for the Enuresis, none of the other Specific Developmental Disorders has a relevant psychochemotherapy. The symptomatic effectiveness of tricyclic antidepressants like imipramine in enuresis is well documented, but there is some question whether it is ever curative and deserves its present position among physicians as the treatment of first choice (see Chapter 7).

CAVEAT

There are many substantive differences between the DSM III and ICD-9 classifications. Since the two systems have been discussed here by contributors to DSM III, there is an inevitable flavor of bias in favor of DSM III in our discussion. Yet we are aware of the fact that often the divergences in the nosology are not based on empirical findings, but rather on the application of different principles. DSM III followed explicit guidelines which favored splitting rather than lumping disorders together. In addition, there was a policy to include a diagnostic category if it generated clinical interest. There is little doubt that not all such innovations will withstand the test of time. However, if some do, then the field of psychodiagnosis will be rewarded by the approach.

There are some childhood disorders which have specific drug treatment responses, for instance the Attentional Deficit Disorder with Hyperactivity, and possibly the Separation Anxiety Disorder. However, even among those groups there are children who, though they may fit the diagnostic criteria for these disorders, fail to respond to the usual pharmacologic compounds. A lack of response to treatment among these children should not be construed necessarily as challenging the accuracy of the diagnostic assignment. It is likely that each of the childhood disorders identified has multiple etiologies, and the clinical picture may be a final common outcome of diverse pathophysiologies and social antecedents. Consequently, even among well-diagnosed groups of children, one can expect that some individuals will not conform to the established treatment effects and these differences offer the possibility of further valid subclassifications.

It is important that the proposed DSM III classification be viewed as a working tool, one which will need alterations and refinement, and not as a set of fixed entities. Research findings in psychopharmacology already have influenced some aspects of psychiatric diagnosis. It is hoped that future knowledge in psychopharmacology will contribute further to the validity of the pediatric nomenclature.

II.
INDIVIDUAL DRUGS

6

STIMULANTS

DENNIS P. CANTWELL, M.D.
and
GABRIELLE A. CARLSON, M.D.

Introduction

The psychomotor stimulants are those drugs which in man possess as their principal action *excitation* of the central nervous system (CNS). *Motor* effects of the stimulant drugs are more obvious than excitatory effects in animals where stereotyped movements and increased goal-directed behaviors may be more prominent.

This chapter will discuss primarily the sympathomimetic drugs—amphetamines (Benzedrine, Dexedrine), methylphenidate (Ritalin) and pemoline (Cylert)—since they have been used most extensively in children. Relevant studies of caffeine, a xanthine derivative, which is somewhat functionally similar to, though structurally different from the amphetamines, will also be discussed. A third type of stimulant, deanol (Deaner), differs both structurally and functionally from the amphetamines as its actions are mediated by a cholinergic rather than a catecholaminergic mechanism. Deanol will be mentioned only briefly since its pharmacokinetics have not been well elucidated and its clinical usefulness in children seems limited.

Since the central stimulant actions of the sympathomimetics, and to some extent caffeine, may cause a brief elevation in mood, these drugs are sometimes called antidepressants, but since they do not exert any long-term therapeutic benefit in the treatment of depressive disorders, this use of the term is inappropriate (see Chapter 7, 10).

Structures

The *sympathomimetic drugs* contain a benzene ring and an amino nitrogen separated by 2 carbon atoms; they are thus structurally similar to endogenous (body produced) cathecholamines. With children, methylphenidate, racemic (Benzedrine) and d-amphetamine (Dexedrine) have been ultized the most. L-amphetamine, now withdrawn from the market, is less potent than its d-isomer with the same degree of unwanted clinical effects (Arnold et al., 1972) and would appear to be used more in research designed to clarify the mechanism of action of amphetamines. *Pemoline* is recently developed and not as widely studied.

Caffeine is a xanthine related to purine and uric acid, and in addition to its occurrence naturally in a number of beverages is available in pure pharmacological form.

Deanol is an organic salt of 2-dimethyl amino-ethanol, a precursor to acetylcholine.

The chemical structures of all these drugs are set out in Figure 1.

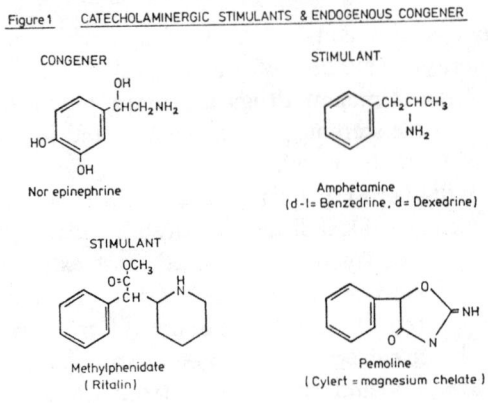

PHARMACOLOGY

Absorption Distribution Metabolism and Active Principles

All of the *amphetamines* and amphetamine-like drugs as well as *deanol* are well absorbed by mouth and cross the blood brain barrier easily (Modell et al., 1976). The absorption of *caffeine* from the GI tract is somewhat unpredictable and may cause gastric irritation (see physiologic effects).

The metabolism of *amphetamine* and its rate of excretion vary with urinary pH, and in an acid urine and normal renal clearance, one third to one half of the drug is excreted unchanged (Saunders, 1974). Oxidative deamination of the aminoalkyl group ultimately to benzoic acid and, to some extent, hippuric acid provides the major metabolic pathway. Parahydroxy-amphetamine is a very minor metabolite (Ebert et al., 1976). None of these products is felt to be metabolically active.

Methylphenidate is principally de-esterified to ritalinic acid though a smaller amount is hydroxylated to p-hydroxymethylphenidate, and the remainder to oxoritalinic acid and oxomethylphenidate. Almost all the drug is metabolized with none appearing unchanged in the urine (Dayton et al., 1970). This reaction does not appear to be pH dependent. There is some evidence that p-hydroxymethylphenidate is more potent than the parent drug, and the oxoderivatives considerably weaker (Faraj et al., 1974).

Pemoline is excreted largely unchanged (50%) in the urine. Its metabolites, which include pemoline dione, conjugated pemoline and mandelic acid, are only weakly active.

Caffeine is metabolized by oxidation to 1-methyluric acid and by demethylation to 1 methyl-xanthine. These by-products are excreted along with about 10% of the unchanged drug. Complete demethylation does not take place so there is no conversion to or increase in uric acid excretion (Goodman & Gilman, 1975).

Half Life and Excretion

Given a urine pH between 6 and 7.5, the mean plasma half life of *d-amphetamine* for 8 adults was $19.6 \pm 4:9$ hrs (Ebert et al., 1976), the peak plasma level occurring at about 2½ hours after an oral dose of 30 mg. In a group of 25 hyperactive children given 10 mg, the mean half life was one third the value for adults, i.e., 6.54 ± 2.54 hours (urinary pH between 5 and 6.5) though there was a wide range of individual response (3-13 hours) (Brown et al., 1977).

Methylphenidate disappears so rapidly from plasma after oral administration that plasma half life is difficult to determine. Measuring a 20 mg dose of C^{14} methylphenidate revealed peak levels in adults at about 2 hours with a T½ (see Chapter 1) from 2-7 hours. The C^{14} consisted of metabolites (Faraj et al., 1974), almost all of which appeared in the urine by 72 hours.

Oral administration of 75 mg of *pemoline* produced a peak serum level in children at 2-4 hours with a T½ of 12 hours and excretion of about 75% of the dose in the urine by 24 hours.

A therapeutic dose of 150 mg of *caffeine* (the amount in 1 cup of coffee or tea) produces peak effect between 30 minutes and 2 hours in adults.

Site and Mode of Action

It is postulated (Arnold et al., 1972) that *amphetamine* and its related drugs work by *enhancing catecholamine effects*, particularly neurotransmitter actions, both centrally and, insofar as there are peripheral effects, peripherally. This enhancement is achieved by blocking catecholamine re-uptake into presynaptic nerve endings and thus preventing inactivation by monoamine oxidase. In respect of which particular catecholamines are involved, there is evidence to suggest that the variety of amphetamine effects can be specifically explained by both dopamine (e.g., motor coordination, psychotomimetic effects) and norepinephrine enhancement (locomotor activity in rats).

There is evidence that *caffeine* effects two changes at the cellular level. One is to increase intracellular cyclic AMP by inhibiting phosphodiesterase, the enzyme responsible for cyclic AMP destruction. The other is to translocate calcium intracellularly. The importance of these or other mechanisms in the responses of individual tissues to caffeine, however, is uncertain (Goodman & Gilman, 1975).

Dose Response and Time Action Relationships

Despite the extensive clinical use of amphetamines and methylphenidate (pemoline has been developed much more recently), pharmacologic data, especially as applied to children, are scanty. This is especially evident for dose response and time action relationships. The reason for this paucity of information is at least threefold:

>1) The *magnitude* of catecholamine release rather than a specific action of the drug seems to be responsible for the actions of amphetamine (and probably its related drugs). Precise pharmacologic measurement of catecholamines intrasynaptically has not been possible.

STIMULANTS

Furthermore, only recently have measurements of serum amphetamine and methylphenidate been possible.

2) Rigorous *definition and measurement* of target behaviors in children are conspicuously lacking in most studies (see Chapter 2, 3).

3) The psychomotor stimulants *affect a variety of behaviors*—some more immediately (e.g., certain cognitive changes) and some over several weeks (behavioral improvement); hence, dose, response and time are all co-varying simultaneously.

In two studies (Ebert et al., 1976; Brown et al., 1977) correlating behavioral variables (euphoria/activation, activity/behavior on Conners rating scale) with plasma level, subjective effects were found to peak between 1½ to 3 hours whereas plasma effects peaked between 2 and 3 hours. In one study (Swanson, et al., in press) measuring the effect of methylphenidate on a paired associate learning task in children, responders reached their peak of accuracy at 2 hours and began returning to pre-drug levels of performance at 3 hours.

Two studies designed to determine optimal dose of *methylphenidate* found that outpatient hyperactive children performed a picture recognition test best at 0.30 mg/kg but long term behavioral changes measured by the Conners Parent Rating Scales required 0.70 to 1.00 mg/kg (Werry & Sprague, 1974) for optimal response. Further studies are necessary to clarify optimal dose for desired response over the short and long term in children (see Sprague & Sleator, 1975).

CLINICAL EFFECTS

General difficulties in evaluating psychopharmacologic agents in pediatrics have been discussed elsewhere in this volume (see Chapters 2-5). Two such difficulties with the literature on stimulants should be mentioned here, prior to a discussion of their clinical effects.

The first problem is *definitional* and comes from multiple usages of the same term by different people. For example, as discussed in Chapter 2 and 5, the word "hyperactivity" is often used to mean conduct problems or socially disapproved disruptive behavior, while in other cases it is used to refer to motor activity. This type of confusion makes it very difficult to compare studies.

Secondly, while terms may be used similarly by different investigators, again as pointed out in some detail in Chapter 2, the *measurement techniques to quantify the same dimension may be quite different*. For example, *hyperactivity*, in many cases, is measured by a global assessment made by a physician. In other cases it may be measured by use of systematic teacher rating scales. Yet in other cases it may be done by the actual measurement of motor activity by various types of measuring devices. Thus different results may be explained simply by differences in measurement techniques.

This confusion is eloquent testimony to the need for a new nosology of the characteristics of DSM III (see Chapter 5) and for the standardization of measurement argued in Chapter 2.

Most of the work with stimulants in children has been done with the amphetamines (Benzedrine, Dexedrine) and methylphenidate (Ritalin). Their clinical effects are similar. Much less work has been done with caffeine, pemoline (Cylert) and other stimulants. The clinical effects discussed below will be discussed for all of the stimulants. When the effect of one stimulant seems to differ from another, it will be remarked.

Physiological

CENTRAL NERVOUS SYSTEM

The major central nervous system effects of *amphetamine* (and probably of *methylphenidate* and *pemoline* which have been studied less extensively) are secondary to the *location and degree of arousal produced*. Those effects can be summarized as follows:

1) Excitation of the *respiratory center* in the medulla produces an increased rate and depth of respiration said to be observable in man only when respiration has been previously depressed by centrally acting drugs. In children there is one report of increased respiration (Aman & Werry, 1975a) though most reports are negative (Ballard et al., 1976; Barkley, 1977; Barkley & Jackson, in press; Boileau et al., 1976). *Caffeine*, too, stimulates the respiratory medulla though the effects are significant only with parenteral administration (Goodman & Gilman, 1975).

2) Activation of the *reticular arousal system* by *amphetamine* is probably responsible for improved task performance (by improving motivation and reducing sense of fatigue), for improved attention span after prolonged sleep deprivation (possibly by reducing the occurence of miscrosleeps that impair task performance) and for the hyper-aroused, jittery symptoms which affect some children. Insomnia is the undesired extension of this activation. *Amphetamine* (and to a lesser extent methylphenidate and pemoline) substantially alters sleep patterns by reducing to one half the percentage of time spent in REM sleep and by diminishing stage 4 sleep as well. With cessation of the drug, compensatory REM sleep (with concomitant increased dreaming, often nightmares) not only appears more rapidly in the sleep cycle, it also occupies a greater percentage of it. In some in-

dividuals several months elapse before the sleep pattern returns to normal (Safer & Allen, 1976).

Caffeine also increases alertness, concentration, appreciation of sensory stimuli and diminishes reaction time. A feeling of depression may follow large doses of caffeine but the exact effects of the 150 mg dose in a cup of coffee is still controversial.

3) Appetite suppression is possibly secondary to *amphetamine* effects on the *lateral hypothalamic feeding center*. Although some tolerance may develop to the anorexia and diminished food intake, the resultant retardation of growth may be a problem (see Treatment Emergent Effects). There is some compensatory growth with cessation of drug treatment and the overall effect on growth is probably related to frequency and duration of drug administration (Safer & Allen, 1975). *Methylphenidate* anorexia is reported less frequently. This issue is discussed more fully later. Since *pemoline* also produces anorexia, it might be expected also to have some effect on growth and this has been reported (Page et al., 1974). There is some suggestion that 1-amphetamine is less anorexiogenic than its d-isomer; since these isomers are postulated to effect dopaminergic and adrenergic systems differently (Arnold et al., 1972), it would be interesting to see if degree of growth retardation remains the same.

CARDIOVASCULAR SYSTEM

The most significant peripheral effects of the central stimulant drugs in children are on the cardiovascular system. There are reports with *methylphenidate* that find small but significant increments in systolic and diastolic blood pressure (Barkley, 1977; Safer & Allen, 1976) and increments in pulse rate at rest and with exertion (Aman & Werry, 1975a, b; Ballard et al., 1976; Barkley, 1977; Boileau et al., 1976). There is controversy regarding the clinical significance of these changes (Katz et al., 1975). Some long-term studies over several months suggest that tolerance may develop (Safer & Allen, 1976), while others refute this (Ballard et al., 1976; Boileau et al., 1976). Those investigators who found significantly increased pulse and blood pressure changes, especially with exercise, noted that these changes were more pronounced with increasing dosage. Although these pulse and blood pressure responses returned to pre-drug levels almost immediately upon cessation of methylphenidate, minimizing the possibility of cardiovascular changes by administering the smallest effective dose of the drug seems sensible.

Although clinical experience with *pemoline* is not as extensive, significant changes in pulse and blood pressure have not been reported.

Although *caffeine* exerts a direct stimulant action on the myocardium, the medullary vagal stimulation is greater with resultant slight bradycardia or no change in heart rate. With very large doses, however, tachycardia and even arrythmias may result. In coronary, pulmonary, and systemic blood vessels, therapeutic doses of caffeine, acting directly on vascular musculature, produce vasodilation, though this effect is not great enough to be useful clinically. Furthermore, stimulant action on the myocardium, increasing the work of the heart, makes its use in coronary heart disease controversial. Blood pressure effects are unpredictable. Caffeine produces vasoconstriction in the cerebral circulation which may be responsible for its therapeutic efficacy in headaches especially of hypertensive etiology.

MUSCULOSKELETAL SYSTEM

Stimulant drugs have been reported to affect facets of motor behavior including "soft" neurological signs. Increased motor steadiness, motor coordination, and increased speed of task performance have been noted (Knights, 1974; Lerer & Lerer, 1976; Schain & Reynard, 1975; Sprague et al., 1970; Spring et al., 1976; Wade, 1976). However, some experiments designed specifically to measure or quantify these changes have been unable to find significant changes from placebo. Attentional and motivational factors may account for the improved performance and accuracy noted in motor tasks (Conners & Werry, in press). *Caffeine* has been found to enhance certain skills (e.g., typing), though fine motor coordination per se does not seem to improve. The capacity for muscular work increases (Weiss & Laties, 1962).

SMOOTH MUSCLE

In adults, bronchial muscle relaxation occurs with both *amphetamines* and *caffeine* but is not sufficient to be of clinical use; although bladder sphincter contraction is reported, well-controlled studies of therapeutic value of *amphetamines* for enuresis in children are conspicuous by their absence. Although abdominal pain may be a side effect, amphetamine effect on the GI tract is unpredictable (Goodman & Gilman, 1975).

RENAL SYSTEM

Direct action on the renal tubule with increased sodium and chloride excretion is responsible for the mild diuresis produced by *caffeine*.

STOMACH

Caffeine increases gastric secretion of both acid and pepsin normally; and in ulcer prone individuals the response seems to be exaggerated.

METABOLIC SYSTEM

Amphetamines have been found to increase plasma concentration of free fatty acids, increase metabolic rate and decrease growth hormone secretion. A 10% to 25% increase in BMR has been reported following 0.5 g of caffeine and in sufficient quantities, caffeine stimulates gluconeogenesis, glycogenolysis and lipolysis (Goodman & Gilman, 1975). *Methylphenidate* has been found to increase blood levels of plasma dopamine-B-hydroxylase (Rapoport et al., 1974a) but not to affect blood 5-hydroxyindole levels (Greenberg & Coleman, 1976). Both drugs can produce a release of growth hormone similar to that obtained with levodopa (Aarskog et al., 1977).

Activity

Activity as used here refers solely to motor activity. As noted in Chapter 2, a number of methods have been tried objectively to quantify activity level including ballistographic, mechanical, photoelectric and ultrasonic devices; telemetry and motion pictures; direct observation; and rating by observers (Cantwell, 1975).

Apparent contradictions in the literature regarding the effects of stimulants on activity in children can thus probably be partially explained by these differences in techniques. Differences also arise depending on the type of motor activity being measured (i.e., seat movements, ankle movements) and on the situation in which the activity is being measured (i.e., in a free field situation or during performance of laboratory tasks) (Sroufe, 1975; Whalen & Henker, 1976). Some studies (Ellis et al., 1974; Millichap & Boldrey, 1967; Conners, 1971) suggest an *increased* activity in free field situations, even in the face of behavioral improvements as reported by parents and teachers (Millichap & Boldrey, 1967). However, there are equally consistent reports of a *decreased* activity level and a decrease of irrelevant behavior during performance on laboratory tasks which measure attention, cognitive style and concept attainment (Cohen et al., 1971; Millichap et al., 1968; Spraque et al., 1970; Sroufe et al., 1973; Juliano, 1974; Sykes et al., 1971; Werry & Aman, 1975). The study by Knobel and Lytton (Knobel et al., 1959) suggested that methylphenidate resulted in a *decrease* in the total amount of motor activity and an increase in the amount of motor activity which was goal directed. The available literature thus supports the idea that stimulants may affect the quality of motor activity at least as much as, if not more than, the quantity (Whalen & Henker, 1976).

In sum, there is little evidence of consistency of drug effects on children's motor activity across situations (Conners & Werry, in press; Routh et al., 1974; Sprague & Sleator, 1973). Depending on the situation in which the child is tested, on the type of motor activity being measured, and the measuring instrument, stimulants may increase or decrease activity. *However, in the usual clinical situation the effect on motor activity is a beneficial one.*

Psycho- and Electrophysiological Effects

A variety of psycho- and electrophysiological measures have been noted as a result of stimulant drug treatment. In an early study Cutts and Jasper (1939) found that *amphetamine* did not have a definite effect on the EEG of children with behavior disorders. However, other investigators have reported a decrease in abnormal EEG patterns and an increase in alpha activity in certain areas as a result of treatment with stimulants (Lindsley & Henry, 1941; MacKay et al., 1973). Shetty (1971) produced an increase in alpha wave activity of the EEG with the administration of *dextroamphetamine*. He interpreted this finding to indicate that stimulants increased CNS inhibitory mechanisms to help the child filter out irrelevant stimuli.

More recent studies of the EEG have involved averaged evoked responses (AER) of the EEG. Both auditory evoked responses and visual evoked responses have been studied. Several investigators using different methods (Satterfield et al., 1972; Saletu et al., 1973; Buchsbaum & Wender, 1973) have found that responders to stimulant drug treatment were characterized by a reduction of the averaged evoked response of the EEG. Results of similar studies, however, are not entirely consistent (Conners, 1975a; Halliday et al., 1976; Sroufe, 1975; Weber & Sulzbacher, 1975) and some of the discrepancy may lie in heterogeneity within diagnostic groups (Conners, 1975a; Halliday et al., 1976). A very early study by Laufer et al. (1957) reported that hyperactive children had lower photometrazol (i.e., excitation) threshold of the EEG and also that these lowered thresholds were raised by the administration of stimulant medication. This important study apparently never has been replicated.

Studies of skin conductance are somewhat inconsistent. Some investigators have found basal skin conductance to be increased by stimulant drugs (Cohen et al., 1971; Satterfield & Dawson, 1971; Zahn et al., 1975) while other reports are negative (Spring et al., 1974; Montagu & Swarbrick, 1975). The effects of stimulants on nonspecific galvanic skin responses (GSR's) are also inconsistent. Some studies (Satterfield & Dawson, 1971; Spring et al., 1974) have found nonspecific GSR's to be increased by the administration of stimulants while others have failed to replicate this finding (Barkley & Jackson, in press; Cohen et al., 1971; Zahn et al., 1975).

The electropupillogram (EPG) has also recently been used in studies with stimulants (Knopp et al., 1973; Yoss, 1975; Yoss & Moyer, 1971). In an elaborate study, Knopp was able to relate changes in behavior to changes in the EPG after stimulant drug treatment. While many of the other electrophysiological measures reviewed above suggest that *some* hyperactive children may be under-aroused and stimulants serve to increase their arousal level (Conners, 1975a; Satterfield et al., 1972), Knopp's finding with the EPG suggests that both under-aroused and over-aroused hyperkinetic children may respond positively to stimulant medication.

One putative psychophysiological correlate of attentional processes is heart rate deceleration (Sroufe et al., 1973). Sroufe found that methylphenidate increased the magnitude of this measure in anticipation of a stimulus. However, his results were not replicated by Cohen et al. (1971) whose methodology was slightly different. Some of this confusion may be due to the fact that heart rate changes in attention are probably biphasic —initial deceleration followed by acceleration. Porges et al. (1975) showed that methylphenidate in hyperactive children decreased *both* these effects and variability in the response.

In reviewing this area of research Barkley (1977) has suggested that the findings indicate that the stimulants may be acting to increase CNS inhibitory activity, thus enabling the child to screen out distracting stimuli. At the same time the stimulants may facilitate certain excitatory systems enabling the child to focus his attention on a task. More research is needed in this area, with careful replication, using homogeneous populations and the same measurement instruments and methodology. Diagnosis is particularly important since evidence suggesting heterogeneity of psychophysiological state and response to stimulants in children presently diagnosed as hyperactive is compelling (Conners, 1975a; Halliday et al., 1976).

Cognitive Function and Performance

An impressive body of evidence exists suggesting that stimulant medication of all types positively affects cognitive functions such as attention, perception, and memory, as well as influencing cognitive style and other *laboratory measures* of learning (see Chapter 3).

GENERAL COGNITION

As noted in Chapter 3, there is no clear evidence that stimulants improve performance on *general* cognitive measures such as tests of intelligence, reading achievement, language skills and complex learning (Douglas, 1974; Gittelman-Klein & Klein, 1976; Rie et al., 1976; Whalen & Henker, 1976). While there are some studies indicating that stimulants produce improvements in both verbal and performance IQ (Conners, 1971; Douglas, 1972; Epstein et al., 1968; Greenberg et al., 1972; Knights & Hinton, 1969; Lewis & Young, 1975), there are just as many studies suggesting that stimulants do not affect these measures (Conners & Rothschild, 1968; Conners et al., 1969; Conrad et al., 1971; Rapoport et al., 1974b; Werry & Sprague, 1974).

SPECIFIC COGNITIVE FUNCTIONS

However, when more *specific* laboratory measures are used, there is consistent evidence that stimulant medication enhances *attention, memory* and *learning*. The studies of the Montreal group are models in this area. Sykes (Sykes et al., 1971, 1972) showed that *methylphenidate* produced significant improvement on choice reaction time and on serial reaction time tests and also on a visual and auditory continuous performance test. Methylphenidate also produced significant improvement in a continuous performance attention task while at the same time decreasing motor restlessness and distractibility. Cohen et al. (1971) found that methylphenidate decreased variability and increased the speed of reaction time while also decreasing task irrelevant motor responses. In a study of cognitive style Campbell et al. (1971a) found that methylphenidate led to longer reaction times and fewer errors on the Matching Familiar Figures tests. No significant difference was obtained on the Embedded Figures Test of Field Dependence/Independence. Douglas (1972, 1974) summarized the results of these Montreal studies and suggested that methylphenidate exerted its effect by helping the hyperactive child sustain attention and control impulsive behavior.

Conners (1975a; Conners & Rothschild, 1968) has also shown that dextroamphetamine and methylphenidate reduce errors on the continuous performance test while increasing latency, i.e., made children less impulsive. They also showed improved learning on a paired associate learning task. In an earlier study by Conners et al. (1964) utilizing dextroamphetamine with a paired associate learning task, there was no drug effect on the learning task, but there was a positive effect on IQ.

In an important study Swanson and Kinsbourne (1976) studied 32 hyperactive and 16 non-hyperactive children performing a paired associate learning task while being treated with *methylphenidate* or with placebo. Significant drug-related facilitation of the performance on the learning task was found for the 32 hyperactive children. The 16 non-hyperactive children did not demonstrate this facilitated performance. On the second day of testing three questions were considered. Did an overall drug induced facilitation occur? Was performance state-dependent during the drug test? Was performance state-dependent during placebo test? The results indicate that for the hyperactive children there was indeed an overall drug-induced facilitation of performance on learning tasks. Moreover *state-dependent learning* (see Chapter 3) was demonstrated both during the active drug and placebo conditions. No statistically significant evidence of positive or negative effect for the 16 non-hyperactive children were shown on the second day of testing although there was a trend toward an impairment of performance resulting from treatment with methylphenidate. There was also a trend towards state-dependency. Based on these findings Swanson and Kinsbourne (1976) suggest that hyperactive children being treated with medication should be treated consistently so that their behavior would be constantly normalized and thus provide full benefit. Other investigators, however, (Aman & Sprague, 1974) have failed to demonstrate such a state-dependent learning effect with stimulants (see also Chapter 3).

In a similar study of hyperactive children who were "good responders" and "poor responders" to methylphenidate Swanson et al. (in press) demonstrated a time response effect on a paired associate learning task. Those children who were good responders to the methylphenidate had a peak enhancement of their performance on the learning task about 2 hours after taking the medication, after which the performance decreased. Those who were poor responders had a decrement in their performance which also peaked about 2 hours after the medication. Moreover, those favorable responders at lower doses could be "overdosed" and performance on the learning task would decrease. This U-shaped curve with dosage is much as posited and demonstrated behaviorally by Sprague (Sprague & Sleator, 1975; Werry & Sprague, 1974).

Conners et al. (1972) found significant effects of stimulants consistently on the Porteus Maze. Conners hypothesizes that stimulants produce a positive effect by allowing the child to selectively inhibit, plan, and control his responses and that Porteus Maze is a measure of this effect. He postulates that much of the improvement obtained in other tests result from this particular drug effect.

Sprague et al. (1970) looked at reaction time, correct response on a one trial learning and recognition tasks and activity as measured by a stabilometric cushion coupled with observer ratings of classroom behavior in 12 emotionally disturbed, underachieving boys. *Methylphenidate* was found to decrease reaction time, improve performance on the learning tasks, and reduce activity level. Werry & Sprague (1974) investigated methylphenidate in another group of emotionally disturbed children. A visual picture recognition task was used as an index of short term memory and it was found that there was a significant improvement in this task at dosage levels up to 0.3 mg/kg. In another study Werry & Aman (1975) found an improvement in both attention, as measured by the Continuous Performance Test (CPT), and the short term memory test of Sprague, though, interestingly, improvement in the latter occurred only when performance was falling off. After that there was a decrement in performance. Both dextroamphetamine and magnesium pemoline were found not to affect the continuous performance task in a comparative study (Conners et al., 1972).

Caffeine was found to improve attention in a similar manner to sympathomimetic stimulants in hyperactive children in one study (Reichard & Elder, 1977), though this stands in contrast to the lack of behavioral effects (see below). In the only adequate study extant, *deanol* also improved reaction time (Lewis & Young, 1975).

SUMMARY

In situations where sustained performance is required in laboratory settings, stimulants have led to a significantly greater reduction in errors of omission (Campbell et al., 1971a; Conners & Rothschild, 1968; Sykes et al., 1971, 1972). In vigilance tasks and in tasks requiring immediate and delayed perceptual judgment, an increase in accuracy has been found as a result of the stimulants (Campbell et al., 1971a; Conners & Rothschild, 1968; Sprague et al., 1970; Sprague & Werry, 1971, 1974; Sykes et al., 1971, 1972; Werry & Aman, 1975). In tasks where rapid responses are required stimulant drugs have been shown to reduce response latency and decrease reaction time (Sprague et al., 1970; Sykes et al., 1971, 1972). On laboratory tasks where speed is not an issue and less impulsive responding is desired, the stimulants lead to a more deliberate response (Campbell et al., 1971a). Stimulants have been found to reduce variability of reaction time tasks and to positively affect performance on both simple and choice reaction time (Sroufe, 1975). These results may be interpreted as showing that stimulants improve performance on tasks requiring sustained attention particularly under conditions of stress, paced tasks, and failing performance (Conners, 1975a; Douglas, 1972, 1974; Werry & Aman, 1975). Douglas has made a persuasive case for the fact that the children who improve on stimulant medication have an *attentional deficit* which is improved by the use of stimulant medication. Thus the available evidence indicates that *all stimulants have a positive effect on certain aspects of cognitive function-*

ing. However, there is little or no evidence to support the contention that learning in a classroom situation, reasoning, or problem solving ability are positively affected by the stimulants (Rie et al., 1976; Werry, 1977; Whalen & Henker, 1976). The effects of drugs on cognitive function are discussed in more detail in Chapter 3.

Academic Achievement

The effect of stimulant drugs on academic achievement of children has been reviewed by Barkley and Cunningham (in press) (see also Chapter 3). Out of 120 drug studies reviewed, only 17 used objective measures of academic achievement. These 17 studies involved 52 objective tests. Barkley and Cunningham found few positive drug effects on these measures. Moreover, they felt that any improvements on the tests were better attributed to improvement in attention and concentration during the test taking performance rather than on actual change in academic achievement. They also reviewed 6 follow up studies of hyperactive children who had been treated with stimulant medication over a period of 2 to 10 years. All of the follow up studies were unanimous in suggesting that stimulants have little if any impact on the long term academic outcome. However, it is the authors' opinion (consistent with that in Chapter 3) that a proper study evaluating the effects of stimulants on actual academic achievement in the classroom has not been carried out.

Such a study presents a difficult methodological problem. First, the *time frame* must be long enough for actual achievement in the classroom to have occurred.

Secondly, the effect the stimulants have must be *singled out* from a combination of other factors that may affect achievement.

For example, Satterfield and Cantwell (1977) have recently reported changes in the reading comprehension and recognition, arithmetic and general information subtests of the Peabody Individual Achievement Test in a group of children intensively and consistently treated with methlyphenidate over a one-year period. No such improvement was determined for the group in spelling. However, these children were also receiving a wide variety of other forms of treatment including individual psychotherapy, group therapy for the children, family therapy, and some were in individual educational therapy; thus the effects of these various treatment modalities cannot reliably be separated out from the effects produced by stimulant medication alone.

Third, the measurement of such academic changes *presents difficulty*. The question to be answered is whether or not an individual child makes as much or more progress in a subject over a year's time than would be predicted for him. Prediction for an individual child probably needs to be done by using a multiple regression equation involving intelligence, chronological age, and academic achievement. (This measurement issue is discussed in more detail by Rutter and Yule, 1973 and in Chapter 3).

SUMMARY

Currently there is no positive evidence that actual academic achievement in the classroom is facilitated by the use of stimulant medication. However, there is also no research which definitely and conclusively proves that it is not.

Behavior

Of all the effects of stimulant drugs, those on the social behavior of problem children are the most well documented. Since Bradley's original report (1937) there have been a large number of well controlled, methodologically sound studies confirming the original finding that the behavior of children referred for treatment is rated as improved following treatment by the stimulants other than caffeine and deanol. There are a number of well written reviews which detail the various controlled studies that support this finding (Barkley, 1977; Conners, 1971; Conners & Werry, in press; Gittelman-Klein, 1975; de la Cruz et al., 1973; Lambert et al., 1976). As pointed out in Chapter 2, while the majority (75% of 31 studies reviewed by Barkley, 1977) of such reports attest to an overall or global improvement (Barkley, 1977; Conners & Werry, in press; Knights, 1974), a rather more important question is what *particular types of behavior* are positively affected by the use of stimulants? To a large extent these depend on the type and quality of measures used. Most of the best work with the stimulants has relied on factored teacher and parent rating scales, notably Conners (1973b) Teacher and Parent Questionnaires (TQ and PQ) yielding four or more dimensions. Discussion of such scales is to be found in Chapter 2 and in Quay (in press).

Most consistently factors I and IV on the TQ (Conduct Disorder and Hyperactivity) are those which have been shown to improve with stimulant drug treatment. The other two factors (Attention Disorder and Anxiety-Oversensitivity) have not been as consistently affected by stimulant medication, but there are studies which do report positive effects on attention disorder, though infrequently on anxiety (Arnold et al., 1972, 1976; Conners & Werry, in press; Conners et al., 1972; Huestis et al., 1975; Garfinkel et al., 1975; Rapoport et al., 1971, 1974b; Safer & Allen, 1976;

Schleifer et al., 1975; Satterfield & Cantwell, 1977; Werry & Sprague, 1974; Winsberg et al., 1974b).

Conners PQ has eight factors: conduct problems, anxiety, impulsive/hyperactive, learning problems, psychosomatic, perfectionism, antisocial and muscular tension. As with drug effects in general (see Chapter 3), the PQ has been much less consistent in detecting stimulant-produced changes in behavior than the TQ. Satterfield and Cantwell (1977) reported significant positive changes at the end of one year on all eight factors while other investigators have found only some factors to be positively affected by the stimulants and others none (Arnold et al., 1972, 1976; Conners et al., 1972; Finerty et al., 1971; Gittelman-Klein & Klein, 1975; Hoffman et al., 1974; Rapoport et al., 1974b; Werry & Aman, 1975; Werry & Sprague, 1974).

However, as pointed out in Chapter 2, there is considerable doubt about the validity of hyperactivity as measured by rating scales and its distinctiveness from disruptive behavior executed motorically. Six items of behavior on the TQ make up the *hyperactivity* factor: constantly fidgeting, hums and makes other odd noises, restless or overactive, excitable/impulsive, disturbs other children, and teases other children and interferes with their activities. It can be seen that only one or two of these items are *related purely to activity level*.

Besides teacher and parent rating scales, physician, psychologist, observer, and parent *observational methods* (see Chapter 2) have also been used. Generally speaking such methods have been less sensitive to any effects of drugs in general and to stimulants in particular. However, those that have shown effects of stimulants have supported the rating scale effects in showing a reduction in *disruptive behavior*, especially of a motoric kind (Arnold et al., 1976; Gittelman-Klein & Klein, 1975; Gittelman-Klein et al., 1976a, b; Rapoport & Benoit, 1975; Rapoport et al., 1974b; Schleifer et al., 1975; Sprague et al., 1970).

Thus the evidence from the best controlled and methodologically sound rating scale studies suggest that *the most consistent positive effect of the stimulants* (other than caffeine and deanol) *is on behavior, particularly of the type perceived by teachers as disruptive and not socially appropriate.* Caffeine has not established itself as affecting behavior (Conners, 1975b; Garfinkel et al., 1975; Gross, 1975; Huestis et al., 1975) and deanol is really untried except in one positive study (Lewis & Young, 1975). There is little evidence from these studies that emotional symptoms (escape/avoidance behavior such as phobias, etc.) are affected positively by stimulant medication. In Fish's (1971) view those children who respond best to stimulants among the behavior disordered group include those with a predominance of *anxiety and neurotic mechanisms* and those predominantly manifested by *negativism, belligerence and aggressive behavior*. She feels that these two groups correspond to the Over-anxious Reaction and the Unsocialized Aggressive Reaction in DSM II. Support for her view as far as Over-anxious Reactions are concerned can be seen in the study by Arnold et al. (1976).

In their comprehensive review, Conners and Werry (in press) also concluded that, while stimulant drugs exert their positive effects chiefly on *socially disruptive impulsive behavior* manifested primarily in schoool, there are occasional reports of positive effects on shy children who are stimulated to more active outgoing behavior. They make the point that the reports of positive effects on conduct disorder are made in children who are brought for treatment because they manifest those types of symptoms. Possibly the shy type of child is less seen for drug treatment because shy, withdrawn behavior is less disruptive to adults, and the current climate in child psychiatry favors psychotherapy for this type of child. They suggest that stimulants may produce changes in both types of children, overcontrolled and undercontrolled, depending upon which set of symptoms is severe enough to show changes. Further research is needed on this report.

Personality

As with most of pediatric psychopharmacology (see Chapter 2), systematic research on the effect of stimulant medication on the child's personality structure is lacking. Conners et al. (1967) used the Cattell to study the effects of stimulants on personality structure. "A vigorous and energetic" approach to tasks was the factor on the Cattell most affected by dextroamphetamine. This is one of the few studies of its kind. However, clinically it is well recognized that in some children the use of stimulants radically transforms the personality, so much so that parents state, "he's not my child," "he's a different boy," "I don't have the same boy I used to have." Bradley (1937) in his very early studies commented on some changes in personality of the patients he treated with the amphetamines, and it has been noted informally since (e.g., Schain & Reynard, 1975). In some cases the authors have found these effects on the personality to be so significant that both the parents and the children wanted the medication to be discontinued, even in the face of an otherwise positive response.

Mood

The effects of stimulants on mood in children have not only been inadequately studied but statements are made which go far beyond the available data. For example, some (Safer & Allen, 1976) including a U.S. Government "Blue Ribbon Committee" (Freedman, 1971) state that stimulants do not cause euphoria in children and conclude from that that this is probably the reason why therapeutic use of stimulants in hyperactive children does not lead to a later drug dependence.

However, very little in the way of systematic research is available to support such a statement. Moreover, what research has been done tends if anything to suggest the opposite. As noted above, Bradley described a generalized euphoria in some children as well as a *zestful*, energetic approach to tasks. This euphoric reaction was confirmed by Bender (Bender & Cottington, 1942) in her clinical studies and the literature since is full of informal reports of behavior suggestive of, if not euphoria, some positive mood change. In one of the few formal studies the Clyde Mood Scale completed by parents of children who had been treated with dexedrine also indicated that the children were judged as being happier while on the medication (Conners et al., 1965). However, Rapoport et al. (1974b) failed to detect any change on a self-concept scale but this instrument is, of unknown drug sensitivity (see Chapter 2).

There is also some evidence that the stimulants may cause depression rather than elevation of mood in some children. However, Ounsted (1955) is one of the few to report a significant number of children responding with a *depressive* reaction to treatment with stimulants whereas the more usual reports are of an occasional child showing fearfulness, sadness or, more frequently, irritability (see Barkley, 1977). However in this study children all had epilepsy as well as the hyperkinetic behavior disorder.

In summary, informal and a few formal reports suggest that both elevation and depression of mood may occur in children, though, as Barkley's (1977) review shows, dysphoria is much more frequent. However, positive mood change is particularly difficult to detect in children (Rapoport, 1976), but both have been inadequately studied.

Summary of Clinical Effects

The above review indicates stimulants may have clinical effects in many areas. The bulk of these effects have been noted in children referred for treatment for certain disorders. Whether these same effects are peculiar to disturbed children, as often suggested, to specific diagnostic groups, or would be obtained in non-referred, "normal" children is unknown. Apart from one or two contentious areas such as reduction of motor activity and the infrequency of positive mood changes, most of these are consistent with the pharmacological actions of catecholamine potentiation and similar to those observed in normal adults (Weiss & Laties, 1962), best described as an increase in alertness, efficiency and compliance.

Predicting Clinical Response

It is not uncommon to find statements about various clinical, historical, neurological or socioeconomic factors as predictive of a good (or poor) outcome with stimulants. Probably the greatest consensus relates to that diagnostic category of hyperkinetic (now called attention deficit) disorder, but there is reason to believe that this diagnosis often may be adapted to fit the treatment rather than vice versa and there is also reason to believe that the responses of other diagnostic groups have not been fully explored. This is discussed in more detail below.

Barkley (1976), in the most comprehensive review of this area, concluded that variables, independent of any particular type, which measure *attention span* are the best predictors while other measures were of no or of unestablished value. Others (see Conners, 1975a; Satterfield, 1976) hold that *underarousal* is the best criterion but, in general, *inattention appears inversely correlated with level of arousal in children with attention deficits* so the two are actually facets of the same explanation. The only question is which comes first or do they both reflect a common underlying pathophysiological or psychopathological disorder?

Treatment Emergent (Side) Effects

As with all psychoactive drugs the *potential* side effects of stimulants are numerous. Perusal of the Physician's Desk Reference will indicate possible effects in almost every system in the body. However, there is a paucity of *published* reports of significant side effects. This offers at least indirect evidence that significant side effects are relatively uncommon.

Short-term Effects

In his review of 29 studies reporting this type of data Barkeley (1977) found that almost all reported insomnia and decreased appetite while weight loss, abdominal pain and headaches were reported in about half. However, in most instances these side effects occurred in a minority of children and were minor, temporary or easily dealt with by reducing dosage. Other side effects such as drowsiness, sadness, increased talkativeness, dizziness and more dramatic ones such as dyskinetic episodes and a toxic psychosis can occur but are considerably less common (Barkley, 1977; Conners, 1971; Conners & Werry, in press; Greenberg et al., 1975; Shader & Di Mascio, 1970) and likewise seem temporary and/or dose dependent.

In *summary*, the current opinion is that the *short-term side effects* of the stimulants are generally temporary and of minimal clinical significance. They very rarely are enough of a problem to cause the medication to be stopped (Shader & Di Mascio, 1970; Safer & Allen, 1976). However, whether the anorexia and accompanying weight loss are in fact ordinarily simply temporary side effects which the children adjust to over time is still an open question (Werry, 1976a). Also, although there are claims for fewer side effects with certain stimulants (Safer & Allen, 1976) there appears to be little hard evidence to choose between the amphetamines and methylphenidate in this regard (Werry, 1977).

Long-term Effects

With regard to the question of *long-term* side effects the safest statement that can then be made is that this area requires a great deal of further research. There does not seem to be any clear tendency for children who have been treated with stimulants to become abusers of drugs later in life (Beck et al., 1975; Denhoff, 1973; Freedman, 1971; Weiss, 1975). However, caution in this area is still necessary since most of these studies have failed to locate a significant number of subjects at follow-up (Werry, 1977).

The one long-term side effect that is currently of concern is the possible *depression of growth rate* which can occur with both the amphetamines and methylphenidate, although the amphetamines seem to be more implicated (Safer & Allen, 1976). However, there is one meticulous prospective follow-up of hyperactive children who were treated with methylphenidate for one year in which neither height nor weight in the treated children differed from the control children (McNutt et al., 1977). Similarly Gross (1976) was unable to find evidence of growth retardation with stimulants. Thus the exact frequency of this side effect is unclear.

It has been assumed that the effects on growth are related to the *anorexia* caused by the medication through its effects on the hypothalmus (see Clinical Effects), but a metabolic effect has not been completely ruled out. Greenhill et al. (1977) reported a study of seven children on chronic amphetamine treatment for 6 months. While no growth hormone (GH) change occurred with either acute or chronic amphetamine usage, there was a significant difference for prolactin after six months of treatment with d-amphetamine. Chronic d-amphetamine therapy appeared to significantly suppress prolactin during sleep. Since prolactin has been implicated as a growth stimulating agent the authors hypothesize that one mechanism for growth retardation secondary to amphetamine *might* be through prolactin suppression, but further work is needed to establish this. Aarskog et al. (1977), however, did find alterations in GH, notably a raised resting level and reductions in amphetamine-produced release. The significance of the finding is unclear.

Studies with pemoline indicate that weight loss returns to the normal curve after 3 to 6 months (Page et al., 1974). The evidence also suggests that the effects of methylphenidate and the amphetamines on height and weight are dose dependent (in excess of 20 mg daily or about 1 mg/kg of methylphenidate), are strongest in the first year (Safer & Allen, 1973, 1976) and that there is a rebound effect when the children are taken off medication. Thus the children not only return to previous growth patterns, but actually gain more in both height and weight than would be predicted while they are off medication (Safer & Allen, 1976; Satterfield & Cantwell, 1977). The actual long-term effect of this growth depression, when and if it occurs, is not known, in particular whether the rebound when children are taken off medication is enough to completely restore any growth depression. Further research is needed with children followed over longer periods of time, particularly through the period of the growth spurt in early adolescence. Obviously, this potential treatment emergent effect calls for the minimum dose possible for the shortest period practicable and the use of drug holidays at weekends or school vacations whenever clinically feasible.

In *summary*, serious side effects of stimulants with children are most infrequent. However, more careful long-term work needs to be done, particularly in the area of growth suppression, and possible drug dependence, especially when the stimulants are continued into the high-risk stage of adolescence. Also, the effects on the cardiovascular system, noted above, suggest this system might also be scrutinized.

Drug Interactions

Greenblatt and Shader (1975) define drug interaction as occurring when one pharmacologic agent alters the therapeutic or toxic effects of another pharmacologic agent. The various ways that one pharmacloogic agent can interact with another have been discussed in Chapter 1 and include the following: 1) altering the gastro-intestinal absorption of another drug; 2) influencing a drug's metabolism; 3) competing for the same metabolic site in the liver or for the same binding site on serum protein; 4) preventing a drug from reaching or acting at the receptor site.

Certain classes of drugs seem to be affected by the concurrent administration of stimulants.

1) *Hypnotics*: Stimulants such as methylphenidate, caffeine, and the amphetamines antagonize the effects of the hypnotics though paradoxically they also increase their toxicity in overdosage (see Chapters 9 and 10).

2) *Tricyclic antidepressants*: Methylphenidate increases the blood levels of tricyclic antidepressants (see Chapter 7) and thus may potentiate their clinical effect. It appears to do so by impairing the metabolism of the tricyclics in the liver.

3) *Monoamine oxidase inhibitors*: Adrenergic crises have been reported due to the interaction of amphetamines and methylphenidate with MAO inhibitors (see Chapter 7).

4) *Anticoagulants*: Methylphenidate inhibits the metabolism of ethyl biscoumacetate thus pontentiating its clinical effect.

5) *Anti-inflammatory agents*: Methylphenidate has been shown to inhibit the action of phenylbutazone.

6) *Antipsychotics*: In the only study of its kind, Gittelman-Klein et al. (1976b) found that thioridazine enhanced the effect of methylphenidate in hyperactive children.

For a fuller discussion of this area see Greenblatt and Shader (1975) and Dayton et al. (1973).

In summary, while there are possible interaction effects of stimulants with other classes of drugs, any actual clinical significance of such interactions is minimal. Only in rare instances would stimulants be prescribed concurrently with one of the above classes of drugs.

Interactions with Other Treatments

Many therapeutic interventions are available in child psychiatry: individual and group therapy for the child, various forms of behavior modification, educational therapy, family therapy, etc. Considering that some or all of these therapies are likely to be used in combination with stimulants in treating children, as pointed out in Chapter 3, it is somewhat surprising that there is so little research comparing stimulant treatment alone to stimulants combined with another form of therapy, to that form of therapy alone.

There have been a few attempts in studies of hyperactive children to compare drug treatment in combination with other forms of therapy. In an early study Christensen and Sprague (1973) compared 6 children receiving methylphenidate plus behavior modification to 6 children receiving behavior modification plus placebo. Seat activity, as measured by a special device, was found to be lower in the group of children who received the active medication plus behavior modification than in the group of children who received behavior modification plus placebo. The authors also looked at the number of correct answers in daily quizzes and found that there were no significant differences between the two groups on this measure. In a later study Christensen (1975) studied 13 hyperactive children over a 4-week period of time. For one 2-week period the children received behavior modification combined with placebo and for the other 2-week period they received behavior modification combined with methylphenidate. The study was conducted in a special experimental classroom setting. There were a wide variety of measures used including observation of classroom behavior, the Conners Teacher Questionnaire, seat activity, and measurement of academic output and accuracy. Results indicated that the behavior modification alone seemed to account for most, if not all, of the significant differences over the baseline ratings. However, this study was conducted with a group of mentally retarded hyperactive children who were institutionalized and it is not known if this finding can be generalized to other hyperactive children, or would be true of less optimal learning situations.

Conversely, in a very sophisticated, direct comparative study of behavior modification and methylphenidate Gittelman-Klein et al. (1976b) compared 34 children receiving behavior modification alone, behavior modification plus methylphenidate and methylphenidate alone. They were studied in a wide variety of ways using rating scales and observational methods. Evaluations were done by the teacher, by parents, and by psychiatrists. Classroom observations were also carried out in a systematic fashion. Results indicated that at the end of 8 weeks all three groups had improved over baseline ratings. However, behavior therapy alone was significantly less effective than either behavior modification plus methylphenidate or methylphenidate alone. There was no significant difference between the latter two treatments.

Conrad et al. (1971) attempted to assess the effect of tutoring and medication in a group of 68 hyperactive children who were matched for intelligence and degree of hyperactivity. There were 4 experimental groups. One received dextroamphetamine alone, one received tutoring and a placebo, one received placebo alone and one received both dextroamphetamine and tutoring. All four groups made a disappointing amount of progress in that only 3 of the 68 progressed to the point that they no longer needed remedial educational help at the end of one year. Moreover, there was no evidence that the tutoring added significantly to the improvement produced by the medication alone.

In contrast again, in a well designed study of hyperactive children in a special class (Wolraich et al., in press), behavior modification and medication were found to be effective in different situations (group v. individual) and on different behaviors (attention v. motor and verbal overflow).

The contradictions in these studies are difficult to explain though some may relate to the *behavior* concerned and the type of *situation*. The behavior (and attention) of overactive children is relatively easily brought under control in small group situations and stimulant effects are revealed only in failing situations (see Chapter 3). Thus, the interaction with other treatments needs above all to be tested in naturalistic ways and situations.

There have been a number of reports of the use of stimulants to treat enuretic children, not only alone, but in combination with conditioning treatment. However, the most comprehensive review (Blackwell & Currah, 1973) indicates that there is no controlled study of the efficacy of the amphetamines in the treatment of enuresis so it is at a disadvantage right at the outset. Only two studies have attempted to look at whether amphetamine could be used as an adjunct to treatment with the conditioning treatment (bed-buzzer) (Kennedy & Sloop, 1968; Young & Turner, 1965). Unfortunately neither of these was a blind study but the results were disappointing. Young and Turner (1965) studied three groups of children with enuresis. One received conditioning alone, one received conditioning plus dextroamphetamine and one received conditioning combined with methamphetamine, the latter being slightly superior. However, at follow-up the highest rate of relapse was associated with the combination of conditioning and drug treatment. Kennedy and Sloop (1968) failed to show that methamphetamine facilitated the conditioning process in enuretic children.

Clinical Indications and Contraindications

The diagnostic classification of the psychiatric disorders of childhood according to DSM III has been discussed in Chapter 5. That classification scheme will be used to discuss the clinical indications for the use of stimulant drugs in children. Since most of the work has been done with methylphenidate and amphetamines, most of what is said will apply to those drugs. There has been some work with pemoline, caffeine and deanol (and some work with deanol with children with other forms of learning disabilities). These will be mentioned separately.

Established Indications

ATTENTION DEFICIT DISORDER WITH HYPERACTIVITY

This condition, formerly called hyperkinetic reaction, is that par excellence for the use of stimulants and is the best example of a specific indication in pediatric pyschopharmacology. Following early clinical reports by Bradley (1937) and Bender and Cottington (1942) there have been numerous well-controlled clinical studies of both the amphetamines and methlyphenidate indicating that they are effective for the treatment of children with Attention Deficit Disorder with Hyperactivity.

This literature has recently been reviewed by Barkley (1977). Fifteen studies of children treated with *amphetamine* involving 915 subjects revealed 74% improved and 26% were unchanged or worsened. In 14 studies with *methylphenidate* involving 866 subjects, 77% improved and 23% were unchanged or worsened. In two studies involving 105 subjects treated with magnesium *pemoline*, a mean percentage improvement of 73% was obtained with 27% unchanged or worsened. In contrast, the results obtained with *placebo* in 8 studies involving 417 subjects revealed a 39% improvement rate and a 61% figure for those unchanged or worsened. Clearly then, these three types of stimulants are the drugs of choice for this condition* and are quite effective. There is little to choose between the three major groups of stimulants regarding percentage of children showing improvement, although pemoline does come in a longer acting form which need only be prescribed once a day. As noted above (Treatment-Emergent Effects), there is some evidence that it may not have quite as strong effect on growth as do the amphetamines and methylphenidate.

With regard to *deanol* favorable reports from open clinical studies have not been replicated by systematic controlled studies except in one recently (Lewis & Young, 1975). Conners (1973) reviewed the literature on deanol and concluded that studies to that time did not support its effectiveness in the treatment of this disorder. However, Campbell and Small (1976) felt that its possible positive effects on behavior and performance

---

* This makes the assumption that most children in all the studies reviewed by Barkley (1977) would have received this diagnosis using DSM III criteria, a point which could be disputed, though another review by Barkley (1976) which pinpoints inattention as the best predictor of drug response is supportive of this diagnosis (Ed.).

(as later shown by Lewis & Young) plus the suggestion of milder side effects warranted it more definitive study. Conners and Werry (in press) suggest that its unique pharmacological action also makes it of interest.

One report (Schnackenberg, 1973) suggested *caffeine* might be efficacious in children with Attention Deficit Disorder with Hyperactivity. However, controlled clinical studies (Conners, 1975b; Garfinkel et al., 1975; Huestis et al., 1975) failed to substantiate this clinical effect.

However, from all of the studies it is quite clear that *only a certain percentage* of children with this syndrome will respond positively to stimulant medication. Clinically it would be useful if it could be predicted whether an individual child is likely to respond positively. Predictors have been recently examined by Barkley (1976), Cantwell (in press), and Conners and Werry (in press) who conclude that clinical, physical and neurological, laboratory, and familial predictors all have been looked at but with little in the way of success except in one or two areas. Barcai (1971) found performance on a finger twitch test to be a useful clinical predictor but his work is unreplicated. The subclassification of Attention Deficit Disorder children according to *organic* or *non-organic* or to other subcategorization has not been found to be consistently helpful. There are some studies indicating that the presence of an abnormal EEG and/or the presence of minor abnormalities on neurological examination are predictive of a good response to stimulant medication but these results are often as not contradicted by other studies. There are no direct laboratory predictors although vigorous present research in the biochemical and neurophysiologic area indicates that such predictors ultimately may be found, particularly since they are closer to the locus of drug action. There have been some investigators who have found a relationship between family interaction pattern and a positive response to medication, while others have not found such a correlation. The presence of mental illness in a family member likewise has been found to predict a negative response in some studies, but not in others. Barkley (1976) concludes that the best predictor is inattention, however measured, which is consonant with the new DSM III terminology. For complete reviews see Barkley 1976; Cantwell, in press).

However, despite the fact that there is very strong evidence for the *short-term efficacy* of stimulants with this disorder, a review of follow-up studies of children treated with stimulant medication over a number of years indicates that there is very little evidence for a positive effect at the time of follow-up that can be attributed to stimulant medication (see Barkley, 1977; Cantwell, in press).

Possible Indications

CONDUCT DISORDERS

While there are some investigators who feel that severely antisocial children (who may resemble somewhat children with attention deficit disorder) do not respond to stimulant medication (Katz et al., 1975) there is actually some clinical evidence suggesting the contrary. As early as 1947 Hill reported a positive response of some delinquents to amphetamine. Eisenberg et al. (1963) also found that dextroamphetamine was effective for delinquent boys in a residential training school. Maletsky (1974) studied 14 delinquents on dextroamphetamine and found a significant positive effect compared to placebo. However, there was a strong relationship between a history of attentional deficit disorder with hyperactivity in the past or the presence of such traits concurrently and a favorable clinical response. As pointed out in Chapter 2, one of the difficulties about assessing the value of stimulants in Conduct Disorders (or indeed in Attention Disorders) is the inextricable association of these two clinical features in many children in most studies. Clear separation diagnostically is elemental to any future work.

ATTENTION DEFICIT DISORDER WITHOUT HYPERACTIVITY

This is a new category created by DSM III (see Chapter 5). Theoretically it makes sense that children with attentional deficit disorders without excess motor activity should in fact respond positively to stimulant medication since the studies reviewed under Clinical Effects above indicate that the main effects of stimulant medication seem to be on attentional processes and these are the best predictors of drug response. Barkley (1977), Fish (1971), Dykman et al. (1971) suggest that such children do respond positively to stimulant medication, but definitive controlled studies have not yet been carried out.

SPECIFIC DEVELOPMENTAL DISORDERS

As discussed in Chapter 3 and above (under Clinical Effects), there exists no current evidence to suggest that actual *academic achievement* in the classroom is positively affected by stimulant medication. However, as noted, there is abundant evidence that certain cognitive functions and laboratory learning are positively affected, and that all studies of naturalistic learning are, so far, methodologically less than satisfactory. If a properly conducted study were to be carried out, it may be that academic achievement would be improved. For example, Satterfield and Cantwell

(1977) have demonstrated an improvement in reading recognition and comprehension and mathematics over a one year period of time in children treated with methylphenidate. However, the children were also involved in a variety of other treatment programs. A properly controlled study of the effect of stimulant medication on learning disabled children over a sufficiently long period with adequate measures of learning (compare Gittelman-Klein, & Klein, 1976; Rie et al., 1976) has not yet been carried out.

MENTAL RETARDATION AND PERVASIVE DEVELOPMENTAL DISORDERS

While no medication has any effect on the core symptoms of retardation, there is some evidence that *certain symptoms* in retarded children such as short attention span and hyperactivity can be positively affected by the use of stimulant medication. With the Pervasive Developmental Disorders (or psychoses) the issue is roughly the same (see also Chapter 8). Rutter (1967) has reviewed evidence suggesting the stimulants may be effective in a limited way for symptoms such as short attention span and hyperactivity in children with infantile autism.

Contraindications

The use of stimulants is contraindicated in depression, anorexia nervosa, motor-verbal tic disorder (Fras & Karlavage, 1977), and in the pervasive developmental disorders which resemble adult schizophrenia. The Bellevue group (Campbell, 1973) feel that psychotic symptoms are exacerbated in children who present with an adult-type schizophrenic picture. Medical contraindications also exist such as with hypertension or other conditions or symptoms treated with drugs which would preclude sympathomimetic activity.

Non-indications

The rest of the conditions listed in chapters on diagnostic classification have not been shown to be positively affected by the use of stimulant medication. However, there is some controversy, as mentioned above (Clinical Effects—Anxiety), on the question of overanxious children and their response to stimulants. In the authors' opinion there is no controlled study which would firmly support their use in this condition, though Bradley's (1937) initial observations and the study by Arnold et al. (1976) are supportive.

CLINICAL USAGE OF STIMULANTS

A general discussion of clinical procedures is to be found in Chapters 1-4. What is presented here is a personal view.

In considering the use of a stimulant for any psychiatric disorder the first thing to be done, of course, is a *comprehensive diagnostic evaluation* of the child. Components of this evaluation should include: a detailed interview with the parents, a detailed psychiatric evaluation of the child, physical and neurological examinations of the child, obtaining information from the school, and obtaining appropriate laboratory studies including psychological tests (Cantwell, 1975; see Chapters 2, 3). Information from the schools is probably best obtained by the use of a systematic rating scale, such as the TQ developed by Conners (1973). Phone contact with the school is also very helpful. In the physical examination stress should be placed on recording of baseline height and weight. In addition a screening of all body systems should be done, at least by interrogation. The central nervous system should be particularly emphasized and a *screening neurologic examination* carried out (Cantwell, 1976). The pediatric psychopharmacologic package presented as part of FDA and NIMH ECDEU packages offers helpful guidelines in this area (see Chapter 2).

Baseline blood count, urinalysis and a screening battery such as the SMA-12 are probably all that need to be done initially in the way of laboratory studies. Children do not like blood tests and they really only need to be done if there are clear clinical indications that toxic effects have developed as a result of the stimulant drug use.

It is important for the physician to insure that *proper baseline assessments* have been made of the *target functions* that he will attempt to modify with the use of the stimulants. The relevant behaviors to be modified are probably best assessed by the Conners Parent and Teacher Questionnaires and by the clinical global *impressions* rating made by the physician himself (see Chapter 2).

As mentioned above, it is also important to have *some measure of learning and academic achievement* as a way of assessing the effect of the stimulant medication. The techniques developed by Swanson and Kinsbourne (1976, Swanson et al., in press) appear to hold the promise for ordinary clinical practice but this matter is discussed in detail in Chapter 3. *Baseline assessments* should also be made routinely of the *possible toxic and side effects* that may develop. These can also be done by the use of patient, parent and physician rating scales which are part of the ECDEU package, discussed in Chapter 2.

Once the decision to use a stimulant has been made by the physician, after a comprehensive diagnostic evaluation has been completed, the next step is *counseling with the parents and with the child*. The physician should try to help the child understand the nature of his difficulties and how the use of the stimulant is intended to help the child help himself. This is often a very neglected part of the use of stimulants with children. In addition to the work with the child, a great deal of work must also be done with the parents. In an individual child it is highly likely that either the type of stimulant, the dosage, or both will have to be changed over a period of time. This often must be done in order to find the optimal dose of the optimal drug. If the physician invests time right from the beginning in a detailed preparation of the parents for a rational trial of medication, when this change in dosage or drug occurs the parents will not feel that the doctor is "shotgunning." The parents' cooperation will make any drug trial easier and more meaningful. The physician should tell the parents that one stimulant may help a particular child, but not help another one. Also one dose of a particular stimulant may help one child, but have little or no effect on another child of roughly the same age and body weight. Parents also should be told that there is no definite way of predicting which stimulant might work for which child, if in fact, any stimulant will be effective at all. Moreover, the physician should explain in great detail that if a stimulant is effective, it will exert only certain effects. If the parents are expecting their children to be "model" children after the use of stimulants, they are likely to be disappointed if only one or two behaviors are changed. Possible side effects should be discussed in detail, and parents should be encouraged to observe their child carefully for any likely side effects.

The third step in the use of stimulants is *establishing good rapport with the school*. Direct contact should be made with the child's teacher, either in person or by phone, and the importance of her or his cooperation emphasized. Since most stimulants are prescribed so that they are only effective throughout the school period, the teacher is likely to be the only person who sees the child regularly on an effective dose of medication. Moreover, she has a unique position in the sense that she sees him in a setting where he can be compared with other children doing roughly the same tasks. Thus she has somewhat of a ready-made "control group" to compare the child's behavior with on and off medication.

The next step is for the physician to *select the stimulant* that he wishes to use. Obviously the selection should be made primarily on the basis of the clinical evidence in the literature of its efficacy and safety. However, for the usual child to be treated, the physician will have little to guide him in the current literature for choosing which drug to use within the group of stimulants.

As a general rule, an *older drug* which has been around for a number of years should be used in place of a new drug unless there is overwhelming evidence for the clinical superiority of the new drug. This is because with increasing usage over a number of years more evidence about positive and negative effects is available. This would mean that for the stimulants, the amphetamines and methylphenidate should be given a thorough trial before considering the use of pemoline.

Another general principle is to use the smallest dosage possible for the initial trial. Some authors (Werry, 1976a, 1977) advocate using one-half of the minimum dosage ordinarily recommended. Knowledge of the *duration of action* of any medication is obviously necessary to know how often to prescribe it. In theory, the regular tablets of amphetamine would probably need to be prescribed every 4-6 hours to insure effectiveness, whereas the longer acting form of the amphetamines may be effective throughout an entire school day and could thus be prescribed on a once-a-day basis. Clinically, however, many children seem manageable on once-a-day dosages of simple, short-acting forms. The physician should begin with the lowest dose possible of the medication as described above and then titrate the dosage, increasing dosages until a positive clinical effect is obtained or until side effects prohibit an increase. If improvement occurs after a medication has been started, the patient needs to be followed at regular intervals. The same ratings of behavior that were taken initially at baseline should be made at these regular intervals. This would include information from the parents, from the teacher, and from the child himself about any positive and/or negative effects. Any other appropriate assessments such as measurement of learning should be done on a regular basis. If improvement seems to occur initially, but disappears with time, the *dosage should be increased as tolerance* to stimulants may develop.

The *total amount* of medication required by an individual child is very idiosyncratic and only rough guidelines can be given for optimal dosage on a milligram per kilogram basis. The matter of dosage for the stimulants is a very controversial area. For example, the American Academy of Pediatrics (1975) recommends 2 mg/kg of methylphenidate or 1 mg/kg of dextroamphetamine as an average daily dose for a child. Wender (1971) has advocated a high dose of 1.5 mg/kg per day of dextroamphetamine and a high dose of 4.6 mg/kg per day of methylphenidate. However, Sprague and his colleagues have conducted laboratory studies showing that teacher ratings show an increasing improvement in behavior up to doses of 1.00 mg/kg per day of methylphenidate. However, this dosage is

Table 1

Dosage Range

Drug	Number of Daily Doses†	Range for Single Dose (mg/kg)
Amphetamines		
Amphetamine	1 - 3*	0.15 - 0.50
Dextroamphetamine	1 - 3	0.15 - 0.50
Methamphetamine	1 - 3	0.15 - 0.25
Methylphenidate	1 - 3	0.3 - 1.0
Magnesium Pemoline	1	0.5 - 2.0
Deanol	1 - 3	1.0 - 3.0

Not all of the above are recommended for children below the age of 6.
* Long acting forms of the amphetamines need only be given once daily.
† Only in exceptional cases will 3 doses need to be given.

double that at which the peak enhancement of cognitive performance seems to occur (Sprague & Sleator, 1973, 1975). Werry and Sprague (1974) failed to show much difference in effectiveness between different doses of methylphenidate once 0.3 mg/kg was attained but there were more side effects at higher doses. (More details on dosages of the individual stimulants are given in Table 1).

How many times a day and how many days during the week a stimulant should be given is also somewhat controversial. The duration of action of the regular form of the stimulants, dextroamphetamine and methylphenidate, is around 4 hours. This should indicate that if the drugs are to be effective throughout the school day, they probably would have to be given in the morning and at noon. And some practitioners, including the authors, find this to be true in the great majority of cases (see also Swanson et al., in press). However, there are others (Safer & Allen, 1973, Werry, 1976a, 1977) who find that many children can be managed on one dosage of the stimulants per day.

Likewise, it is felt by many that the drug should be given 5 days a week when the child is in school, not on the weekends, not on holidays, and not during summer vacations. This probably makes sense from the standpoint of side effects, if nothing else, in that there probably is a relationship between total dosage and certain side effects such as the suppression of height and weight. However, others (Swanson et al., in press) based on studies of the effects of stimulants on learning, feel that methylphenidate tablets probably should be given 3 times a day and 7 days a week at least until such time as the "ideal drug" is developed.* The "ideal drug," in their view, would be one that would last 8-10 hours a day, have an immediate onset and immediate endpoint and have no long-term side effects. The likelihood of such a drug being created in our lifetime seems remote.

Should a child receive a negative, equivocal or neutral response to stimulants, the type of stimulant will probably have to be changed. One might also be considered if a positive response is obtained, but side effects are bothersome. Clinical evidence for *clinical superiority of one stimulant over another is generally lacking*—if a child responds to one stimulant he is likely to respond to another. But there are idiosyncratic children who have a positive response to one stimulant but do not respond as well to another or who have equally positive responses to one stimulant but have more side effects with one but not the other. So it is worth trying to find the optimal dose of the optimal drug for an individual child.

At the present time there is no perfect way of determining when a child should be *taken off the medication* completely. All children who are on stimulants chronically should be given a drug-free trial sometime during the course of the year. This is probably best done near the end of the school term and usually no more than a week off the medication is needed for this purpose. This is probably best done by placebo substitution which should be done without child's or the teacher's knowledge, though parents will, of course, have to know. If the substitution of placebo is followed by deterioration of behavior, the medication should be reinstituted. If no change is noted, the child should probably be maintained on placebo and watched a bit more closely over time.

It is the authors' feeling that each child should *start school each new school year in a new class with a new teacher without any medication*. Then after a week or so of school to allow for a "honeymoon" period, new ratings should be obtained from the parents and the teacher to compare with ratings obtained at the end of the previous school term. If the ratings off the medication appear to be no different from those obtained at the end of the previous school term while on stimulant medication, the child should be followed closely to see if behavior deteriorates over time.

There is no definite age when stimulant medication should be stopped. Stimulants should be used when the clinical picture indicates that the

---

* This is an extreme view based upon the extrapolation of laboratory findings to the naturalistic situation and ignores the lack of evidence for any long-term benefit, social or educational. Arguments for drug holidays and minimum administration to prevent tolerance and metabolic changes seem more compelling.—(Ed.)

child continues to require and benefit from their use in the absence of significant side effects. However, there has been little systematic research done on the question of when children can actually be taken off medication. Sleator et al. (1974) reported on a continuous long-term placebo-controlled follow-up of hyperactive children. There were 42 children who were on methylphenidate, generally during the school days. Conners PTQ ratings were obtained at the end of every school month and a placebo trial was instituted during one month of the school year. Thirteen patients were followed up for two years, 29 for one year. Seventeen patients showed deterioration of behavior during the placebo trial. These were called the "drug benefited group." Of these 17, 7 needed an increased dosage to maintain previous level of improvement, while the other 10 remained at the same level of improvement without an increase in the dose. However, *26% (11 children) of the total could be taken off the medication at the time of follow-up.* These subjects were called the "remission group." This study would make it seem likely that many more children can be taken off the long-term stimulant medication than usually occurs in clinical practice if regular placebo substitutions are made.

Ethical and Social Considerations

As pointed out in Chapter 4, probably no treatment in child psychiatry has aroused as much controversy in the public press as the use of stimulants for behavior disordered children. This is despite the fact that one could make a strong case that *this form of therapeutic intervention for children with Attention Deficit Disorder with Hyperactivity has more empirical evidence to support it than any other therapeutic intervention in child psychiatry for any other condition.*

There are a number of issues involved in this debate (see Chapter 4). These include the training of chlid psychiatrists, the place of pyschopharmacologic agents compared to other therapeutic modalities, and most importantly the *antimedication* viewpoint delineated by a small, but vocal, band of individuals in the public media.

It is an unfortunate truth that in settings where child psychiatry training takes place, those doing the training are often unskilled in the use of psychopharmacologic agents, and thus do not consider them in the differential therapy of the patient. This attitude is passed on consciously or unconsciously to child psychiatry trainees. If a trainee does not become comfortable with and proficient in the use of psychopharmacologic agents in training, it is unlikely that he will do so in later life. Also, there is often the unspoken notion that psychopharmacologic treatment is *second rate treatment compared to insight oriented psychotherapy or, lately, to behavior therapy too.* The authors feel that, rather, stimulants and other drugs should be considered as only one of several possible therapies and as part of an overall multimethod treatment program. Their considerable cost/benefit advantages when properly used, to say nothing of the uncertain efficacy of alternatives preferred *a priori*, should also be noted. These problems are minor though, compared to the vocal views put forth by those who feel that stimulant medication should not be used under any condition (Schrag & Divoky, 1975; Walker, 1974). The argument put forth is that drugs are *chemical straitjackets* which are used to control the natural exuberance and activity of children who come into conflict with the system. They argue for changing the system rather than helping the child to come to grips with his difficulties. However, this argument reflects a great deal of political naivete and medical ignorance. Those children who are properly treated with stimulant medication are not controlled robots, and are actually freer than when unmedicated in the sense that they are freer to respond to the internal and external stimuli as they wish rather than being at the mercy of all and every passing stimulus. Neither is it correct that such children are the way they are because of the "System" rather than because of the systems within.

This does not mean that serious thought must not be given to the long-term use of stimulant medication in children. First, there still is not clear evidence that the effect on the suppression of height and weight is only a temporary one. Longer term studies are needed before it can be said that no permanent effects occur even after stimulant use is discontinued. Secondly, the use of these drugs with potential for abuse or dependence in older children and adolescents must be approached with caution since this is the age of maximum risk of development of drug abuse and dependence. However, the long-term follow-up studies to date do not support the idea that drug abuse and dependency might be an outcome of treatment with stimulant medication in childhood. As with any other treatment in medicine a cost benefit analysis must be done. The potential benefits obtained from the use of stimulant medication must be weighted against the possible risks. This can only be determined by careful, ethical, empirical research. Ethical, legal and social issues, raised here are discussed in more detail in Chapter 4.

Summary and Conclusions

Of all of the psychopharmacologic agents in child psychiatry, central nervous system stimulants are the most established. Both *methylphenidate* and the *amphetamines* have been found to be effective in children with Attention Deficit Disorder with Hyperactivity. In this condition, these two drugs seem to affect the attentional processes and possibly secondarily decrease motor activity, particularly task irrelevant motor behavior.

This disorder can be serious if untreated. What is known about the long-term untreated outcome indicates that these children often, though by no means always, grow up to have significant social and psychiatric pathology as adults. The type of pathology that they sometimes demonstrate as adults, such as alcoholism and sociopathy, are conditions which are not easily treatable in adulthood. It is entirely possible that the proper use of catecholaminic stimulant medication in childhood might help prevent such outcomes though to date no such evidence for the long-term preventive efficacy of stimulant medication with Attention Deficit Disorder or any other disorder exists. This is an area which requires much further research as does the question of whether or not the known effects on laboratory learning and cognitive function can be translated into actual improvement in academic achievement in the classroom.

Short-term side effects tend to be relatively minor and rarely lead to discontinuance of the stimulant. However, the long-term side effects, particularly on height and weight and on the cardiovascular system, remain to be conclusively determined.

The usefulness of the catecholaminic stimulants in psychiatric disorders other than Attention Deficit Disorder with Hyperactivity is unproven as yet, but there is some suggestion that they may also be useful with Conduct Disorders, Attention Deficit Disorder without Hyperactivity, and possibly for Specific Learning Disabilities, and for selected *symptoms* in children with Mental Retardation and Pervasive Developmental Disorders (psychoses). Also unproven is any usefulness for caffeine and deanol though the latter, being related to acetylcholine rather than catecholaminergic, is of theoretical interest.

The exact mechanism of clinical action of the stimulants is unknown, with some neurophysiological evidence suggesting that they may be acting to increase CNS arousal mechanisms and cortical inhibition in some way.

Finally, with an individual child it is impossible to predict *a priori* whether or not he will respond positively to stimulants—only an empirical trial will establish this. Much more research in the future should be directed toward these areas of ignorance.

7

ANTIDEPRESSANTS

JUDITH L. RAPOPORT, M.D. and
EDWIN J. MIKKELSEN, M.D.

DEFINITION

The term antidepressant is used to cover the so-called tricyclic and quadricyclic drugs and the monoamine oxidase inhibitors (MAOI). The tricyclics have had the greatest attention up to the present time but there may well be increasing use of quadricyclics in pediatric psychopharmacology and so these are covered in some detail too in this chapter.

INTRODUCTION

MAOI's are reviewed only briefly here because of their limited use to date in psychopathological symptoms and disorders of childhood.

The tricyclics are somewhat similar chemically to the phenothiazines and share some of their properties, such as long action and atropine-like side effects. However, they do not share the antipsychotic effects, nor, except in rare instances, do they produce extrapyramidal side effects. Quadricyclics are a new class of chemical compound, having been synthesized and put into clinical use only recently. They are generally similar to the related tricyclics in their action but may differ in particular behavioral effects. For example, in animals, maprotiline (Ludiomil), a quadricyclic, possesses anti-aggressive properties not seen with tricyclics.

These drugs are able to relieve severe depression in some adult patients. Because the adult type of depression which constitutes the original and main use of the antidepressants and which gave them their name is rare in childhood (Rapoport, 1976; see also Chapter 5), the antidepressants

---

The authors would like to thank William Potter, M.D., Laboratory of Clinical Science, NIMH, for helpful discussion of this chapter.

have been used in pediatric psychopharmacology principally for a variety of other conditions such as enuresis, school phobia and conduct disorders, which makes the unavoidable name antidepressant incongruous.

TRICYCLICS AND QUADRICYCLICS

Classes and Chemical Structure

The tricyclics, like the antipsychotic phenothiazines (see Chapter 8), are 3-ring structures with a pharmacologically critical side chain attached to the central ring structure. Unlike the phenothiazines, however, the central ring lacks a sulphur atom, its place being taken by a 2-atom substitute (usually both carbon) to produce a 7-atom central ring. This side chain is also less variable being always a 3-carbon straight chain (propyl) terminating in a nitrogen radical.

Imipramine (Tofranil) and amitriptyline (Elavil) are two widely used and typical tricyclic antidepressants, the basic chemical structure of which can be seen in Figure 1.

The demethylated derivative of imipramine, desmethylimipramine, a normal metabolic product of imipramine, is also a pharmacologically

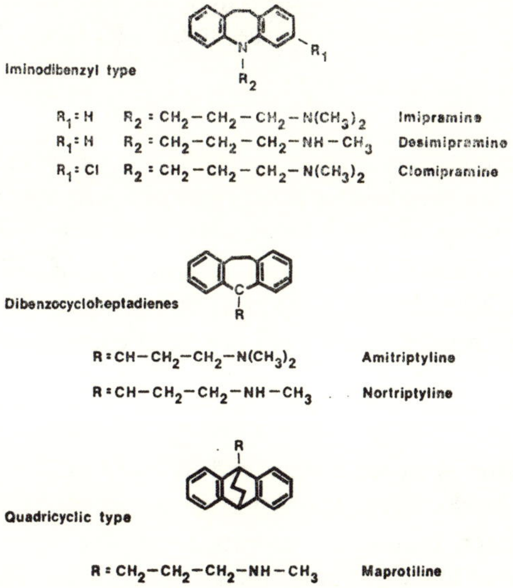

Iminodibenzyl type

$R_1 = H \quad R_2 = CH_2-CH_2-CH_2-N(CH_3)_2$ Imipramine
$R_1 = H \quad R_2 = CH_2-CH_2-CH_2-NH-CH_3$ Desimipramine
$R_1 = Cl \quad R_2 = CH_2-CH_2-CH_2-N(CH_3)_2$ Clomipramine

Dibenzocycloheptadienes

$R = CH-CH_2-CH_2-N(CH_3)_2$ Amitriptyline
$R = CH-CH_2-CH_2-NH-CH_3$ Nortriptyline

Quadricyclic type

$R = CH_2-CH_2-CH_2-NH-CH_3$ Maprotiline

Fig. 1. Tricyclic and quadricyclic antidepressants in clinical pediatric use.

active agent marketed as desipramine (Pertofrane, Norpramin). Amitriptyline has a carbon substituted for the nitrogen in the central ring structure and the side chain is attached to the ring by a double bond. Quadricyclics resemble tricyclics but have a fourth ring created by a bridge across the centre ring.

Maprotiline belongs to a new chemical series, the dibenzo-bicyclo-octadienes, while a newer, less well studied quadricyclic is mianserin hydrochloride, a piperazino-azepine compound.

Pharmacology

The fate of tricyclics in the body has been the object of many investigations and is, therefore, relatively well understood. The newer quadricyclics have, of course, been studied much less.

ABSORPTION

Orally administered tricyclics are relatively rapidly absorbed from the intestine although the anticholinergic effect of high doses may influence absorption due to the inhibition of peristalsis. The quadricyclic maprotiline has been less extensively studied, but intravenous vs. oral dose pharmacokinetic studies in humans suggest that like the tricyclics the oral dose is relatively fully absorbed (Riess et al., 1972).

SERUM HALF LIFE

Peak plasma levels of imipramine occur 1½ to 3 hours after an oral dose on continuous treatment, with a half life in children that may range from 10 to 17 hours using available methods (Winsberg & Perel, 1974). In adults, maprotiline has a significantly longer half life (52 hours) and a slower rise to peak levels (6 hours) after an oral dose (Riess et al., 1972). Kinetic studies of quadricyclics have not been carried out in children.

DISTRIBUTION

Some imipramine is stored unchanged in body cells while metabolites, largely formed in the liver, are found in extracellular fluid and in the gastrointestinal tract. Imipramine and its metabolite desipramine cross the blood brain barrier but their polar metabolites do not (Bickel & Weder, 1969). Maprotiline does not differ significantly from the tricyclics in its distribution, the only distinctive feature being its affinity for the zona reticularis of the adrenal (Hansson & Cassano, 1966).

DIFFERENCES IN CHILDREN

These have been discussed in detail in Chapter 1. Children differ significantly from adults in pharmacokinetics; children have a smaller adipose compartment, and lipid soluble drugs are not taken up, redistributed and stored in inactive lipid-storage sites to the same extent as in adults. There are also reported differences in children in the degree of drug binding to plasma albumin (Pruitt & Dayton, 1971; Winsberg et al., 1974a). Imipramine binding in umbilical cord and adult plasma average 74% and 86% respectively, indicating 26% free drug in the neonate and 14% free medication in the adult. At age 13, adult binding values are obtained. It has been suggested, that children are more susceptible to imipramine side-effects because of this relatively greater amount of circulating free drug (Winsberg et al., 1974a). These authors also suggest that with chronic administration, a single daily dose may have a bolus effect and thus have the pharmacokinetics of an intravenous dose.

EXCRETION/DETOXIFICATION

Tricyclics undergo biotransformation along multiple pathways by the oxidative drug metabolizing enzyme system located chiefly in the endoplasmic reticulum of the liver. The principle pathways of imipramine metabolism are shown in Figure 2. Excretion is rapid; studies with C^{14} imipramine show 40% in the urine in 24 hours and 70% during the first 72 hours. A small proportion can be recovered as unchanged drug or as the active desmethyl derivative. The greatest portion is excreted as the N-oxide or as the 2-OH derivatives.

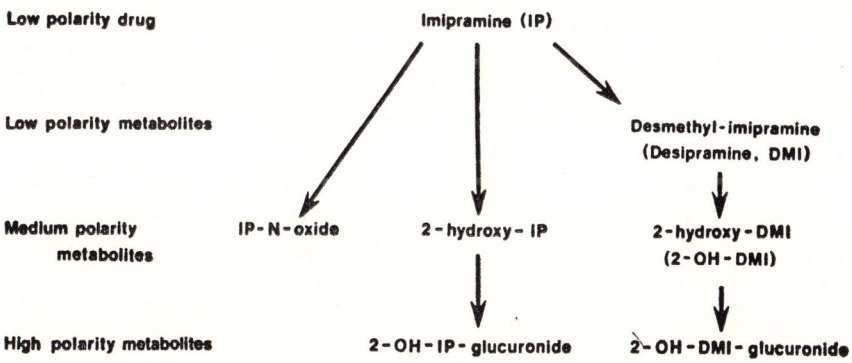

Fig. 2. Pathways of imipramine metabolism (adapted from Bickel, 1976)

As noted in Chapter 1, except for newborns, the rate of drug biotransformation by the liver in children tends generally to be enhanced, probably due to a relatively higher amount of liver tissue. This property could result in the enhanced production of some metabolites, but there is little actual information about differential metabolic or excretion rates and patterns for tricyclics for children compared with that for adults. One recent study (Klutch & Hanna, 1976), however, reports that children excrete a higher portion of 2-hydroxylated imipramine which may have relevance to the cardiotoxicity of tricyclics in children discussed below. Excretion patterns for quadricyclics in adults are similar to those of the tricyclics, but have not been studied in children (Riess et al., 1972, 1975).

ACTIVE PRINCIPLES

The tricyclics and their low polarity desmethyl derivatives such as desipramine cross the blood brain barrier and are clinically active while the 2-hydroxymetabolites of higher polarity do not cross and are inactive clinically psychotropically though not peripherally (e.g., on cardiac tissue). Active metabolites of quadricyclics are unknown.

SITES AND MODE OF ACTION

The tricyclics are thought to owe their therapeutic effect in the treatment of depression to the inhibition of transmitter reuptake back into monoaminergic neurons in the brain where most of it is normally inactivated, presumably thus increasing transmitter effectiveness (Carlsson, 1966). It must be stressed that reuptake of several monoamines such as dopamine, norepinephrine as well as the indoleamine, serotonin, are inhibited by tricyclics although some compounds may show more specificity in this respect. For example, clomipramine (Anafranil) is thought to have a relatively specific effect on serotonin (Meek et al. ,1970), while desipramine shows relative specificity for noradrenaline (Waldmeier et al., 1976).

The quadricyclic maprotiline is thought to be the most specific inhibitor of noradrenaline of all the commercially available antidepressants (Waldmeier et al., 1976; Greengrass et al., 1976) while mianserin may have a greater effect on serotonin (Raiteri et al., 1976).

The tricyclics also have anticholinergic effects both centrally and peripherally. The peripheral anticholinergic effects, generally regarded as unwanted or side effects in adult patients, have been thought to provide the basis for the efficacy of tricyclics in enuresis (see below). A recent review of the relative potency of the various tricyclics in blocking muscarinic type acetylcholine receptors indicates considerable variation between compounds in this action (Snyder & Yamamura, 1977); amitriptyline is the most potent and desipramine the least potent, with imipramine intermediate between these two.

Both the quadri- and tricyclics also have the property of potentiating peripheral alpha adrenergic activity by sensitizing alpha receptors to the effects of norepinephrine (Sigg, 1959); however, they have some antagonist effects at alpha-adrenoreceptors as well. The sympathetic nervous system may be critically important in control of urination by providing a balance between detrusor contractility and involuntary urethral sphincter tone. The alpha adrenergic system, in particular, is involved in maintaining the bladder sphincter muscle tone. As imipramine inhibits bladder neck response to noradrenaline in laboratory studies, this action, rather than the anticholinergic one, has been also postulated as the basis for clinical effectiveness in enuresis. Additionally, tricyclics have local anesthetic properties and a resultant direct cocaine-like action on the muscle membrane, decreasing resting muscle tension, has been described for imipramine (Labay & Boyarsky, 1973), although it is questionable whether this effect occurs within the therapeutic dose range used in enuresis.

DOSE RESPONSE DATA

Unlike in adults, there has been little study of dose-response relationships of tricyclics with children. While there have been several studies in depressed adults indicating relationship between plasma levels of tricyclics and clinical effect, it is far from simple. In most studies, only total plasma concentrations (protein bound plus free) was measured although only the free fraction is considered pharmacologically active and thus the variation in individual differences in the plasma protein binding may be responsible for some of this complexity (Glassman et al., 1973; Glassman & Perel, 1974). In a series of studies with nortriptyline, it has been shown that on the same oral dose, adult patients develop widely differing individual plasma levels (Asberg, 1976; Kragh-Sorensen et al., 1976a, b), and the relation between plasma level and observed clinical response is not simple; further there may be a "therapeutic window" above which (e.g. 150 ng/ml of nortriptyline) there may be decreased or even adverse effect in the clinical treatment of depression.

The only studies in children, (Winsberg et al., 1976, 1977) suggest that, as in adults, serum levels of the drug attained after similar doses are highly variable across children, (a sixfold difference was obtained from a given oral dose) but that clinical response in behaviorally disordered children parallels roughly the serum level.

In adults, fourfold differences in steady state serum concentrations with maprotiline have been obtained on the same oral dose (Reiss et al., 1975) suggesting dose/response characteristics similar to the tricyclics.

TIME RESPONSE DATA

The clinical effects of tricyclics in enuresis and behavior disorders are seen within hours or a few days of the start of treatment (Blackwell & Currah, 1973; Yepes et al., 1977). This is in contrast to the 2-4 week delay in the clinical response of depressed adults, and to the 3-6 week delay in the response of school phobic children (Gittelman-Klein & Klein, 1971). This difference in time response, if replicated in future studies, is important as it suggests different mechanisms of drug action in these different clinical conditions. In adults, quadricyclics appear to show clinical effects more rapidly than tricyclics but more data are needed (Trick, 1975; Fleischhauer & van Reizen, 1974).

Clinical Effects

ELECTROENCEPHALOGRAM (EEG)

In adults, imipramine decreases the percentage time of alpha and total electrical activity on the electroencephalogram (EEG) but increases both theta and fast beta activity (Fink, 1959). Quadricyclics have a similar effect on EEG (Misurec et al., 1973).

In adults, tricyclics produce a prolonged sustained reduction in REM sleep as seen on the EEG; this is an immediate effect, and though some tolerance to it does develop, this is incomplete (Mendelson et al., 1977). Similar effects have been reported for enuretic children (Ritvo et al., 1969). Such changes in REM time and associated dreaming and the rebound increase in both upon cessation of the drug could, in theory, be associated with some psychological discomfort. It is of interest that these EEG and sleep changes are similar to those produced by sedatives and antipsychotics (see Chapters 8 and 10) rather than one of stimulation suggested by other clinical data.

AUTONOMIC NERVOUS SYSTEM

As noted above, tricyclic antidepressants possess cholinergic blocking properties, effective particularly against the muscarinic actions of acetylcholine. Some of the side effects seen clinically, such as blurred vision, dryness of mouth, constipation and urinary retention, can be attributed to this atrophine-like effect. The quadricyclics are said to be less active than tricyclics in this regard (Vogel et al., 1976). The cholinergic rebound upon stopping these drugs, especially when done suddenly after high doses, may explain the withdrawal symptoms sometimes seen (vomiting, sweating, colic) (Byck, 1975).

The peripheral action of imipramine on autonomic control of bladder functioning described above (under site of action) may provide the basis for its therapeutic efficacy in enuresis. There are conflicting reports on the effect of imipramine on the micturition reflex in the treatment of neurogenic bladder. One study (Diokno et al., 1972) found no effect on the cystometrogram 45 minutes after 75 mgm of imipramine administered intramuscularly. On the other hand, Cole (1972) reported a significant effect of imipramine in a similar population following one week of an oral daily dose of 50 mgm. Mahoney et al. (1973) reported increased involuntary (internal) sphincter tone in the bladder is about 50% of a group of 73 enuretic children who received treatment with 25-50 mg/day of imipramine. The authors cite a slightly higher percentage (59% compared to 44%) in the markedly improved group compared with nonresponders. However, these group differences are small, did not reach significance and do not correspond well with observed clinical outcome. It is possible then that the change in vesical tone simply reflects blood levels of the drug which may vary considerably among children and which may not relate to clinical effect at all. The authors do raise the interesting possibility (which their data fail to support) that imipramine in enuresis may act via its action on alpha adrenergic nerves rather than anticholinergic action. However, a recent study by Shaffer and co-workers (1977) showed that an alpha blocker drug had no deleterious effect on enuresis, suggesting that the therapeutic action of imipramine is unlikely to be due to any alpha adrenergic action.

CARDIOVASCULAR SYSTEM

Imipramine obtunds various cardiovascular reflexes and hence can lower the blood pressure, the degree depending mostly on dosage, but there is also individual variation. Paradoxically, clinical studies of tricyclics in children which have addressed themselves to this issue (Rapoport et al., 1974b: Greenberg & Yellin, 1975; Werry et al., 1975a) have all revealed if anything slight increases in blood pressure (as well as the expected increase in heart rate). Toxic doses of imipramine may produce serious cardiac arrhythmias and tachycardia, which can result in death in accidental and deliberate poisoning. In adults, EKG changes following the use of imipramine consist of inversion or flattening of the T waves and prolongation of the PR interval. The possibility of relatively greater cardiotoxicity of imipramine in the pediatric age group has been suggested in recent reports (Robinson & Barker, 1976; Saraf et al., 1977; Winsberg & et al., 1975) in which EKG change of prolonged PR and QR intervals and T wave changes including first degree AV block were observed at doses in the 5 mgm/kg range in children with behavior disorders.

Quadricyclics may be less cardiotoxic than are the tricyclics and this may prove of future importance for their use with childhood disorders (Reace & Motolese, 1975; Selvini et al., 1976).

ACTIVITY

Tricyclics and quadricyclics produce depression of spontaneous motor activity in laboratory animals. Tricyclics have seen reported useful in the treatment of hyperkinetic behavior disordered children, but, in contrast to the stimulants (see Chapter 6), there have been only two studies of effects of tricyclics on motor activity in children. Werry et al. (1975a, 1976b) found evidence of reduction in motor overflow during a sedentary task using a specially designed seat. Effects on disruptive behavior are discussed below.

CENTRAL NERVOUS SYSTEM

The frequent reports of insomnia and euphoria and the occasional induction of seizures in psychiatric patients indicate that tricyclics and quadricyclics can have a stimulant-like action under certain circumstances (see Chapter 6). This is said not to occur in normal or non-depressed adults in whom sedative-like effects predominate (Byck, 1975). This has been questioned by Werry et al. (1975a) who claim most of the adult data are based on only single or a few doses and while a sedative-type action does occur with many tricyclics (even in depressed patients), it is characteristically short-lived and superseded by a stimulant-like action. This needs further study.

COGNITIVE FUNCTIONING (SEE ALSO CHAPTER 3)

There are few studies of cognitive effects of tricyclics in children compared with the vast literature for the stimulants (see Chapter 6). However, these studies are of considerable theoretical importance as they may provide indirect evidence for the mechanisms of action of the drugs.

Rapoport et al. (1974b) found imipramine in relatively low doses (2-3 mgm/kg), given to behavior disordered children, to have a stimulant-like effect increasing vigilance (Continuous Performance Task) and decreasing impulsivity as measured by the Porteus Maze Test. There was an increase in latency, but not a decrease in errors in the Kagan Matching Familiar Figure test, presumably a test of cognitive "impulsivity." This finding, in combination with the side effects (appetite, weight loss, increased blood pressure), suggested a stimulant-like action of tricyclics in children. Similar effects for amytriptyline, also with behavior disordered children, have been reported (Yepes et al., 1977, Kupietz et al., 1976), in which the absolute score and correct detections improved on the CPT and omission errors were decreased to an extent comparable to that for methylphenidate.

The cognitive effects of imipramine (and other tricyclics) have rarely been examined in enuretic children. In the only studies on this subject Werry et al. (1975a, 1976b) likewise found weak stimulant-like effects on motor overflow and less certainly directly on cognitive function. These latter reports are of particular interest as most of their sample of enuretic children were regarded as normal and so this represents a rare opportunity to observe the effects of tricyclics in normal children; there is need for more such work.

ACADEMIC ACHIEVEMENT (SEE CHAPTER 3)

There have been no reports of beneficial effects of tricyclics on academic achievement in naturalistic settings. One study failed to find any difference between the Wide Range Achievement Test scores in Arithmetic or Reading between hyperactive children who had been treated for a year on imipramine and a comparable group of children who had dropped off medication during the year because of adverse side effects (Quinn & Rapoport, 1975). It remains unknown, therefore, whether or not academic improvement can be produced by antidepressant medication. Since laboratory tests which are assumed to be learning related have tended to show improvement with tricyclics, these tests are clearly not sufficient measures for predicting adequate scholastic performance (see Chapter 3).

A study of academic achievement and antidepressant treatment could be of considerable interest in validating the disputed diagnostic entity of "masked depression" evidenced by learning disability and poor self-esteem (see Rapoport, 1976).

BEHAVIOR

Imipramine has been reported useful for the treatment of school refusal in a double-blind study (Gittelman-Klein & Klein, 1971). Imipramine treatment (mean dose of 152 mgm/day) of nonpsychotic school phobic children in the context of a multidisciplinary treatment program produced significant drug-placebo differences at 6 weeks (not present at 3 weeks). Several points emerge from this study. This is the only study of clinical effects of imipramine in children for which the effects are shown to be delayed as in adults in contrast to immediate effects found in enuresis and conduct disorders. In addition, separation anxiety, but not anticipatory anxiety, was felt to be improved in the phobic children, suggesting a different substrate for those symptoms associated with school phobia.

The authors are careful to point out that they do not interpret the response of these phobic children to antidepressant drug as reflecting an underlying depression in this group (Gittelman-Klein & Klein, 1973). Rather, they feel that a separate biological phenomenon may be involved, i.e., one that related to separation anxiety; this thinking is a continuation of their work on drug responsive anxiety states in adults also thought to be an independent phenomenon from that for depressive illness.

Imipramine has been found to decrease conduct problems such as restless, aggressive and impulsive behavior in children (Winsberg et al., 1972; Rapoport et al., 1974b; Waizer et al., 1974). In contrast to a true antidepressant effect, this is immediate, occurring within hours after the first dose. In some children however, there is exacerbated conduct disturbance, with hyperirritability as discussed below. This has also been noted for quadricyclics (Kuhn & Kuhn, 1972).

MOOD

Adult-type depression, i.e., disorders characterized by persistent dysphoric mood, self-depreciating thoughts, insomnia, weight loss and motor retardation, is rare in children. This subject has been reviewed extensively elsewhere and will not be elaborated here (Conners, 1976b; Graham, 1974; Rapoport, 1976).

As a consequence, few controlled studies have been interested in the effects of imipramine on mood in children. Werry et al. (1975a) reported a positive mood effect as rated by psychiatric interview with the mother after 3 weeks of treatment with 25/50 mg of imipramine daily in enuretic children. This study does not conclusively demonstrate a direct effect on mood, however, as a change in mood secondary to achieving continence cannot be entirely ruled out. Indeed, in an attempted replication of this study, Werry et al. (1976b) failed to find any mood changes. In their study of school phobia, Gittelman-Klein and Klein

(1973) noted universal reports of "feeling better" which took several weeks to develop.

Several clinical studies with enuretic children report that a minority of children may be restless and irritable even with doses of tricyclics as low as 50 mgm/day (see Blackwell & Currah, 1973, Werry et al., 1975a). In higher doses, the dysphoric effect may be striking, necessitating discontinuation of the drug.

Maprotiline has been reported to improve "depression" in pediatric populations in two uncontrolled studies, which are discussed in more detail below.

Treatment Emergent (Side) Effects

SHORT-TERM EFFECTS

Until recently, the therapeutic use of imipramine was considered safe in children. Di Mascio and Solty (1970) found the prevalence and severity of side effects similar to those reported in adults—namely minor annoyances like dryness of mouth, drowsiness, lethargy, tremors, appetite disturbance, nausea and sweating. While agranulocytosis has been reported in adults, none has yet been reported in children. However, in the past few years, there has been increasing concern about the vulnerability of children to tricyclics, especially as higher doses than those used in enuresis have become more common. Seizure threshold, lower in children in any case, appears to be reduced particularly. Several cases of seizures in children aged 3 to 6 years, previously seizure free, were recently reported with doses ranging from 150 to 225 mgm (about 7-10 mg/Kg) of imipramine daily (Brown et al., 1973). This has also been observed in children receiving maprotiline (Kuhn-Gebhardt, 1972).

There has also been particular concern about the possible cardiotoxicity of tricyclics in children. The sudden death of a 6-year-old following a bedtime dose of 300 mgm (14 mg/kg) for school phobia (Saraf et al., 1974) may have resulted from cardiotoxicity. EKG abnormalities (increased heart rate, increased PR interval and nonspecific T wave changes) were found to be produced by imipramine in doses of 5 mgm/kg given over 24 hours (Winsberg et al., 1975). As a result the Food and Drug Administration in the U.S. has cautioned against the use of doses in excess of 5 mg/kg and advised EKG monitoring as this level is reached (Hayes et al., 1975). As noted previously, it has been speculated that the 2-hydroxy metabolites of imipramine (2-hydroxyimipramine and 2-hydroxydesmethylimipramine) are responsible for this effect as these metabolitets show binding affinity to cardiac tissue.

Weight loss has been reported for children after 3-6 weeks of tricyclic treatment (Rapoport et al., 1974b; Waizer et al., 1974; Werry et al., 1975a, 1976a). It is interesting that maprotiline is said to produce weight gain in children and adults (Kuhn-Gebhardt, 1972). Two reports have noted mildly increased distolic blood pressure in behavior disordered children (Rapoport et al., 1974b; Greenberg, et al., 1975) and two in enuretic children (Werry et al., 1975a, 1976a).

In contrast to therapeutic uses, poisoning with tricyclics is much more likely to prove life threatening. Delirium, drowsiness, flushing, tachycardia, arrhythmias, coma and cardiovascular collapse may result. Bickel (1975) has recently discussed reported poisoning with tricyclic drugs in an exhaustive review. The dosages for severe intoxication in adults were found to be a minimum of 7 mgm/kg and maximum of 127 mgm/kg with a mean of 38 mgm/kg. For fatal cases, the values were 10 and 210 respectively with a mean of 66. The values for children under 7 years were even higher than those for adults, arguing against the assumption that the children *are more sensitive* to the toxic effects of tricyclics than are adults. Nevertheless, it should be pointed out that the smaller body size of young children makes the possible *absolute* fatal dose quite small; the lowest dose reported to result in the death of a child was a mere 250 mg (Sidiropoulos & Bickel, 1971), or only 10 tablets of commonly used antidepressants.

If tetracyclics continue to prove less cardiotoxic than tricyclics, they may find special use in some childhood conditions. There is also some evidence that doxepin may be less cardiotoxic than other tricyclics (Davies et al., 1975).

LONG-TERM EFFECTS

It has been suggested that dyskinesia may occur following chronic administration of tricyclics in adults (Fann et al., 1976); while these have not yet been reported for children, the possibility should be considered during long-term administration of this group of drugs.

In view of short-term effects noted above, other possible long-term effects to be monitored are those on growth and on the cardiovascular system.

DRUG INTERACTIONS

Tricyclic antidepressants have clinically important interactions with several agents (Miller, 1975). Combined treatment with methylphenidate increases the serum levels of antidepressant, and there may be a synergistic effect with phenothiazines and other sedatives. Simultaneous treatment with monoamine oxidase inhibitors has been reported to result in hyperpyrexia, convulsions, coma and death. Thyroid hormones may increase the antidepressant effect of tricyclics; whether they increase their effectiveness with hyperactive or enuretic children is unknown.

Clinical Indications and Contraindications

ESTABLISHED INDICATIONS

1) *Enuresis.* Following the initial brief report of MacLean (1960) and a controlled clinical trial by Poussaint and Ditman (1965), more than 30 double-blind studies have demonstrated the symptomatic efficacy of tricyclic medication in enuresis in nightly doses ranging from 25-125 mgm. While improvement is noted in 60-80% of most samples, total remissions are reported in only 10 to 50% in a condition which has a significant spontaneous and placebo remission rate. This literature has been reviewed extensively by Blackwell and Currah (1973), who concluded that the case for *cure* of enuresis by tricyclics is not proven. Most children who appear to be cured resume wetting when medication is stopped.

Studies with enuretic children have not used comparable doses, populations or even definitions of the condition. For that reason, it is difficult to make a statement about comparability of different tricyclics or to define "good responders" from the available reports. In general, institutionalized, retarded, older enuretics, and those with daytime wetting seem to show a less favorable response. Interestingly, clinical response to imipramine has been demonstrated in cases with known urinary tract abnormality.

Those enuretic children with associated psychiatric problems may require treatment for these difficulties; it is unclear whether imipramine will provide significant benefit for the variety of psychiatric conditions that show significant association with enuresis (see discussion below).

2) *Conduct and Attention Deficit (Hyperkinetic) Disorders.* Shortly after tricyclics began to be used for enuresis, reports of beneficial effects on hyperactive/aggressive children claimed changes similar to those found with stimulants (Rapoport, 1965; Krakowski, 1965; Huessy & Wright, 1970). More recently, controlled trials have generally confirmed these initial open studies and demonstrated the beneficial effect of tricyclics in doses from 2-5 mg/kg for restless, antisocial behavior (Waizer et al., 1974; Rapoport et al., 1974b, Winsberg et al., 1972; Werry et al., 1977, Yepes et al., 1977). This response appears to be immediate and, in some cases, dramatic. It should be noted, though, that one study (Greenberg

et al., 1975) found no useful clinical effect and side effects were prohibitive on 100 mg daily. Most of these studies too have shown methylphenidate to be superior to tricyclics.

All these studies are short-term (4 weeks or less). The long-term usefulness of tricyclics for these disorders, however, remains controversial. In an open study, Gittelman-Klein (1974) indicated that an initial response to a daily dose of 150-300 mgm of imipramine seen at 2 weeks was not maintained at 12 weeks. Similarly, in a one-year follow-up (Quinn & Rapoport, 1975), significantly more hyperactive children had discontinued tricyclic medication than methylphenidate, even when both groups had shown an initial response after 6 weeks. It is the authors experience that long-term treatment of conduct disordered and hyperkinetic children with tricyclics is unsatisfactory; this point deserves further study.

Unfortunately, studies to date have not used DSM III categories and separated out Attention Deficit Disorders from Conduct Disorders sufficiently clearly to be sure in which or how many of these conditions antidepressants may be useful.

Possible Indications

1) *Separation Anxiety*. A single double-blind study has shown that imipramine benefits the separation anxiety associated with school phobia (Gittelman-Klein & Klein, 1971, 1973). This effect was seen at 6 weeks after the rather high average daily dose of 200 mg. The authors stress that the anticipatory anxiety associated with school return did not seem altered. More studies are needed to confirm the usefulness of tricyclics here—and their safety since the doses said to be required are very high and associated with one fatality.

2) *Depressive Disorders*. The difficulty in defining depressive disorder in childhood has been reviewed elsewhere (Conners, 1976b; Graham, 1974; Rapoport, 1976). Several points emerge from these reviews. As the persistent dysphoria, self-recriminations, and psycho-motor retardation characteristic of adult depression are rare in childhood, there is debate as to the existence and nature of childhood depressive disorder. Clinical reports on childhood depression have included heterogeneous populations with temper tantrums, mood swings, learning difficulties, enuresis and overactivity as presenting problems. The overuse of vague diagnostic labels such as masked depression or depressive equivalent has been detrimental to research in this area.

In uncontrolled studies, imipramine and quadricyclics have been described as useful for a variety of possible depressive symptoms such as learning disabilities, irritability, dysphoria, somatic symptoms such as headaches and stomachaches, insomnia, and nightmares. Some of these studies (Ling et al., 1970; Weinberg et al., 1973; Frommer, 1967) are particularly suggestive of true antidepressant action inasmuch as children, described as having social withdrawal, deteriorating school performance and self-depreciation of recent onset seem to benefit from tricyclic medication. In an uncontrolled study of 100 children and adolescents (Kuhn-Gebhart, 1972) the quadricyclic maprotiline was also reported to produce good or very good results in 60% of cases when used alone. However, these studies often lack clear clinical description, objective behavior ratings, independent diagnostic ratings, or proper controls for time and placebo effects. With the lack of data on latencies of effect and the possibility of alternative pharmacological effects such as stimulant or anxiolytic, these reports must be regarded as only suggestive of a true antidepressant effect. These studies do, however, indicate an area in pediatric psychopharmacology worthy of much closer attention.

3) *Specific Development Disorders (Learning Disabilities)*. Like the stimulants, tricyclics may have some beneficial effect on attentional and cognitive laboratory measures (Rapaport et al., 1974b; Yepes et al., 1977, Werry et al., 1975a) though studies are few. Also, as with the stimulants which these effects resemble, the relationship between these laboratory improvements and improved academic performance in naturalistic setting has yet to be demonstrated. It is thus important that appropriate educational efforts be made in children with learning disabilities even if drug treatment is ongoing for this or other indications (hyperactivity, enuresis, etc.). As with depression, research in this most interesting area is too sketchy to define a positive indication for antidepressants.

Contraindications

The tricyclics are not indicated in psychotic and schizophrenic conditions as they may aggravate the underlying psychotic process; although true manic illness in childhood is contentious, presumably tricyclics would also not be indicated for this condition because of possible worsening of the manic process. It might be expected that anxiety states would contraindicate antidepressants but as discussed above the evidence is actually contrary.

Tricyclics should be used with extreme caution or not at all in children with cardiac disease because of their known cardiac toxicity. In children with glaucoma, tricyclic drugs should be used only with ophthalmologic consultation.

Because of a number of reports of collapse, convulsions and hyperpyrexia in adult depressed patients treated with an MAO inhibitor and a tricyclic antidepressant, a 14-day drug free interval is recommended before discontinuation of either drug and the institution of the other. The necessity for this has been questioned recently (Ayd, 1975) in cases where the drugs are started simultaneously or where the tricyclic has been started first. At the present time, it seems unlikely that pediatric populations will be treated by these agents in combination, but an increase in the use of or indications for these agents with children could make this issue of importance in pediatric psychopharmacology.

Clinical Administration, Dosages and Precautions

ENURESIS

In the treatment of enuresis, a single bedtime dose of 0.5-2.5 mg/Kg is the usual therapeutic range. In some instances where the child is likely to wet very early in sleep, it may be advisable to give the medication earlier in the evening (Alderton, 1967). Imipramine should be started at a dose of 10-25 mgm and the dose increased every other night or so until either there is a clinical response (7 out of 10 dry nights is a recommended criterion), side effects appear, or, at the very most, a maximum dose of 5 mgm/kg is reached. The long-term maintenance treatment of enuresis must include periodic withdrawals (in the authors' practice, every 3 months), to ascertain whether medication is still necessary. At low doses graduated withdrawal is not necessary, but at higher ones it is necessary to prevent cholinergic rebound symptoms. In treating enuresis, however, it is necessary to titrate the essential benignity of this condition against the risks of medication-discomfort and occasional threat to life in the patient or his small sibs who may gain access to the medication. This calls for good clinical judgment.

Conduct Disorders and Attention Deficit Disorders

Tricyclics (imipramine and amytryptiline) are usually given in total daily doses from 2-5 mg/Kg. There is continuing controversy over the clinical benefits of divided doses; it is said that fewer side effects occur with twice or more daily medication schedules. A usual starting dose would be around 1 mg/kg daily, increasing in 23 mgm increments over a period of two weeks. If successful, the response should follow immediately upon attaining the dosage appropriate for that child. Long-term tolerance to the drug effect may be handled by increased dosage in some cases and in other cases by drug holidays. An upper daily dose limit of 5 mgm/kg has been recommended for children (Hayes et al., 1975), which for the average grade school child will not exceed 150 mgm. As with most pyschotropic drugs, side effects are likely to be most troublesome for a few days immediately after dosage increments after which they often lessen to an acceptable degree.

SEPARATION ANXIETY DISORDER (SCHOOL PHOBIA)

Treatment of school phobia will be largely centered around the family and school cooperation with the treating agency, in supporting early school return. On the basis of a single, double-blind report, doses in the range of 100-200 mg/day produced an effect by 6 weeks; the effect was not seen at 3 weeks. For patients receiving doses of imipramine greater than 3.5 m/kg, baseline EKG and periodic EKG monitoring are suggested (Saraf et al., 1977).

For children, Kuhn-Gebhardt (1972) recommends that treatment with maprotiline be initiated with 10 mg tablets and gradually increased to a dosage level employed in adults i.e., 75-150 mg/day, but it is suggested that until more data are available on the use of quadricyclics in children, the same precautions as with the tricyclics be observed.

MONOAMINE OXIDASE INHIBITORS (MAOI)

Definition and Introduction

Historically the MAOIs were first used as antibacterial drugs in the treatment of tuberculosis. It was noticed that one such drug, iproniazid, produced side effects of central nervous system stimulation and euphoria. This observation and evidence that it caused increased concentration of amines in the brain resulted in its introduction as an antidepressant. In contrast to use in adults, there have been few clinical trials of MAOIs in children, and no properly controlled studies. This brief section has been included only for completeness and because there could well be increased use of these drugs.

CLASSES AND CHEMICAL STRUCTURES

The MAO inhibitors are of two chemical types, the hydrazines and non-hydrazines. Iproniazid, the first antidepressant drug of the former type, was introduced originally because of its anti-mycobacterial activity, but was removed from the market as an antidepressant because of toxicity believed to be due to the formation of free hydrazine, a subsequent highly hepatotoxic substance. Later variants of this group have tended toward structures which protect the hydrazide moiety, as in the case of isocarboxazid and nialamide (Hollister, 1972).

An example of a non-hydrazine MAO inhibitor, tranylcypromine (Parnate) bears a close resemblance to dextroamphetamine, having a cyclopropyl, rather than an isopropyl chain. It is this difference which allows it to inhibit monoamine oxidase whereas dextroamphetamine possesses this action only weakly.

Chemical structure of some representative MAOI are given in Figure 3.

Pharmacology

ABSORPTION

Plasma assays for levels of MAOI have not yet been developed for clinical use and accordingly pharmacological activity is generally inferred from physiological effects. These have been observed to begin 30 minutes after oral intake and accordingly absorption would be assumed to be rapid though not necessarily complete (Sulman et al., 1973).

SERUM HALF-LIFE

As MAO inhibitors act as irreversible inhibitors of the enzyme (Plet-

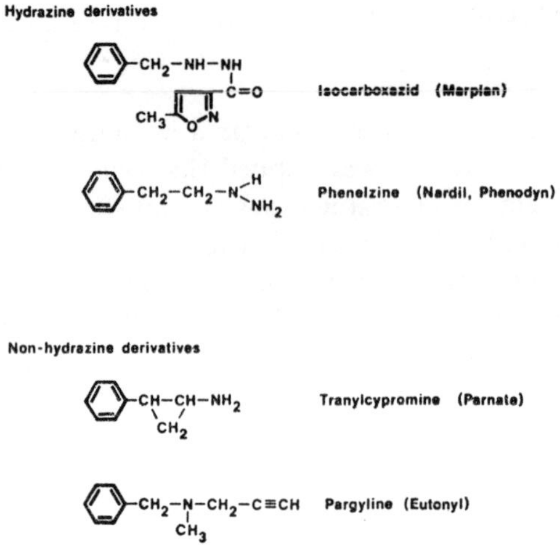

Fig. 3. Monoamine oxidase inhibitors

scher, 1966) there is not the usual interest in studying serum half-life. Also the difficulty in obtaining blood levels has effected research in this area.

DISTRIBUTION

Direct assay of these drugs has not been carried out. MAO inhibitor will cause an increase in endogenous norepinephrine, epinephrine, dopamine, and 5-hydroxytryptophan in various tissues including brain, heart, intestines and blood; it is assumed therefore, that the drugs are widely distributed (Byck, 1975).

EXCRETION/DETOXIFICATION

These drugs are present in the body for only a short time; however, as they produce their effect by irreversible enzyme inactivation, the termination of drug effect depends on the weeks-long process of enzyme regeneration (Byck, 1975). Genetic factors have been shown to have an important effect on the rate at which the drugs are metabolized, with rapid vs. slow acetylators having been identified (Price-Evans, 1965).

ACTIVE PRINCIPLES

The non-hydrazine MAOIs combine directly with the enzyme, while the hydrazine MAOIs are cleaved, resulting in the liberation of the active product (Byck, 1975).

SITES AND MODES OF ACTION

The primary site of action is at the cellular level wherever MAO occurs. There is some variability in organs affected according to the particular MAOI. The drugs are known to produce their effect to some degree in brain, heart, intestines, liver, plasma, and platelets (Murphy et al., 1977).

The drugs work at the cellular level primarily by irreversibly inactivating MAO. There is some evidence that they may prevent the release of norepinephrine from nerve endings by nerve impulses. However, they do not block the release of biogenic amines secondary to the administration of pharmacological agents, such as amphetamine and tyramine, leading to their clinical toxicity (Hendley & Snyder, 1968). It should be noted that they affect MAO which is only one of several monoamine inactivating enzymes each, of course, with its specific substrate or monoamine. They also affect to a varying degree other enzyme systems which, together with their MAOI action, greatly increases their overall toxicity (see Drug Interactions).

DOSE RESPONSE DATA

Due to the irreversible enzyme effect and the difficulty of testing the end result, this variable cannot be as closely examined as with other drugs.

RELATIONSHIP BETWEEN SERUM LEVELS AND EFFECTS

Serum levels of MAO inhibitors have not proved to be a fruitful line of research. However enzyme inhibition may prove to be as useful in correlating drug activity with clinical effect, as have serum levels with most compounds (Raskin et al.,1974). MAO inhibition was found to correlate with clinical effect in a study by Robinson where the dosage of the drug was kept at a level that was sufficient to produce 80% inhibition of platelet MAO (Robinson et al., 1973).

TIME RESPONSE DATA

In general, several weeks are necessary for onset of clinical effect, in spite of the fact that measurable MAO inhibition may be found in tissues within 24 hours (Byck, 1975). It should be noted that other effects of the drugs such as the amphetamine-like action of tranylcypromine and the interference with the inactivation of other drugs may appear immediately (Byck, 1975).

Clinical Effects

CENTRAL NERVOUS SYSTEM

Signs of central nervous system stimulation have been seen in patients receiving pargyline, an antihypertensive MAOI (Byck, 1975), so this effect does not seem to be confined to depression. MAOI have been reported to reduce the frequency of grand mal seizures in a high percentage of epileptic patients (Burns & Shore, 1961). This is further evidence of a general stimulant type activity since it is well known that seizures are commoner in low-arousal states.

ELECTROENCEPHALOGRAM (EEG)

Like the tricyclics, MAO inhibitors supress REM sleep with a rebound following withdrawal (Kupfer & Bowers, 1972). Awake, computerized

EEG profiles produced by the MAOI resemble those evoked by the stimulants, characterized by a decrease in slow waves, and an increase in 7.5-20 cps activities accompanied by a decrease of 40-90 cps in the primary wave (Itil et al., 1975).

CARDIOVASCULAR

MAOIs have been found to lower standing blood pressure in man (Nussbaum et al., 1957) and indeed one MAOI, pargyline, was introduced specifically as an antihypertensive agent. There is also a pronounced postural or orthostatic hypotensive effect which can be a troublesome side effect.

HEMATOLOGICAL AND METABOLIC

MAO inhibitors have been shown to change the permeability of enythrocyte membranes in mentally retarded children (Bichonski, 1973).

Jaundice was a frequently noted problem with MAO inhibitors but is less frequently noted with the non-hydrazines. The MAO inhibitors have been shown to have a significant hypoglycemic action which should be taken into account when prescribing the drugs to diabetic children (Adnitt, 1968).

ACTIVITY, COGNITIVE FUNCTIONING, ACADEMIC ACHIEVEMENT

The effects of MAOI upon these areas of function have not been studied in children.

CLINICAL SYNDROMES

Anecdotal reports have suggested that the MAOI's may be useful in conduct disorders, schizophrenic and autistic children as well as phobic anxiety states and severe obsessive-compulsive conditions (Soblen & Saunders, 1961; Freedman, 1958; Annesley, 1969; Sargant, 1969). Only the studies with obsessional and phobic disorders provide lucid clinical description.

In a retrospective study with adults presenting with severe phobic symptoms or panic attacks, Kelly found 90% improvement at one month and at one year following treatment with 30-60 mg of phenelzine, 10-40 mg of isocarboxazide or 20-40 mg of tranylcypromine either alone or in combination with minor tranquilizers or tricyclics (Kelly et al., 1970). In the same study, 50 severely phobic children were treated with isocarboxazide or tranylcypromine alone and in combination. The doses were not specified. At least 2 of these children were judged to have suicidal thoughts with severe depression. Ninety percent were found improved at one month and at one year; however, only 14 children were seen at one year. Stack (1972) reported similar results in an uncontrolled study of 64 children. Frommer (1967) demonstrated that a combination of phenelzine, an MAOI and chlordiazepoxide was superior to phenobarb in children she diagnosed as phobic or mood-type depressives. Unfortunately, the mixing of one anxiolytic with the MAOI and the use of an entirely different type of anxiolytic as a control procedure makes the interpretation of an antidepresesant effect impossible. Further there was a drug order effect which added to the confusion. As can be seen, data are meager in this area.

MOOD

The first psychiatric use of MAOIs in adults was in the treatment of depression. However, the toxicity of MAOIs, and greater efficacy of tricyclics led to their decline. There is now renewed interest in the use of MAOIs in adult depressives with atypical features.

There has been no controlled sutdy of the effects of MAOIs on mood in children utilizing objective mood ratings, though suggestions from Frommer's (1967) and others' work suggest that they may produce mood changes. This could of course be stimulant-type euphoria rather than a true antidepressant action.

Treatment Emergent Side Effects

SHORT-TERM EFFECTS

In general, MAOIs seem better tolerated than tricyclics, yet their potential toxicity is much greater, and, because of their long action, the risk period is much longer. Though clinical effects may be delayed for weeks, toxic reactions from acute overdosage develop within hours. Effects reported include convulsions, hyperpyrexia, hyperirritability, hallucinations and agitation. Both hypotension and hypertension have been reported. However, fatalities seem unusual. One 2-year, 9-month old girl suffered only lethargy, ataxia and rash following an overdose of 225 mg of phenelzine (Greenblatt et al., 1976). Conservative treatment aimed at maintaining normal blood pressure, electrolyte and fluid balance, temperature and respiration has proven to be the most successful.

Most fatalities have resulted in the course of normal treatment from hypertensive crises due to ingestion of tyramine-containing foods or pressor amines or from drug interactions discussed below. Treatment of hypertensive crisis is achieved by administration of an alpha-adrenergic blocking agent such as phentolamine. Less dramatic side effects include orthostatic hypotension and overstimulation.

LONG-TERM EFFECTS

In adults, reactions following chronic administration of MAOIs include hypomania, hallucinations and confusion as well as convulsions and peripheral neuropathy. Orthostatic hypotension and constipation are common, and hepatotoxicity, though uncommon with current MAOI, still occurs (Byck, 1975). Recently, there has been evidence that drug dependence can develop (Shopsin & Kline, 1976).

DRUG INTERACTION

This is one of the most serious risks with MAOIs, which also interfere with the metabolic degradation of barbiturates, aminopyrine, acetanilid, cocaine and notably meperidine where a hyperpyrexia can result. They also intensify the effects of central depressant agents such as alcohol, of anticholinergic drugs and tricyclic antidepressants. Concurrent use with l-dopa and other sympathomimetic substances can result in a hypertensive crisis. The hazards of potential interactions with stimulants such as amphetamine make the prescription of these drugs more dangerous in depressed, acting out adolescents (Shamsie & Barriga, 1971). The problem then with the MAOIs lies in their sensitizing the patient for a period well beyond actual drug treatment to a wide variety of foods and drugs.

Clinical Indications

ESTABLISHED INDICATIONS

The MAOIs cannot be considered as proven treatments for any childhood psychiatric illness, though they may be useful in other diseases such as narcolepsy or hypertension.

POSSIBLE INDICATIONS

As discussed previously, Kelly et al. (1970) have suggested that MAOIs may be useful in the treatment of children with severe phobic disturbances. This is reminiscent of the possibly effective role of tricyclics in separation anxiety. They may also yet prove to have a role in childhood depression and in conduct disorders, though it is hard to see how they could replace safer drugs like the tricyclics or stimulants.

CONTRAINDICATIONS

Any preexisting or intended other drug treatment calls for consultation with a pharmacologist before proceeding. Cardiovascular, liver or CNS disease and high risk of food tyramine consumption are contraindications.

Clinical Administration, Dosages and Precautions

Pediatric dose ranges have not been established. In two studies using phenelzine with children, the dose was started at 15 mgm q.d. and increased up to 15 mgm tid in larger children. Thus, any administration in children must be regarded as a clinical trial and proper procedures and precautions observed.

ETHICAL CONSIDERATIONS OF ANTIDEPRESSANT USE

The risks incurred from use of psychotropic medication must be weighed against the possible benefits to the children from drug treatment. Enuresis is often an intermittent problem and drug treatment should be used only when the condition is interfering with the child's self-image, social and interpersonal functioning. Behavior disordered children often respond to stimulant drug treatment and, as these medications have been found less toxic than antidepressants (see Chapter 6), they probably should be tried before antidepressants.

Finally, childhood "depression" is, as yet, a poorly defined entity and many dysphoric reactions of childhood are both brief and situational. It is incumbent upon the physician to investigate environmental manipulations and alternate treatment strategies in children with presenting complaints such as anxiety and poor self-image. In view of the toxicity of tricyclics antidepressants, the dose should be restricted to less than 5 mgm/kg unless special circumstances indicate otherwise. Similarly, the high potential toxicity of MAOIs must be considered particularly since, in most instances, safer agents are available. However, some conditions such as severe phobic states, if unresponsive to other treatments, may yet prove to be an occasional indication for MAOI.

SUMMARY AND CONCLUSIONS

The efficacy of antidepressants for childhood psychopathological conditions is still unclear, but most of the possibilities are quite distinctive from those in adults. Even in enuresis, the long-term efficacy and interaction with other treatments have yet to be established (Blackwell & Currah, 1973). For the behavior and mood disorders, there are more questions than answers. The undisputed, immediate, short-term response to tricyclics in hyperactive-conduct disorders is of theoretical interest as these drugs share some properties with stimulants in increasing the availability of central monoamines, and the immediacy of effect suggests a different mechanism of action than that in depression. While the tricyclics may be useful for short periods clinically, their long-term efficacy has not yet been demonstrated for hyperactive and conduct disorders, which usually require long-term management. Neither has any beneficial effect on academic achievement yet been demonstrated, in spite of some improved laboratory performance on cognitive tasks.

The usefulness of antidepressants in childhood anxiety, phobia, depressive and (possibly) obsessional disorders remains an unsettled but interesting area, deserving of further study. Comparison of tricyclics with differing relative specificity for neurotransmitter reuptake (such as chloimipramine for serotonin and desipramine for noradrenalin) may permit pharmacological dissection out of drug-responsive and presumably etiologically distinct subgroups within the at present, meaninglessly heterogeneous population of neurotic children.

The mechanism of action of imipramine in enuresis is still unclear and also deserves further study. The micturition reflex is complex in man; peripheral nerves, spinal cord, brain stem, thalamus and cortex are involved. Because of the complex relation between enuresis and psychiatric disturbance of childhood (Shaffer, 1973), the possible higher central action of imipramine in this condition is particularly interesting. If, for example, a subtle neurotransmitter defect is present, then careful comparison of different tricyclic compounds known to have differential central effects might reveal drug responsive subgroups, or possibly indicate the underlying nature of this disturbance in some enuretic subgroups.

Because of their distinctiveness in children and their clinical and heuristic possibilities, thus, the antidepressant drugs or at least the tri- and quadricyclics are amongst the more interesting drugs in pediatric psychopharmacology.

8

ANTIPSYCHOTICS (MAJOR TRANQUILIZERS, NEUROLEPTICS)

BERTRAND G. WINSBERG, M.D.
and
LUIS E. YEPES, M.D.

INTRODUCTION

Antipsychotics, as their name suggests, are distinguished by their ability to relieve psychotic symptoms (especially those of schizophrenia) or major mental disorders marked by impairment of reality testing and bizarre behavior, in adults. However, like the term antidepressant (see Chapter 7), the term antipsychotic is singularly inappropriate for pediatric psychopharmacology where: 1) the commoner forms of psychoses such as autism appear quite distinctive from those encountered in adults (see Chapter 5); 2) most childhood psychoses do not respond well to antipsychotic drugs; and 3) the indications for the use of these drugs are largely symptomatic, rather than specific, and in non-psychotic conditions. However, alternative terms like neuroleptic, psycholeptic or major tranquilizer are confusing, carry undesirable social connotations or are not widely accepted. Thus, and since it is, after all, an adultocentric world, the term antipsychotic will be used here with the clear understanding that it implies no such clinical action in children.

Chemical Structure and Classes

Antipsychotics are subclassified by their chemical structure into five main groups: 1) phenothiazines, 2) butyrophenones, 3) thioxanthenes, 4) dibenzoxapines (dibenzodiazepines), and 5) dihydroindolones. The chemical structures of the most commonly used antipsychotic agents can be seen in Figure 1.

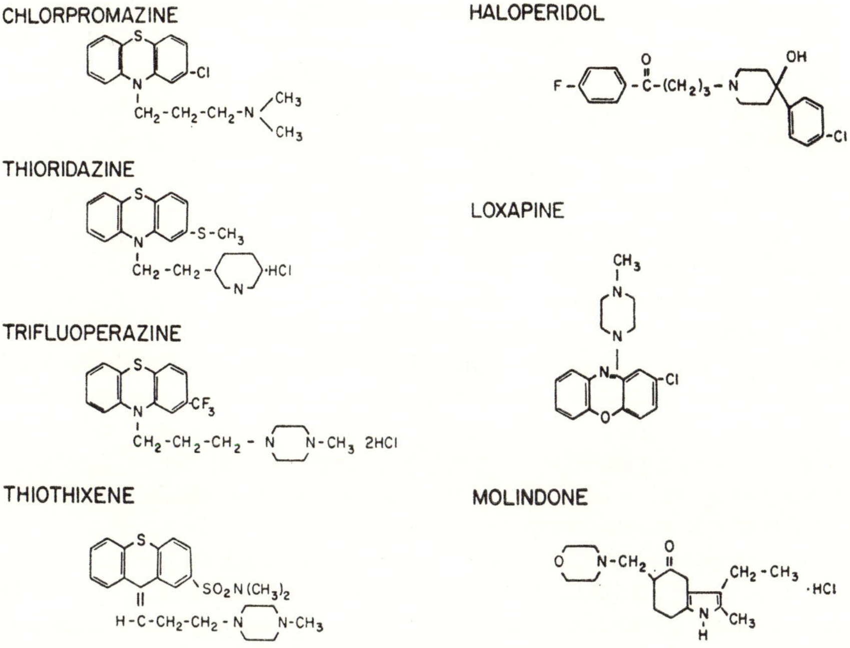

ANTIPSYCHOTICS (MAJOR TRANQUILIZERS, NEUROLEPTICS)

FIGURE 1

While some of the chemical groups are clearly related to each other (for example, phenothiazines and thioxanthines), others appear chemically distinct and their grouping together as antipsychotics depends on their ability to allay psychotic symptoms in adults. Structure/activity relationships have recently been reviewed in detail by Janssen (1976) and McDowell (1974). In addition to their antipsychotic properties, demonstrable only in humans, they usually have the following pharmacological characteristics in animals: 1) decrease motility, 2) selectively inhibit the conditioned avoidance response, 3) antagonize amphetamine-induced stereotopy and apomorphine (dopamine agonism)—induced emesis (vomiting), 4) produce cataplexy, and 5) potentiate analgesic agents.

Although they tend to share all of the above properties to a greater or lesser degree, it is virtually impossible to predict their efficacy or their potential toxicity solely on the basis of their biochemical and physiological properties, which are discussed in more detail in following sections. In the end, antipsychotic activity must be based on clinical trials in humans.

The phenothiazines, usually recognizable from a generic name terminating in *azine*, made their pharmacological debut around 1950 and, as a result, are by far the best understood and most widely used of the antipsychotic agents, with the butyrophenones and thioxathenes a poor second. Most of what follows, then, relates of necessity to the phenothiazines.

As with the tricyclic antidepressants (see Chapter 7), antipsychotic phenothiazines require a 3-carbon (propyl) bridge between the 10-position of the 3-ring structure and the end of the side chain. Reduction of this side chain to a 2-carbon radical results in loss of antipsychotic properties with enhancement of anticholinergic properties. A straight, aliphatic, 3-carbon side or dimethylaminopropyl chain without terminal ring structures, often designated by *prom* in the middle of the generic name of the drug (such as *chlorpromazine*) enhances anticholinergic properties though without loss of antipsychotic ability, while a 3-carbon side chain terminating in a piperidine or piperazine ring structure (often detectable by *per* or *phen* in the middle of the generic name) diminishes autonomic defects but enhances extrapyramidal effects.

Substitutions in the 2-position of the 3-ring structure influence milligram potency particularly, the most potent radical being CF_3 seen in fluphenazine (Anatensol, Permitil, Prolixin, Modicate) and trifluoperazine (Stelazine). When the nitrogen at position 10 (where the side chain is attached) is chained to a carbon with a *double bond* attachment to the side chain, a new class of antipsychotic agent, the thioxanthenes, is produced. For all practical purposes, these are pharmacologically identical to the phenothiazines.

While there are many commercially marketed antipyschotics, there seems little to choose between them in terms of their antipsychotic activity. Decisions are ordinarily made on the basis of the desirability of particular treatment emergent (side) effects and in parenteral use, milligram potency, and duration of action (for example, fluphenazine decanoate). In the case of children, where the therapeutic indications are different from those in adults, a treatment emergent (side) effect such as sedation or motor retardation may become the principal therapeutic action of the drug, rather than any antipsychotic action.

Pharmacology

It must be said at the outset that there are almost no data relating to children and much of what is said is based on assumptions of similarity with adults which may well be quantitatively if not qualitatively unwarranted for children. Where data relating to children are known, they will be stated. As already noted, phenothiazines, and in particular chlorpromazine (CPZ) (Largactil, Thorazine), the first antipsychotic, are the best studied and hence will be taken as the prototype. Where differences of some moment are known to occur in other chemical groups or subtypes, they will be noted but, in general, failure to note a difference, as with children, is much more likely a confession of ignorance than of proven fact.

Absorption and Distribution

This can be variable according to the form of the preparation, the state and pH of the gastrointestinal tract, other medication in the gut, notably, of course, the commonly coadministered anti-Parkinson agents which, being anticholinergic, may slow absorption.

It is worth noting that parenteral preparations of some of the antipsychotics can be highly irritating locally, resulting sometimes in aseptic abscesses. This is most particularly true of the weaker (that is, in terms of milligram potency) antipsychotics such as chlorpromazine and thioridazine (Mellaril) where it is likely that the irritation is as much a function of the large amount which has to be injected as of any particularly irritant nature of the substance itself.

Because, like the antidepressants (see Chapter 7), there is no simple relationship between serum levels and dosage, absorption studies are difficult. Peak blood levels for most of the antipsychotics seem to be attained ordinarily after 1-4 hours. Serum half-lives for CPZ in adults range from 2-31 hours with 80% of subjects in one study falling within 6 hours (Curry, 1968). Figures for thioridazine were somewhat longer, in one study averaging 24 hours (Gottschalk et al., 1975), with haloperidol about the same (12-38 hours) (Forsman & Ohman, 1976a, b), and chlorprothixene rather shorter (Raaflaub, 1975), though these data are based on only one or two studies with varying sizes and number of dosages.

Binding of antipsychotics to plasma proteins (see Levy, 1973, and Chapter 1) is high—in the region of 90% (Curry, 1970; Forsman & Ohman, 1976a, b), but distribution into the brain appears fairly rapid nevertheless, probably because of the high lipoid solubility of the antipsychotics (see Fingl, 1972, and Chapter 1). As a result, brain concentration may be considerably higher than blood levels.

Metabolism and Excretion

While absorption and distribution may be quite rapid, excretion is slow and metabolites may be detected for weeks after cessation of chronic drug administration, presumably because of slow release of tissue-bound forms of the drug. Excretion of CPZ is by way of urine and feces.

The metabolism of CPZ is extremely complicated. A varying but usually small portion of the drug is excreted unchanged. Liver-produced metabolites probably number over 150, over 50 of which have been studied (Curry, 1968, 1973). However, the majority of the drug is metabolised into hydroxylated, glucuronidated and sulphoxidated derivatives. The lipoid solubility of these metabolites and hence their penetration of the blood brain barrier may be considerably less than that of CPZ and it is not known how many are pharmacologically active though the 7-OH derivative does appear to be. These factors may account for some of the disparity between serum levels of CPZ and observed clinical effects. Haloperidol, on the other hand, is metabolised by oxidative dealkylation, oxidation and glycine conjugation and, unlike CPZ, its metabolites seem pharmacologically inactive making the study of the relationship between serum levels and clinical response *potentially* simpler. Loxapine (Loxitane), a dibenzoa(ze)pine, has at least 8 known metabolites, the principal route being hydroxylation and demethylation.

Dose/Response Relationships

As noted, this is very complex and, as with antidepressants, serum levels are highly individualistic and may vary between individuals as much as 10 times. As also noted, pharmacological activity of metabolites may also contribute significantly to this confusion. As a result, no doubt, efforts to relate the plasma concentrations of antipsychotics, particularly CPZ, to clinical response and to neurological side effects in adults have been largely unsuccessful and various investigators have achieved widely differing results (Curry, 1968; Gottschalk et al., 1975; Kolakowaska et al., 1976; Rivera-Calimin et al., 1976; Wiles et al., 1976).

Dose/Time Relationships

While the serum half-life is usually 24 hours or less, the drug may continue to be excreted for several weeks after chronic dosage. The time relationship between onset and decay of clinical activity, on the one hand, and dosage, on the other, are, however, far from clear and depend on the target symptom. Thus sedation and extrapyramidal side effects such as acute dystonias (muscle spasms) may occur within an hour or a few hours of initial dosage, but the antipsychotic action may not be apparent for weeks or, in chronic schizophrenia, months. Relapse following cessation of antipsychotic medication seems to follow a similar time course. However, the dose/time relationships in pediatric psychopharmacology, since they relate to other than the antipsychotic action, may well be different and much shorter.

Pharmacokinetic Data in Children

With the exception of some very preliminary work in our laboratory on CPZ and loxapine, therefore not reportable at this stage, there appear to be no data relating specifically to children, though differences from adults would be expected to be quantitative rather than qualitative (Rane & Wilson, 1976, see also Chapter 1).

Site and Mode of Action

Most of the study of the site and mode of action of antipsychotic drugs has, understandably, centered on the brain, particularly the effect of the drugs on the monoamines thought to be neurotransmitters (dopamine, serotonin, norepinephrine, and, most recently, octopamine), which studies have been mostly executed in rodent brain, particularly the mouse. Attempts to extrapolate such biochemical, animal-derived findings to antipsychotic and extrapyramidal effects in humans must be regarded as highly speculative (see Goldstein et al., 1974; Quinn et al., 1976) and, as yet, of little direct clinical use.

In general, these animal studies have focused on dopamine and its metabolism and two general conclusions appear warranted: 1) Antipsychotic agents appear to cause an initial increase in dopamine turnover which is followed, as tolerance develops, by a return to baseline levels; and 2) chronic exposure of neuronal pools to antipsychotic agents hypersensitizes the receptor neurone to its transmitter. This latter finding has been used to explain the development of adverse treatment emergent effects of an extrapyramidal nature such as tardive dyskinesia and parkinsonism (see below). Recent work in support of a dopamine based activity comes from the demonstration of the relationship between the potency of antipsychotic agents expressed as their average optimal oral dose with their ability to inhibit the stimulated release of dopamine in neonatal rat brain slices (Seeman & Lee, 1976).

Efforts to correlate these animal findings of antipsychotic drug effects upon monoamine metabolism have measured various metabolites in cerebrospinal fluid (CSF) using probenecid to block the active transport mechanisms responsible for their removal. Data derived in this way have led to much speculation about the relationship between the antipsychotic drugs and the monoamines (Chase, 1976), but efforts to differentiate various neurologic and psychiatric diagnostic groups on the basis of monoamine metabolite accumulation have yielded contradictory results. It does appear, however, that antipsychotic drugs do increase the accumulation of monoamine metabolites in the CSF and, similar to the mouse dopamine studies, this apparent elevation is not sustained over time (Post & Goodwin, 1975). However, the relevance of these biochemical studies to the clinical status of individual patients remains obscure.

Perhaps not surprisingly, then, recently attention has shifted away from the monoamine neurotransmitters to mediators such as cyclic adenosine monophosphate (cAMP) (Clement-Cormier et al., 1974; Hornykewicz, 1975; Iverson, 1975; Seeman & Lee, 1976; von Hungen & Robert, 1974), modulators such as prostaglandins (Palmer, 1976) or inhibitors (gamma aminobutyric acid) (Groves et al., 1975; Snyder et al., 1974, 1976) of transmitter action or metabolism (see Calne et al., 1975; Costa et al., 1974; Cuatrecasas, 1975; Ehrenpreis & Kopin, 1974; Friedhoff, 1975a, b).

There has also been some renewed interest in acetylcholine, particularly with respect to drug-related parkinsonism, and recent animal data suggest that antipsychotic drugs' ability to produce extrapyramidal symptoms is inversely proportional to their anticholinergic activity (Fann et al., Snyder et al., 1974).

However, most interest is still centered on dopamine and, to a lesser extent, other monoamine transmitters. Enthusiasm in this area has been encouraged not only by the animal studies described above but by findings of diminished dopamine and serotonin metabolism in patients with Parkinson's disease as well as by the therapeutic efficacy of l-dopa in this condition. The doctor is most interested in extrapyramidal type movement disorders more particularly because of the ominous side effect of antipsychotic drug therapy, namely tardive dyskinesia, which is seen in what may be a transitory form in children as "withdrawal emergent symptoms" (Polizos et al., 1973). There is no scarcity of hypotheses attempting to explain the nature of these drug-induced movement disorders, particularly the relationship to dopamine sensitization (Klawans, 1973; Seeman et al., 1974) but efforts to detect dopamine abnormality in adult patients with tardive dyskinesia have been unsuccessful (Pind & Faurbye, 1970). In our work with children no abnormality of CSF homovanilic acid (HVA), 5-hydroxyindoleacetic acid (5-HIAA), or, indeed, cAMP was found among a group of children showing dyskinetic movements following withdrawal of antipsychotic medication. Preliminary studies on prostaglandins using a radio immuno assay in the

ANTIPSYCHOTICS (MAJOR TRANQUILIZERS, NEUROLEPTICS)

same group of children with withdrawal emergent symptoms also failed to produce easily interpretable results.

Recent work in Australia (Wade, 1977) has suggested that the dopamine blocking effects of antipsychotic drugs may, as far as their antipsychotic action at least is concerned, be simply side effects and that their basic pharmacological activity is related to a relatively unstudied monoamine called octopamine, so-called because it occurs in the venom of octopus. This monoamine is found widely distributed throughout human brain tissue but is concentrated particularly in the temporal lobe, the hypothalamus and the locus caeruleus. This finding may help to explain why one of the most recently developed antipsychotics, clozapine (a dibenzoxapine) is only very weakly dopamine blocking and the only antipsychotic which does not produce extrapyramidal symptoms to any degree. On the other hand, all the antipsychotics, including clozapine, studied by Wade and his colleagues do have octopamine blocking effects and, interestingly, all the psychotomimetics they have studied to date appear to have a chemical configuration resembling that which accounts for the pharmacological activity of octopamine.

In summary, then, the evidence from animal experiments, and to a lesser degree, studies of movement disorders both naturally occurring and drug induced, as well as CSF monoamine studies in humans, are highly suggestive of some effect of antipsychotic drugs upon brain monoamines directly or through the role of intermediary substances, though much of the picture, particularly that relating to the specific monoamine or amines involved, is contradictory and unclear. Dopamine blocking and ultimately sensitizing effects appear to be the best established but that does not preclude other actions as well. Also unclear is the effect on acetylcholine.

CLINICAL EFFECTS

Basic Clinical Actions

From the clinical point of view, the most important pharmacological actions, apart from whatever is responsible for the antipsychotic effect, are a complex admixture of dopaminergic, alpha-adrenergic and cholinergic *blocking* actions on the central and autonomic nervous systems, plus in some cases a weak adrenergic action due to block of reuptake of monoamines qualitatively similar to that which is thought to be the basis of the action of tricyclic antidepressants (see Chapter 7 and review in Gordon, 1967). The extent of these actions varies with the type of antipsychotic drug (see below). In addition to these nervous system mediated actions, there are some minor local tissue effects notably: 1) a local anesthetic action (observed if tablets of CPZ are chewed), of uncertain clinical significance, but possibly involved in quinidine-like effects on cardiac muscle; 2) vasodilatation which is additive to nervous system effects in the production of orthostatic lowering of blood pressure.

These pharmacological actions lead to a set of basic clinical effects (Byck, 1975) *which are seen in many body systems,* so that antipsychotics, like antidepressants, are sometimes referred to as "dirty drugs," an unfortunate term, since most of these effects are mild and not life-threatening. The extent to which they will appear depends on: 1) dosage, 2) individual susceptibility (some of which appears genetic), 3) the particular antipsychotic agent (see below). If the effects are prominent and unwanted they are called side, adverse or, now more commonly, treatment emergent effects, so that the clinical details of most of them are described in that section. These effects are:

1) *Antipsychotic* (see clinical indications).

2) *Sedative* distinguished from true sedation seen with drugs such as alcohol or the barbiturates (see Chapters 8 and 9) in that there is no incoordination, and no behavioral disinhibition and the patient is easily aroused, which features, coupled with a concomitant lowering of emotional tone, are sometimes called *ataraxis* (hence the drug name Atarax for hydroxyzine), rather than sedation.

3) *Antiemetic* which in general is only effective against chemically induced vomiting (Chemoreceptor Trigger Zone).

4) Increase in *heart rate.*

5) Weakening of *postural cardiovascular reflexes* resulting in a variable fall in blood pressure on standing.

6) Reduction of *hypothalamic* and thus in pituitary activity which may lead to lowering of body temperature, decrease in secretion of so-called female sex hormones, growth, prolactin inhibiting and possibly antidiuretic hormones.

7) Interference with *extrapyramidal* function which is described in considerable detail under side effects.

8) *Antihistaminic* though this is weak and not important clinically since far stronger agents exist as by shortening the side chain of the phenothiazines, though with loss of antipsychotic power.

9) Depression of *brain stem* function which becomes important only in gross overdosage where it compounds the cardiac and other effects, and possibly in the suppression of hiccough.

Generally speaking, with the exception of the antipsychotic, antiemetic and extrapyramidal effects, these clinical actions are most pronounced with the dimethylaminopropyl or straight side chain phenothiazines such as CPZ and thioridazine, and with thioxanthines such as chlorprothixene, and least pronounced with the piperazine members of these two groups such as perphenazine, trifluoperazine, fluphenazine and thiothixene, and with the butyrophenones. However, the potentially more serious extrapyramidal effects occur in the reverse order. In general, too, there is a strong tendency to development of tolerance for most of the "unwanted" effects that are due to autonomic blockade, especially sedation.

Electroencephalogram

The effects of antipyschotic drugs on the CNS have been studied by examining electroencephalograms (EEG) and cortical evoked potentials (EP). However, neither has been used extensively for investigating the influence of antipsychotic drugs on the CNS of children. In addition, the functional significance of the reported drug-related EEG and EP changes remains unclear.

ROUTINE EEG

As far as the EEG is concerned, Campbell et al. (1972a) and Korein et al. (1971) reported that the administration of CPZ results in decreases in alpha (8-14 cps) frequency and increases in the amount and/or amplitude of slow (< 6 Hz) activity in some children. Campbell et al. (1972a) also reported that some children showed decreased focal abnormalities with medication, while Korein et al. (1971) found that children who evidenced asymmetries prior to medication showed greater asymmetry when CPZ was introduced. As to the significance of these findings Korein et al. (1971) saw no consistent relation between EEG changes under CPZ and either behavioral change or drug toxicity.

Findings similar to those with CPZ are reported by Saletu et al. (1975a), who noted that the administration of thiothixene, in conjunction with the antiparkinson drug trihexyphenidyl (Artane), resulted in a general slowing of the EEG wave frequencies consistent with a reduction in arousal, namely a decrease in the amount of fast alpha activity, an increase in the amount of slow alpha and theta activity and a decrease in slow beta. In contrast to the work with CPZ, this investigation showed a statistically significant correlation between one aspect of EEG change (increased theta) and clinical improvement, though this study is isolated and unreplicated.

EVOKED POTENTIALS (EP)

EP investigation of brain response to specific stimuli has been used by Saletu and his colleagues to study the effects of thioridazine (Mellaril) (Saletu et al., 1975b), fluphenazine (Anatensol, Modicate, Permitil, Prolixin) (Saletu et al., 1975a), and thiothixene (Navane) (Simeon et al., 1974) on the CNS of children. All three antipsychotic drugs have been reported to increase latencies of the secondary, nonspecific peaks of the visual EP. Since neuropsychiatrically impaired children often show shorter secondary EP response latencies (thought to reflect the clinically observed attention deficits) than do normal children (Saletu et al., 1975a), latency increases occurring in conjunction with antipsychotic pharmacotherapy appear to represent a normalization of the EP response with medication. This notion of normalization is supported by preliminary data from the above EP studies, which indicate that latency increases are correlated with improved behavior as judged by various psychometric scales.

Despite the promising note that these EP data provide for the future electrophysiological assessment of CNS change with antipsychotic drugs, the significance of the findings is weakened because of serious methodological problems in the various studies. For example, in the thioridazine investigation (Saletu et al., 1975b) the doses were so low as to preclude any significant behavioral effect. Consequently the obtained EP changes, even if replicable, are of questionable clinical significance. Regarding both the fluphenazine and thiothixene studies (Saletu et al., 1975a; Simeon et al., 1974), meaningful interpretation of the effects of these drugs on the EP is difficult because trihexyphenidyl (Artane) was administered concomitantly with the antipsychotic medication. This is not a trivial problem since, as the authors clearly demonstrate, trihexyphenidyl alone generates striking secondary EP latency changes which may interact with EP effects of neuroleptics. In summary, the EP changes that have been reported with antipsychotic drugs must be viewed as highly tentative and in need of corroboration.

SUMMARY

Future investigation of the utility of electrophysiological measures of assessing antipsychotic drug effects on the CNS in children must be more carefully executed with regard to dosage and plasma levels of medication, so that both EEG and EP techniques may be more profitably employed.

Activity Level

The consensus of the clinical literature (see below) suggests a reduction in activity level with most antipsychotics, but particularly with the sedative type antipsychotics such as CPZ and thioridazine. However, there are a few reports, especially in psychotic children, of increased activity and interest. Since there are few objective measures of activity level in these clinical studies, it is difficult to be sure of the effects. However, such evidence as there is, coupled with effects observed in animals, is in favor of a reduction in activity level, though as will be seen, unlike with the stimulants (see Chapter 6), this may reflect a general psychomotor slowing or quasi-sedative type effect which could, in certain circumstances, be undesirable (Sprague & Werry, 1971, 1974).

Cognition and Learning

This topic is reviewed in more detail in Chapter 3.

The effects of phenothiazines on such measures as intelligence tests, figure drawing, and paper-and-pencil maze performance have received considerable research attention with adult patients. Although there are some discrepant findings, the bulk of the evidence suggests that patients with thought disorders show improvement with the phenothiazines, whereas normal individuals (e.g., student volunteers) show deterioration (Barker, 1968). For the pediatric psychopharmacologist, the most important question is whether these drugs adversely affect learning in the *classroom*. Here the data are extraordinarily sparse. To our knowledge, only two studies (Freed et al., 1959; Gittelman-Klein, 1977; Gittelman-Klein & Klein, 1975; Gittelman-Klein et al., 1976b) have been conducted on the classroom performance of children receiving neuroleptic drugs.

In an early study Freed et al. (1959) investigated the effects of chlorpromazine and prochlorperazine (Compazine, Stemetil) among 5 matched groups of children who were of normal intelligence and not behaviorally impaired, but who were 3 or more years retarded in reading. The 5 treatment conditions—which covered a 10-week period—were: 1) placebo, 2) placebo and reading instruction, 3) chlorpromazine, 4) chlorpromazine and reading instruction, and 5) prochlorperazine and reading instruction. It was found that chlorpromazine plus reading instruction was superior to reading instruction alone, or chlorpromazine alone. Prochlorperazine also facilitated reading performance. While significant differences in favor of neuroleptics were found in this study, they were not striking; and in our opinion, do not warrant the authors' recommendation that neuroleptics may be useful for treating reading failure. Nevertheless, it is important to note that there was no evidence that classroom learning was impeded by neuroleptic medication.

In a much more recent study Gittelman-Klein (1977; Gittelmen-Klein & Klein, 1975; Gittelman-Klein et al., 1976b) examined the effects of thioridazine (Mellaril), methylphenidate (Ritalin), and placebo on achievement and psychometric test performance in hyperkinetic, reading retarded children. The sample included 155 children assigned to 4 treatment groups: 1) thioridazine, 2) thioridazine and methylphenidate, 3) methylphenidate, and 4) placebo. After 12 weeks of pharmacotherapy, thioridazine (relative to placebo) was found neither to enhance nor adversely affect scores on the various measures, though a number of significant gains were in evidence among the methylphenidate-treated group.

Investigations of drug effects on learning and memory in children, using laboratory measures, have often provided the basis for drawing inferences with regard to clinical effects. Unfortunately, as noted in Chapter 3, the clinical relevance of many such laboratory tasks to learning, attention and impulsivity in naturalistic environments such as the classroom remains undemonstrated. In the area of learning and cognition, most research has been conducted with stimulants. Such work as has been done with the neuroleptics has been reviewed by a number of authors, (e.g. Sprague & Werry, 1971, 1974; Werry, 1970) for different diagnostic groups. Sprague and Werry (1971) and Werry (1970) have concluded that in the laboratory situation neuroleptic drugs have typically been found to 1) increase response latency, 2) deteriorate task performance under conditions where the task is a simple, repetitive motor one, where the level of task difficulty is "optimal," and where memory processes are involved, and 3) have no consistent effect on motor activity. Sprague and Werry (1974) have reported that on various laboratory tasks thioridazine was found to: 1) depress learning, 2) marginally decrease performance on a repetitive task (marble dropping), and 3) decrease the latency of response among retarded children in a 2-choice discrimination task.

Helper et al. (1953) found that chlorpromazine interfered with paired-associate learning and was associated with decrements in Porteus maze mental age scores among a group of hospitalized children. However, in that study, serial learning, digit span tapping, dotting rates, and a number of retention measures pertaining to the paired-associates tasks were not affected. On the other hand, Freibergs et al. (1968) found that chlorpromazine, prescribed in moderate doses (37 to 150 mg/day), did not affect laboratory measures of concept learning among an outpatient group of hyperactive children. Although these investigators used a different learning task from that employed in the study by Helper et al. (1963), the latter researchers also used higher dosage levels (75-450 mg/day). Consequently, the discrepancy in chlorpromazine's effect on learning may have been dose-related. Recently, for example, Werry and Aman (1975) reported that haloperidol (Haldol, Serenace) in low doses (.025 mg/kg) facilitated performance among hyperactive children on measures of attention, memory, and motor activity, while higher doses (.05 mg/kg) produced slight deterioration in performance.

SUMMARY

Apparently, there are as yet insufficient data for drawing any firm conclusions regarding the effects of antipsychotic drug therapy on learning or academic performance of children. However, it is important to note that while laboratory type tests suggest some possible slowing and depression of function, in clinically prescribed doses the drugs do not seem to interfere with classroom learning, though studies are few. This discrepancy may be due to the stressed nature of the classroom, since adult studies suggest a drug x arousal interaction.

Behavior

See Clinical Indications.

Other Systems

See Treatment Emergent Effects.

TREATMENT EMERGENT SIDE EFFECTS

Obviously the distinction between clinical effects and TES is (apart from toxic or idiosyncratic effects) a matter of regarding one set of effects as desirable and others as unwanted.

Short-Term Effects

NERVOUS SYSTEM

1) *Drowsiness.* Transient drowsiness, apathy and lethargy of mild degree are perhaps the most common side effects of the antipsychotic compounds. They seem to be more usual following the administration of CPZ (Engelhardt et al., 1973) and thioridazine, but have also been reported with the piperazine group of phenothiazines, the thioxanthenes, and the butyrophenones. The incidence and the degree of these side effects seem to be dose related. Thus, Werry et al. (1976a) found that of 30 patients receiving a low dose of haloperidol, 4 showed mild drowsiness, while a higher dose of the same medication led to drowsiness in 18 of 30 chil-

dren (in 4 of them, the side effect was moderate to severe). In most children these symptoms will disappear after 2 or 3 weeks without dosage modification, but sometimes a reduction of the dose is necessary.

2) *Anticholinergic effects.* Reports of these effects are less common in children than in adults. Blurring of vision and dry mouth have occurred in children receiving CPZ (Solomons, 1965), thioridazine (Renard et al., 1962), and haloperidol (Werry et al., 1976a). Blurring of vision secondary to trifluoperazine (Stelazine) (Silberstein, 1965) and acetophenazine (Tindal) (Darling, 1963) have also been reported. In the study that most systematically sought side effects, Gittelman-Klein et al. (1976b) found that 22% of the children receiving thioridazine experienced mild to moderate dryness of the mouth, and 6% had nasal congestion. There was a decrease in frequency of these as the treatment continued.

Urinary retention, constipation, and abdominal pain are also probably related to anticholinergic activity. Abdominal pain, which is the most common of these symptoms, has been experienced by more than one-fifth of the children receiving CPZ (Greenberg, et al., 1972) and thioridazine (Gittelman-Klein et al., 1976b).

3) *Extrapyramidal effects.* The antipsychotic drugs can produce disorders of motor function and posturing called extrapyramidal symptoms (EPS) (see American College of Neuropsychopharmacology, 1973), because of their presumed origin in that part of the motor system concerned with muscle tone and modulation of movement. Although most antipsychotic drugs [with the possible exception of clozapine (Snyder et al., 1974)] can produce EPS, the type and frequency of these disorders appear to vary with the medication. Thioridazine seems to produce a smaller incidence both in cases where it has been given in therapeutic doses (Engelhardt et al., 1972) and in cases of intoxication (Engelhardt et al., 1972; Greenblatt & Shader, 1970). Haloperidol and the piperazine group of phenothiazines are believed to cause a higher incidence of akathisia and dystonic reactions. This differential effect has not yet been documented in a well-controlled study, but it is usually accepted by clinicians (Engelhardt et al., 1972), and it can be extrapolated from the findings of well-designed studies with similar populations. Thus, relatively high and clinically effective doses of thioridazine (6 mg/kg/day) produced tremor in 6% of a group of hyperkinetic children (Gittelman-Klein et al., 1976b), while relatively low and marginally effective doses of haloperidol (0.05 mg/kg/day) produced EPS (mainly acute dystonias) in 33% of another such sample (Werry et al., 1976a). It has been postulated (Snyder et al., 1974) that this discrepancy might be explained by

the different anticholinergic blocking potency exhibited by antipsychotic agents at muscarinic receptor sites. Clozapine and thioridazine exhibit relatively high anticholinergic properties, while haloperidol and the piperazine group of the phenothiazines are weaker in this respect. As discussed earlier, it may also be related to striatal dopamine blocking ability, weak with clozapine.

Acute EPS take three common forms:

a) *Dystonic reactions* are characterized by the abrupt contraction of a muscle or group of muscles. Head and neck are more commonly involved, with resulting torticolis (head turned to a side), retrocolis (head turned to back), and jaw pulled to side. There can also be facial grimacing and distortion, tongue protrusion or curling, spasms of throat muscles, with difficulty in speech and swallowing, and occasionally in breathing. Oculogyric crisis (fixed upward gaze), opisthotonos (arching of the back), scoliosis, dystonic gait, and shoulder and leg movements have also been described.

These dystonic reactions are very dramatic and frightening both to the patient and his relatives. They usually appear during the first 72 hours of treatment, and children seem to be more susceptible than adults (Ayd, 1972). Because of the abrupt onset and the dramatic neuromuscular manifestations of the dystonic reactions, they can be mistaken for hysteria, seizures, tetanus, meningitis, encephalitis and poliomyelitis. Patients with these reactions sometimes have been hospitalized and subjected to many diagnostic and treatment procedures which would have been unnecessary had the correct diagnosis been made.

Parents should be forewarned of the possibility of dystonic reactions. If they occur, the treating physician should be informed that the child is receiving an antipsychotic medication so that the proper treatment may be provided. Such treatment consists of antiparkinsonian drugs as outlined in Table 1. For example, the acute episode can be treated with 1 to 2 mg IM of benztropine mesylate (Cogentin) which may be repeated in one-half hour if improvement is not complete. Diphenhydramine hydrochloride (Benadryl) in doses of 25 to 100 mg IM (maximum 5 mg/kg/24 hrs) is also very effective. Lying in a quiet darkened room expedites recovery. During the next 48 hours, oral benztropine (1-2 mg), given every 4 to 6 hours usually controls the symptoms. In an occasional case, the antipsychotic medication has to be decreased or discontinued, but the symptoms are usually benign, shortlived and controllable. After 48 hours, the benztropine should be reduced to 1 to 2 mg, given 2 or 3 times a day, and discontinued gradually over several weeks or as soon as the symptoms allow.

Dystonic reactions have been reported in children receiving CPZ (Ehrlich, 1959) thioridazine (Oettinger & Simonds, 1962), trifluoperazine (Stelazine) (Engelhardt et al., 1972; LeVann, 1959), per-

TABLE 1

Antiparkinson Agents

Name	Available	Oral Dose	Parenteral Dose
Biperidin (Akineton)	Tabs. 2mg Amp. 5mgxcc	2-6mgxday	2.5-5 mg per dose IM
Benztropine (Cogentin)	Tabs. 0.5-1-2mg Amp. 1mgxcc	1-6mgxday	1-2 mg per dose IM
Trihexyphenidyl (Artane)	Tabs. 2-5mg	2-6mgxday	
Procyclidine (Kemadrin)	Tabs. 2-5mg	2-15mgxday	
Diphenhydramine (Benadryl)	Amp. 10-50mgxcc		25-50 mg per dose IM Maximum: 5mg/kg/day or 150mgxday

phenazine (Trilafon) (Bellman, 1974; Eisenberg et al., 1961), fluphenazine (Engelhardt et al., 1972; Shaw et al., 1963), haloperidol (Cunningham et al., 1968; Faretra et al., 1970; Lucas, 1967; Werry et al., 1976a), thiothixene (Navane) (Campbell et al., 1970; Wolpert et al., 1967) and molindone (Campbell et al., 1971b).

b) The most uncomfortable EPS of *akathisia* is characterized by motor restlessness and an appearance of continuous agitation often mistaken for anxiety based restlessness. Common manifestations are inability to sit still, rocking and shifting of weight while standing, and shifting of legs and tapping of feet while sitting. Akathisia is the most common extrapyramidal reaction in adults (Ayd, 1961), most cases being seen in middle-aged females and appearing during the initial 3 months of therapy. Akathisia has been reported in children receiving CPZ (Engelhardt et al., 1972), trifluoperazine (Engelhardt et al., 1972), fluphenazine (Faretra et al., 1970), acetophenazine (Tindal) (Darling, 1963), and thiothixene (Fish et al., 1969b; Wolpert et al., 1967). Hyperactivity or restlessness, which were probably undiagnosed akathisia, have been reported in children receiving trifluoperazine (Hunter & Stephenson, 1963; Shaw et al., 1963), perphenazine (Kaplitz, 1966), thiothixene (Campbell et al., 1970) and molindone (Campbell et al., 1971b). Akathisia can be treated with oral antiparkinson agents; however, if severe it should be managed in the manner described above for dystonic reactions. Antiparkinson medication will probably need to be continued longer than with dystonic reactions.

c) Extrapyramidal *parkinsonian reactions* are clinically very similar to the symptoms occurring with Parkinson's disease, namely tremor, "pill-rolling" movements of the fingers, "cogwheel" rigidity, and stiffness of voluntary movement. This is often associated with masklike facies, shuffling gait, slow monotonous speech and micrographia (small, crabbed writing). The latter may be the first noticeable sign and should be particularly useful diagnostically in children. Symptoms usually appear during the first three months of therapy, occurring more frequently in older patients. They have been reported in children receiving CPZ (Engelhardt et al., 1972; Flaherty, 1955; Hunt et al., 1956), perphenazine (Kaplitz, 1966; Molling et al., 1962), fluphenazine (Engelhardt et al., 1973), thioridazine (Gittelman-Klein et al., 1976b); acetophenazine (Darling, 1963), perphenazine (Suckling, 1966), haloperidol (Faretra et al., 1970; Lucas, 1967), and thiothixene (Campbell et al., 1970). In contrast to dystonic reactions, these reactions are usually mild in children, and they are easily alleviated by the oral antiparkinson agents already mentioned or by a decrease in dosage.

4) *Behavior and Mood.* Various signs and symptoms of mood or behavioral impairment have been described in children receiving antipsychotics. CPZ has occasionally produced increased irritability, excitability, and perceptual distortions (Fish, 1960), excitation, euphoria, and worsening of psychotic behavior (Campbell et al., 1972a), and depression (Fish, 1960; Hunt et al., 1956). One case of irritability, insomnia, and visual hallucinations was observed by the present authors in a child receiving 150 mg/day of CPZ. The symptoms disappeared in less than 24 hours following the discontinuation of the medication. Thioridazine has produced euphoria (Allen et al., 1963), depression, irritability, and outburst of anger (Gittelman-Klein et al., 1976b). Similar mood changes have been described with trifluoperazine (Shaw et al., 1963). Haloperidol has caused depression (LeVann 1969), emotional upset and confusion (Werry et al., 1976a), and visual hallucinations (LeVann, 1971). Impulsivity and worsening of psychotic symptoms have been reported in children receiving thiothixene (Campbell et al., 1970); and euphoria is reported with molindone (Campbell et al., 1971b).

5) *Seizures.* Both grand and petit mal seizures have been reported during treatment with CPZ. In one study (Tarjan et al., 1957) of 82 children with clinical epilepsy and mental retardation treated with CPZ, 12 had a rapid and significant increase in the number of seizures. Hunt et al. (1956) have described a similar problem in 2 patients, who required an increase in the dose of phenobarbital to reestablish adequate control of their seizures. In addition, Fabich (1955) found experimentally induced changes in the EEG of epileptic children and adults with CPZ. Consequently, it seems advisable to use caution in prescribing CPZ for children with a history of epilepsy. There are occasional reports of seizures with

other antipsychotic agents, such as fluphenazine (Arnold & Magnin, 1967), and trifluoperazine (Engelhardt et al., 1972; Hunter & Stephenson, 1963). On the other hand, thioridazine has been less frequently associated with an increase in seizures. For example, in a group of 246 children with both convulsive and behavior disorders, Oettinger and Simonds (1962) found that only one patient showed an increased number of seizures. In another instance, status epilepticus occurred in an epileptic boy receiving thioridazine, though an increase in anticonvulsant medication succeeded in controlling the seizures (Alderton & Hoddinott, 1964). Furthermore, thioridazine has been found to decrease seizures in some children with convulsive disorder (Baldwin & Kenny, 1966; Kamm & Mandel, 1967; Pregelj & Barkauskas, 1967). It would seem that thioridazine is the drug of choice in epileptic patients for whom antipsychotic drugs are indicated.

BLOOD

1) *Agranulocytosis.* This is a potentially fatal complication in which certain white blood cells disappear from the blood, increasing vulnerability to infections. It seems to be less common in adults now than in the past and has most often been associated with the high-dose drugs (e.g. chlorpromazine and thioridazine), being virtually unknown with the more potent antipsychotics (such as haloperidol, fluphenazine and thiothixene). Agranulocytosis occurs typically in middle aged and elderly caucasian women, usually appearing between 20 and 30 days after the initiation of treatment. If it has not occurred during the first three months, it is not likely to occur (Pisciotta, 1971). Despite the pharmacological attractiveness of clozapine, recent reports indicating both fatal agranulocytosis and serious leucopenia make it unlikely that it will find a role in pediatric psychopharmacology (cf. Senn et al., 1977).* The only case reported in children (Eveloff, 1966) was discovered in a 14-year-old schizophrenic girl after 2½ years of treatment with CPZ (400-800 mg/day). She recovered with medical treatment after discontinuation of CPZ.

2) *Leukopenia* (reduced numbers of white cells). This side effect has been described in as many as one-third of adult patients receiving phenothiazines. However, the white cell counts ultimately rise spontaneously to normal levels even when treatment is continued (Pisciotta, 1971). Transitory leukopenia has been reported in 9 of 34 children receiving thioridazine (Baldwin & Peters, 1968). In all cases, there was a return to normal

---

* Clozapine has now been withdrawn by the manufacturer but its unique pharmacological properties justify its discussion.—(Ed.)

within two to four weeks without discontinuing the medication. Transitory leukopenia has also been reported accompanying the administration of thiothixene (Campbell et al., 1970).

3) *Eosinophilia* has been reported in children receiving thioridazine (Baldwin & Peters, 1968).

In contrast to these rare reports of blood abnormalities, many studies have reported no changes accompanying the use of CPZ (Blair & Herold, 1955; Campbell et al., 1972a; Freed & Peifer, 1956; Greenberg et al., 1972; Hunt et al., 1956), thioridazine (LeVann, 1959; Shaw et al., 1963), fluphenazine (Engelhardt et al., 1973; Faretra et al., 1970; LaVeck et al., 1960; Shaw et al., 1963), haloperidol (Burk & Menolascino, 1968; Engelhardt et al., 1973; Faretra et al., 1970; Ucer & Kreger, 1969), and molindone (Campbell et al., 1971b).

Because there is no evidence to suggest that frequent monitoring of the leukocyte count during the first several weeks of treatment (when the abnormalities are most likely to occur) leads to early detection, it has been suggested (Hollister, 1976) that one count prior to treatment and occasional checks are sufficient. However, leukocyte counts should also be taken after the discovery of any physical illness accompanied by fever.

LIVER

In adults, *jaundice* occurs mostly with CPZ and usually appears during the first month of treatment. The laboratory findings are those of obstructive jaundice. Liver function tests such as alkaline phosphatase, bromosulfophthalein retention and serum conjugated bilirubin are all commonly elevated. There are no apparent reports of jaundice following the administration of antipsychotic drugs to children.

Abnormal liver function tests are found more frequently in adults than is frank jaundice. These abnormalities are often transitory, and unless serial examinations show increasing abnormality, it is prudent not to overinterpret them. This is especially true when a single laboratory test is abnormal, as this may be based on laboratory or biological variability (Chalmers, 1965).

Majluf (1957) found that some children receiving CPZ developed abnormal liver function tests without clinical symptoms. LeVann (1971) reported slight elevation in serum alkaline phosphatase in about 80% of a group of patients receiving CPZ or haloperidol. There were no clinical signs of hepatic dysfunction, and on retesting only about 30% of the patients had abnormal results, most of which were within two or three units of normal. The author speculated that this high prevalence of abnormal results might be secondary to hemolysis. Ucer and Kreger (1969) noted that 2 patients receiving haloperidol and 2 receiving thioridazine showed slight transient elevation of glutamic pyruvic transaminase. Many studies which have included liver function tests have reported no abnormality with CPZ (Campbell et al., 1972a; Greenberg, et al., 1972; Hunt et al., 1956; Miksztal, 1956), trifluoperazine (Hunter & Stephenson, 1963; LeVann, 1959), fluphenazine (Engelhardt et al., 1973; Faretra et al., 1970; LaVeck et al., 1960), haloperidol (Burk & Menolascino, 1968; Engelhardt et al., 1973; Faretra et al., 1970; LeVann, 1969), thiothixene (Campbell et al., 1970), and molindone (Campbell et al., 1971b).

In short, liver effects do not seem to be common or important in children.

URINARY SYSTEM

Symptoms ranging from frequency, urgency, and polyuria to enuresis and incontinence have been reported in children receiving antipsychotic agents (Engelhardt et al., 1972). In one study involving 5 different neuroleptics, thioridazine produced the highest incidence of these symptoms (Engelhardt et al., 1972). Gittelman-Klein et al. (1976b) also found that, in a group of children receiving thioridazine, mild to moderate enuresis was the most frequent and troublesome side effect, reaching a frequency of 34% at the end of the fourth week (mean dose = 193 mg), and decreasing to 17% at the end of the twelfth week (mean dose = 160 mg). Renshaw (1971) reported 2 cases of urinary incontinence (day and night) with thioridazine, which disappeared 3 days after the medication was discontinued.

Fluphenazine (Engelhardt et al., 1972; Serrano & Forbis, 1973) and haloperidol (Serrano & Forbis, 1973) have also produced enuresis. On the other hand, some children who were enuretic stopped their bedwetting while receiving thioridazine (Engelhardt et al., 1972).

CARDIOVASCULAR EFFECTS

Antipsychotic drugs produce fewer cardiovascular problems in children than in adults. Severe tachycardia, secondary to the use of CPZ, was reported by McLaughlin (1964), but other studies have reported normal pulse and blood pressure in children receiving CPZ (Miksztal, 1956) and thioridazine (LeVann, 1961). Aman and Werry (1975), in a well-designed study, found that consistent with claims in adults (Ayd, 1972), haloperidol (0.035 mg/kg) produced little or no effect on cardiovascular function in children, apart from a slight and transient increase in heart rate. Electrocardiographic changes have been reported in adults receiving thioridazine (Wedkos, 1967). However, Wolpert and Farr (1975) did not find any electrocardiographic changes in children receiving thioridazine, CPZ, perphenazine and chlorprothixene (Taractan).

SKIN REACTIONS

Rashes of an allergic type are the most common skin disorders caused by antipsychotic drugs, but are not at all frequent. They have been reported in children receiving CPZ and perphenazine (Fish, 1960), thioridazine (Wallinga, 1963), fluphenazine and haloperidol (Faretra et al., 1970), and thiothixene (Campbell et al., 1970). Other allergic reactions have been reported with CPZ, such as edema of tongue, glotis and lips, needing the administration of cortisone (Fish, 1960), edema of face and ankles (Horenstein, 1957; Hunt et al., 1956) and urticaria (Hunt et al., 1956). Urticaria has also been reported with fluphenazine (Denhoff & King, 1965). Photosensitivity has been reported following the administration of CPZ (Werry et al., 1966) and thioridazine (Engelhardt et al., 1972). This latter reaction can be prevented by the use of sun screen lotions.

Long-term Effects

WEIGHT CHANGE

Increase of appetite with resulting weight gain is a common problem in children receiving antipsychotic drugs. Thioridazine was found to produce weight increase more often than CPZ, trifluoperazine, and fluphenazine in one study (Engelhardt et al., 1972), but in another, in a group of children receiving CPZ for eight weeks, 93% gained up to 11 lbs in weight (Greenberg et al., 1972). Thiothixene and haloperidol have also produced this side effect (Engelhardt et al., 1973; Wolpert et al., 1967).

In a study on the effects of prolonged phenothiazine intake (McAndrew et al., 1972), the weight of children receiving thioridazine, CPZ or trifluoperazine was compared to that of unmedicated controls. After 3 months, 29 out of 30 children receiving thioridazine had gained weight (median gain = 10.5 lbs), and this gain was statistically significant ($p < .001$). Although many children receiving CPZ also gained weight, some lost weight and the median increase (4 lbs) did not reach significance. In the group receiving trifluoperazine, half of the children gained while the rest lost weight.

Weight changes are thus not uncommon, especially weight gain with thioridazine.

MOVEMENT DISORDERS

There are 7 reports of persistent movement disorders associated with neuroleptic therapy in children. Angle and McIntire (1968) describe the case of a brain damaged 10-year-old child who suffered irreversible torticollis, scoliosis secondary to dystonia of the neck and back, and dystonia of the arms and facial muscles following the accidental ingestion of a phenothiazine. Dabbous and Bergman (1966) report the case of a 5-year-old who was ingesting phenothiazines chronically when he developed dystonic symptoms. Shields and Bray (1976) describe persistent severe dystonia and opisthotonos in a 5½-year-old child who received haloperidol for Sydenham's Chorea. Unlike acute extrapyramidal symptoms, these reactions persisted despite antiparkinson therapy—suggesting some similarity etiologically to *tardive dyskinesia* in adults. This condition, consisting of stereotyped involuntary movements of a choreo-athetotic nature, such as lipsmacking, tongue protrusion, etc., most often in facial muscles but sometimes involving the extremities, is an irreversible neurological disorder, possibly due to damage in the basal ganglia, appearing usually in patients on long-term, high dose antipsychotic medication, though a few instances have been reported after short-term or relatively modest dosage. It is said to be commoner in older, female patients, particularly where there is already some brain damage (e.g., senility). It can be masked to some extent by the antipsychotic medication causing it, becoming apparent only after cessation. It is thought to be due to post synaptic dopamine sensitization and there is an unsubstantiated belief that it may be commoner with drugs more prone to cause acute extrapyramidal symptoms.

McAndrew et al., (1972), and the Engelhardt group (Engelhardt, 1974; Polizos et al., 1973) have described a more formal syndrome of dyskinesia in children associated with the cessation of neuroleptic treatment. In the study by McAndrew et al., 10 institutionalized children, of a total of 200 on medication, developed dyskinesias after phenothiazines were discontinued. Dyskinetic symptoms were noted from 3 to 10 days after discontinuation of the drugs, and unlike tardive dyskinesia they subsided in 3 to 12 months. The prominent movements, which again differed from those typical of tardive dyskinesia (see above), involved the upper extremities, were rhythmical and myoclonic-like, and more evident distally than proximally. Six of the children had facial tics during the first month post-treatment and akathisia was also often present. As with adult patients showing tardive dyskinesias, these children had been on high doses of antipsychotics for long periods of time.

Polizos et al. (1973) report that 14 of the 34 children on phenothiazines and haloperidol developed dyskinetic symptoms within 15 days after drug withdrawal, whether this was done abruptly or slowly. Involuntary movements analogous to those seen among adults with tardive dyskinesia were observed in the children; however a number of differences were noted: 1) there was only one instance of oral dyskinesia in the 14 children; 2) there were ataxia and choreiform movements such as those found in Huntington's Chorea; 3) children showed myoclonic and hemiballistic-like movements (body torsion), posturing, body and head rocking; and 4) these children had received relatively brief neuroleptic therapy. In half of the group that exhibited these symptoms, administration of a new neuroleptic agent resulted in disappearance of the movements. In the other half, the symptoms resolved spontaneously. Fluphenazine (Anatensol, Modicate, Prolixin, Permitil) was the drug most implicated (8 of 10 children on that compound developed the withdrawal syndrome). The least implicated drug was thioridazine (Mellaril) (1 of 9 children affected). Other drugs causing the withdrawal syndrome among these children included haloperidol (Haldol, Serenace) (2 of 6), trifluoperazine (Stelazine) (1 of 3) and thiothixene (Navane) (2 of 6).

In a more recent communication, Engelhardt (1974) reported 141 instances of drug withdrawal during the treatment of 47 children involving 9 different neuroleptics. After therapy was discontinued, neurological withdrawal symptoms were observed in 48% of the children. When they occurred, symptoms were manifest during the first 29 days post-medication. Oral dyskinesia, the most common symptom in adult patients, occurred in only 16% of the children, whereas ataxia was found in 52 of the 68 instances of drug withdrawal. The mean latency period for the occurrence of symptoms following drug withdrawal was found to be 12 days. In 38% of the children, the symptoms remitted spontaneously, the mean duration of the dyskinesias being 15 days, with a range of 5 to 85 days. In the remaining children, a new neuroleptic agent had to be instituted due to the severity of the withdrawal symptoms or their psychiatric condition. Within two weeks after the reinstitution of neuroleptic therapy, these children showed a remission of withdrawal symptoms. With regard to the relative toxicity of the drugs, fluphenazine was implicated in 79% of withdrawal instances, followed by haloperidol (62%), thiothixene and mesoridazine (50% each), trifluoperazine and thioridazine (33% each), and chlorpromazine (31%). In the above study, the mean treatment duration prior to drug withdrawal was 32 weeks.

Because of the symptomatological differences, its invariant relationship with drug cessation and the reversibility in children, Engelhardt has suggested the term Withdrawal Emergent Symptoms (WES) rather than tardive dyskinesia when referring to this condition. Its relationship to tardive dyskinesia of which it might be prodromal remains to be clarified.

Recently Paulson et al. (1975), reported a 4-year followup of 21 children with mild to moderate symptoms of true tardive dyskinesia. All patients had received at least intermittent doses of phenothiazines during the intervening years. Five patients were lost to follow-up. The remaining patients all continued to show the pattern of tardive dyskinesia typical of adults. These authors caution that because of the widespread use of phenothiazines among children, a substantial public health risk of tardive dyskinesia may exist.

EYE AND SKIN COMPLICATIONS

Corneal edema and haziness were found in a child treated chronically with CPZ (Geiger & Lesser, 1967). Reduction in dosage resulted in almost complete reversal of ocular findings within a short period of time. One case of corneal pigmentation and slight blue skin coloring in an 11-year-old patient was reported by Goldman (1968). The child had been receiving CPZ until 6 months prior to the discovery of the symptoms, had also received thioridazine and other unspecified phenothiazines.

Lens and corneal stippling has been found in 5 children who had been chronically treated with phenothiazines (McAndrew et al., 1972). These changes are generally mild and do not produce impairment of vision. Nevertheless, it would seem advisable to perform slit lamp examinations in children who receive high and long-term doses of phenothiazines.

Skin discoloration similar to that seen in adults has been mentioned in children receiving CPZ (Goldman, 1968; Majluf, 1957).

INTERACTIONS WITH OTHER DRUGS

The interactions between pharmacologic agents is an area of increasing clinical concern. Drugs may interfere with the hepatic metabolism of other drugs or displace each other from tissue binding sites. This occasionally results in toxicity reactions or diminished therapeutic efficacy. The pharmacotherapist will require a handbook of drug interactions such as that by Swindler (1971) for consultation when ideally infrequent polypharmacy is required. In the following only some of the more important interactions of antipsychotic drugs are identified.

Antipsychotics (Major Tranquilizers, Neuroleptics)

CNS Depressants

Antipsychotic drugs potentiate the action of other central nervous system depressants. Thus they should be used cautiously in patients who receive drugs such as anesthetics, antihistaminics, analgesics, barbiturates, hypnotics, narcotics, sedatives, and other tranquilizers.

Anticholinergics

Antipsychotic drugs have atropine-like effects which are additive to anticholinergic drugs. Therefore, their combination can produce or aggravate blurred vision, dry mouth, urinary retention, and *narrow angle* glaucoma. However, they do not affect wide angle glaucoma which is more common in children. They can also produce atropinic or belladonna poisoning type psychosis, manifested by delirium and hallucinations, accompanied by tachycardia, wide pupils, and flushed face.

Tricyclic Antidepressants

In general, both groups tend to lower the seizure threshold, and their combination should be used with great care in epileptic patients.

Vasopressor Agents

Antipsychotic drugs block part of the effect of epinephrine and metaraminol (Aramine) and the combination can aggravate hypotension. Norepinephrine (Levophed) does not have this problem and is therefore the drug of choice in any hypotensive state where the child is on antipsychotics.

Diuretics

Thiazide diuretics given to a patient on phenothiazines can cause severe hypotension and shock.

Antihelmintics

The combination of piperazine and phenothiazines can cause convulsions. This interaction is obviously one of the more important in children.

Anticonvulsants (see Chapter 9)

The antipsychotic drugs potentiate the sedative effects of phenobarbital but not their anticonvulsant action. Therefore, phenobarbital should not be decreased when antipsychotic drugs are prescribed. CPZ and prochlorperazine (Compazine, Stemetil) have been found to increase the plasma levels of phenytoin sodium (Dilantin) in a few patients (Kutt & McDowell, 1968). The authors have observed a case of phenytoin intoxication in a child who was receiving thioridazine.

CLINICAL INDICATIONS

The antipsychotic drugs have been found to be useful in the treatment of the following clinical syndromes.

Pervasive Developmental Disorders
(Childhood Psychoses)

It is difficult to interpret the studies of antipsychotics in the childhood psychoses because of poorly defined diagnostic and clinical criteria and inconsistent terminology. Most often, psychotic children are of necessity given the catch-all diagnosis of *childhood schizophrenia*, because this is the only category in the current (1977) American and International Diagnostic Classifications, though this will soon change (see Chapter 5).

The studies rarely separate the commonest *early infantile autism* from the other rarer childhood psychoses, whereas evidence suggests that it is quite distinctive from psychoses after 18 months and before 5 years and after 5 years (Kolvin, 1970). It is more than possible that the various psychoses have different etiologies or pathophysiologies, and, as has been suggested (Fish et al., 1966), differential responses to pharmacotherapy. This suggestion awaits documentation in a well-designed and controlled study. Despite these problems, it would seem that the combined findings of the studies (both uncontrolled and controlled), which are reviewed below, strongly suggest that these medications are safe and effective for the *behavioral management* of these severely impaired children, though not *antipsychotic* in the sense of controlling the disease as they are in adults.

Very soon after its introduction in 1952, CPZ was used with children. In a placebo-controlled study, Freedman et al. (1955) found improvement in 57% of a group of schizophrenic children treated with 30 to 100 mg of CPZ, while only 38% of those receiving placebo had a similar result. He suggested that the drug was especially useful in the hyperkinetic or agitated psychotic child. Other early uncontrolled studies confirmed the usefulness of CPZ (Hunt et al., 1956; Miksztal, 1956). However, Hunt found that adolescent schizophrenics with an acute onset responded much better to the drug than did a chronic subgroup whose illness had started in childhood.

As other antipsychotic medications became available, they were applied to the treatment of children. Fish (1960), after treating schizophrenic children with various antipsychotics (chlorpromazine, prochlorpromazine, perphenazine and trifluoperazine) in private practice, reported that drug therapy was a safe and useful *adjunct* in the treatment of such patients. However, Fish (1960) noted that a subgroup who showed mental retardation, hyperactivity, and features of early infantile autism became too easily sedated by even low doses of CPZ (1 mg/kg). In contrast, trifluoperazine (Stelazine) in average doses as low as 0.02 mg/kg, had a stimulating effect, occasionally accompanied by marked improvement in some cases.

In an uncontrolled study, Silberstein et al. (1965) reported that through the use of trifluoperazine they were able to prevent the hospitalization of psychotic children. Similarly, uncontrolled studies with other medications, such as acetophenazine (Tindal) (Darling, 1963), haloperidol (Haldol, Serenace) (LeVann, 1969) and thiothixene (Navane) (Fish et al., 1969b) have found these compounds useful for children and adolescents diagnosed as having schizophrenia.

Engelhardt et al. (1972), reported 5 single-blind studies in which various phenothiazines were administered to severely impaired outpatient children who received diagnoses of either childhood schizophrenia or early infantile autism. These studies, although not truly blind, used very systematic observations, involved relatively long periods of treatment with each drug (4-5 months), and employed a regimen of increased doses until effectiveness was achieved or toxicity outweighed improvement. The mean daily doses were 214 mg for CPZ, 288 mg for thioridazine, 35 mg for trifluoperazine, 20 mg for prochlorperazine, and 12.5 mg for fluphenazine. The investigators concluded that optimal daily doses for psychotic children seemed to be the same as those used with adult schizophrenics. They found that the drugs were effective in improving the following discrete areas of functioning: activity level, frustration tolerance, eating and sleeping habits, movement, and affect. There were some differences between drugs, but the different number of trials for each of them made it inadvisable to draw any final conclusions. Nonetheless, CPZ seemed to be less and fluphenazine more effective than anticipated. This supports the experience of Fish and her collaborators (Campbell et al., 1972; Fish et al., 1966) as to the superior effects of the piperazine group of drugs over CPZ. Essentially, *the action of the antipsychotic agents in the population of severely impaired children treated by Engelhardt et al. (1972) was to make them more manageable and easier to live with, not to cure the underlying psychosis.*

In another long-term, uncrossed placebo-controlled study, Ojeda (1970) administered thioridazine (average 250 mg) to a group of emotionally disturbed inpatient children, most of whom were diagnosed as having schizophrenia. The drug-treated group showed greater improvement than the placebo group in adjustment to school and to hospital. At the end of the study, only 20% of the drug-treated as opposed to 50% of the placebo group were still in the hospital.

The effectiveness of antipsychotic drugs has continued to be demonstrated in better controlled investigations. In a double-blind study by Fish and Shapiro (1965) three groups of diagnostically mixed hospitalized children, matched for age and symptoms severity, were treated with CPZ, the antihistamine diphenhydramine hydrochloride (Benadryl), and placebo. While none of the more severely impaired children (many of whom were autistic) improved in placebo, 80% demonstrated positive changes on CPZ. Of the less severely impaired patients, 43% showed improvement on placebo, and 60% responded to CPZ.

Similar results were obtained in another double-blind study (Fish et al., 1966), where trifluoperazine (mean dose = 0.1 to 0.7 mg/kg/day) was administered to preschool children diagnosed as retarded, autistic and schizophrenic. A control group received increasing doses of amphetamine, but when irritability appeared, placebo was substituted. The most severely impaired drug-treated children showed significantly greater increase in the rate and degree of improvement than did those in the control group. However, in the milder group (whose speech was better) this was not the case, and 2 of the 4 speaking children treated with trifluoperazine became even worse. It was also found that the children without speech (presumably autistic) tolerated higher doses of trifluoperazine (mean = 0.7 mg/kg) than did those who had speech (mean dose = 0.2 mg/kg).

Two double-blind studies have evaluated the effectiveness of both fluphenazine and haloperidol in psychotic children. The results will be discussed for each drug separately. Faretra et al. (1970) treated 60 inpatient children with pyschotic symptoms, most of whom had received the diagnosis of childhood schizophrenia. The children were randomly assigned to either fluphenazine or haloperidol treatment groups. Of the *fluphenazine* treated group (maximum dose = 3.75 mg), 67% showed some overall improvement, but in only half of these was this moderate or marked in degree. Of the symptomatic clusters evaluated (anxiety, regressive behavior, assaultiveness, provocativeness, and autism) only *anxiety* improved significantly. In the other double-blind study (Engelhardt et al., 1973), outpatient children with a diagnosis of schizophrenia (19 of whom were diagnosed as autistic) were randomly assigned to either fluphenazine or haloperidol for 12 weeks. In the *fluphenazine* group (mean dose = 10.4), 93% were rated as very much improved or much improved on the Clinical Global Improvement rating scale (see Chapter 2). On a 23-item children's psychiatric scale, this group was rated as "significantly improved" on 13 items.

The results obtained with *haloperidol* in the 2 above studies were basically similar. Faretra et al. (1970), using 0.75 to 3.75 mg/day of haloperidol, found that 57% of the children improved, and in 24%, this improvement was marked or moderate. Anxiety, autism, and provocativeness improved significantly while assaultiveness and regressive behavior did not. Engelhardt et al. (1973) found that 87% of the children in the haloperidol group (mean dose = 10.4 mg/day) received global ratings of much improved or very much improved, and that on over half the items of the children's psychiatric scale they were rated as significantly improved. Another butyrophenone found effective in psychotic children is trifluperidol (Campbell et al., 1972b; Fish et al., 1969a). However, this drug has a very narrow therapeutic index, and it is not presently available in the United States.

Thiothixene (Navane), a member of the thioxanthene group, has been found to be a safe and effective agent in the treatment of psychotic children (Campbell et al., 1970; Fish et al., 1969b; Simeon et al., 1974; Waizer et al., 1972; Wolpert et al., 1967). Optimal daily doses have ranged from 1 to 30 mg (mean doses from 2 to 16.9 mg/day). Side effects were similar to those found with the phenothiazines.

The only study with children in which the dihydroindolone, molindone, was used suggests that this drug might be useful in the treatment of childhood psychosis (Campbell et al., 1971b). Stimulant effects were seen at therapeutic levels (mean dose = 1.5 mg/day), and all anergic children showed increased motor vigor and initiative.

SUMMARY

While it seems that antipsychotic drugs effective in the treatment of schizophrenic adults may serve a useful role in the management of the psychotic child, as in adults, superiority of any particular compound has not been well demonstrated. Two double-blind comparisons have found that overall effectiveness was similar for haloperidol and fluphenazine (Engelhardt et al., 1973; Faretra et al., 1970). In a third such study, trifluoperazine and thiothixene were also found to be equally effective (Wolpert, 1967). Less well-controlled research has suggested that *autistic* children might respond better to the more potent drugs such as trifluoperazine (Fish et al., 1966), thiothixene (Campbell et al., 1970), molindone (Campbell et al., 1971b), and perhaps fluphenazine (Engelhardt et al., 1972). It has also been suggested that CPZ is too sedative and perhaps less effective for the same group of children (Fish, 1960). Since these differential effects are based more on clinical experience than on controlled studies, no final conclusions can be drawn at present. *In conclusion, it should be reiterated that the antipsychotics appear useful only in the management of psychotic children, making them less withdrawn, less overactive, less anxious, less agitated and more tractable, but do not seem truly antipsychotic.*

Behavior Problems in Mentally Retarded Children

The behavior problems of the mentally retarded child are difficult to treat, because they are often complicated by social immaturity, physical handicaps and socio-familial rejection. Many drugs have been tried but it would seem that the sedative phenothiazines (CPZ and thioridazine) are the most commonly used. This was clearly demonstrated in a survey of the use of drugs in institutions for mentally retarded persons (Lipman, 1970) which revealed that 51% of the residents were receiving pyschoactive medication, with CPZ and thioridazine predominating. Excellent reviews of the literature on the use of drugs with retarded populations have been provided by Freeman (1970) and Sprague and Werry (1971, 1974). In the present discussion, only some of the most typical or the better-designed studies will be described.

In one of the earliest studies, Bair and Herold (1955) administered CPZ to 10 institutionalized children with difficult management problems, and employed a matched control group. It was concluded that 90% of the drug-treated group improved in behavior. Craft (1957) found CPZ to be significantly better than placebo in reducing hyperactivity and improving social behavior in mentally retarded children. Other uncontrolled or poorly designed studies have reported high rates of improvement with CPZ in retarded patients (Esen & Darling, 1956; MacColl, 1956; Rettig, 1955; Tarjan et al., 1957).

Another group of uncontrolled studies compared CPZ with the now generally disused (because of side effects) reserpine in mentally retarded children with severe behavior problems. Both drugs were found equally effective (Horenstein, 1957; Johnston & Martin, 1957; Sprogis et al., 1957; Wolfson, 1957). In a double-blind study, Adamson et al. (1958) treated 40 mentally retarded patients, ranging in age from 8 to 40 years with CPZ, reserpine, and a combination of the drugs. A placebo group matched for age, sex, mental age, etiology, and type of management problem was used as a control. Although all groups, including the placebo group, improved in behavior, the drug-treated groups improved somewhat more. There were no changes on intelligence tests.

In another controlled study using placebo, Hunter and Stephenson (1963) treated severely subnormal children with CPZ and trifluoperazine. They found significant improvement in hyperactivity and abnormal behavior. In a more recent study (LeVann, 1971), CPZ was found significantly less effective than haloperidol with mildly to moderately retarded children.

The effects of CPZ on motor behavior in retarded children have been explored very carefully by Hollis. In his first study (Hollis, 1968), he found that CPZ stopped rocking behavior in one institutionalized retarded female without interfering with a ball-pulling behavior that had been taught to her. In a second study Hollis and St. Omer (1972) found that acute doses of CPZ depressed conditioned motor behavior (ball-pulling and leg manipulanda) as well as the patellar reflex. Greater doses had greater depressant effects. Although only 4 subjects were involved, this study was very sophisticated and well controlled.

Thioridazine also has been widely used with retarded children, and favorable effects have been reported (Abbott et al., 1965; Badham et al., 1963; Baldwin & Kenny, 1966; LeVann, 1961; Kamm & Mandel, 1967; Oettinger & Simonds, 1962; Pregelj & Barkauskas, 1967).

In a double-blind study, Allen et al. (1963) treated 30 mentally retarded patients with thioridazine (50-250 mg/day) and placebo. Thioridazine was no better than placebo, as measured by a rating scale which assessed toileting, bathing, dressing, feeding, and socialization. However, ratings of *global behavior* by the treatment staff indicated that about 50% of the drug-treated group improved, as compared to 4% of the placebo group. Also, patients with higher IQ improved significantly more than those with lower IQ. In another double-blind study Ucer and Kreger (1969) randomly assigned 50 children (IQ 40 to 70) to thioridazine (mean dose = 53 mg) or haloperidol (mean dose = 2.25 mg) for 8 weeks. Thioridazine produced less improvement both in global behavior and in target symptoms (hyperactivity, anxiety, aggressivity and impulsiveness). Based on our experience, we feel the doses used were not equivalent, and this factor might have contributed to the differential effect.

In one of the better double-blind investigations, Alexandris and Lundell (1968) compared the effects of thioridazine and amphetamine in mentally deficient children (IQ 55 to 85). Twenty-one subjects were randomly assigned to 3 groups (placebo, amphetamine, and thioridazine) for 6 months. The following behaviors were rated: hyperkinesis, concentration, attention, aggressiveness, sociability, interpersonal relations, comprehension, mood, work interest, work capacity, reading, spelling, arithmetic and class standing. Thioridazine (mean dose = 95 mg) was found to be significantly superior to placebo in all areas with the exception of reading, spelling, and arithmetic. Amphetamine (mean dose = 52 mg) was significantly superior to placebo only on comprehension and work interest, and it was never superior to thioridazine. Placebo did not produce any significant changes. This study also investigated the effect of the test drugs on Bender-Gestalt, Goodenough Draw-A-Person, and WISC scores, but no significant differences were found. The effects of thioridazine on the stereotyped behavior of 9 mentally retarded children were investigated in a study with excellent methodology by Davis et al. (1969). As compared with placebo, no-drug and methylphenidate, thioridazine significantly reduced stereotypy without affecting other behaviors.

Trifluoperazine has also been used with mentally retarded patients (Beaudry & Gibson, 1960; Fine, 1964; Himwich et al., 1960; Lawlis, 1958; Lowther, 1960; Rettig et al., 1958; Rudy et al., 1958). It seems useful in the management of behavior problems of mentally retarded children. For example, LeVann (1959) reports improvements in the following symptoms: head banging, assaultiveness, self-injury, feeding difficulties, and hyperkinesis. Trifluoperazine has been found effective in two better controlled studies (Sharpe, 1962; Hunter & Stephenson, 1963). In the latter study, where it was compared to CPZ, both were found to be equally good.

Fluphenazine has been less well studied in mentally retarded children. Most of the studies that are available (Arnold & Maginn, 1967; Burness, 1968; LaVeck & Buckley, 1961; Waites & Keele, 1963) are not very well controlled. In a double-blind study, LaVeck et al. (1960) compared fluphenazine (25 to 40 mg/day) and placebo in profoundly retarded children. The evaluation of improvement seemed to be rather impressionistic. Although more children improved in the fluphenazine group, the difference did not reach statistical significance.

Haloperidol was studied by Burk and Menolascino (1968) employing 50 retarded patients (aged 5 to 21) in a double-blind design. The patients were randomly assigned to haloperidol (0.2 to 7.8 mg) or to placebo for 8 weeks. Fifty-four percent of the drug-treated group showed moderate or marked improvement in the areas of hyperactivity, assaultiveness, impulsivity, and self-injury. On the other hand, only 12.5% of the placebo group manifested moderate improvement. In a more recent study LeVann

(1971) compared haloperidol and CPZ using a double-blind technique. Evaluation of drug effectiveness was based on global improvement and on reduction in the severity of target symptoms. Improvement in global ratings occurred in 95% of the patients receiving haloperidol (mean maintenance dose = 2 mg/day). In reducing the severity of the target symptoms (impulsiveness, hostility and aggressiveness), haloperidol also seemed to be more effective than CPZ.

As already noted, while Ucer and Kreger (1969) found haloperidol superior to thioridazine in mentally retarded children, the interpretation of this difference is made difficult by the proportionally higher dose of haloperidol used in that study.

SUMMARY

It would seem that antipsychotic drugs are useful in controlling some behavior problems, notably *hyperactivity, assaultiveness, destructiveness, self-injury and stereotypies* in mentally retarded children. However, the possibility that this may be a quasi-sedative type action resulting in general psychomotor slowing and impairment of cognitive functions makes caution necessary in their use.

Attention Deficit Disorder with Hyperactivity
(Hyperkinetic Syndrome)

There are many problems associated with the diagnosis of the hyperkinetic syndrome, principally the confusion between conduct problems and true hyperactivity. These have been well described elsewhere (Klein & Gittelman-Klein, 1975; Wender, 1971; Werry, in press b; and Chapter 5), and they make it difficult to interpret many of the studies of the use of antipsychotic drugs in treating hyperactive children. The major problem with the studies to be described below is lack of diagnostic clarity.

Very early after the introduction of the phenothiazines, CPZ was found to be an effective and useful inhibitor of hyperactivity by Hunt et al. (1956) and Freed and Peifer (1956). However, these two investigations suffered from many methodological problems, and, more importantly, they were conducted with groups of children of mixed etiology. Garfield et al. (1962), however, reported no improvement in activity in a group of hyperactive children receiving CPZ. Furthermore, Helper et al. (1963) reported impairment in attention span, in paired-associate learning, and on the Porteus Maze Test among those children treated by Garfield et al. (1962).

More recent evidence for the effectiveness of CPZ in the hyperkinetic syndrome has been provided by a well-designed study by Werry et al. (1966). In this double-blind investigation, 39 outpatient children of normal intelligence who had displayed "chronic, severe, pervasive hyperactivity" were assigned to either CPZ (N = 24, mean dose = 106 mg) or placebo (N = 15) for 8 weeks. Overall change in the child (as perceived by the mother) revealed a significant difference in favor of CPZ. While half of the placebo group improved, this improvement was of a minimal nature, and, in contrast to those of the active medication group, very few placebo subjects achieved the 2 higher levels of improvement on the global scale of improvement. With regard to individual target symptoms, a 3-point rating scale revealed that the drug produced a significant improvement in hyperactivity, but not in distractibility, aggressivity, or excitability. Neither a positive history of events indicating possible brain damage nor an abnormal EEG influenced the drug's therapeutic effect. In addition, ratings of mother-child relationships or the presence of emotional disturbance and added psychopathology did not significantly facilitate or interfere with the drug's effectiveness. In general, both active and placebo groups exhibited improvement due to practice effects on various tests of intelligence, learning, attention, motor development, and perceptual-motor skills. However, there was a slight superiority in the placebo group, suggesting possible depression of psychomotor function.

In another publication, Werry (1970) summarized a group of studies (many employing CPZ and thioridazine) performed by him and his colleagues. The general findings were that, in a clinical or naturalistic situation, the phenothiazines cause hyperactive, aggressive children to be perceived as globally "improved" by mothers and recreation workers, but less so by teachers. With regard to specific symptoms, the mothers noted positive change in inappropriate motor behavior-hyperactivity. In some studies, the effects of these drugs in the classroom, playroom or residential treatment center were inconsistent both for motor behavior and for deviant behaviors of all kinds. In other studies, the phenothiazines were found to significantly reduce positive teacher-pupil interaction.

Perphenazine (8-16 mg/day) was administered to a group of hyperkinetic children in a well-controlled study by Eisenberg et al. (1961). The drug-treated children did not improve significantly more than a placebo control group.

Haloperidol, in doses varying from 0.025 to 0.1 mg/kg/day, has also been used for hyperkinetic children. In general, it has been found to be effective for the target symptoms of hyperactivity and aggressivity (Ayd, 1972; Barker & Fraser, 1968; Cunningham et al., 1968; Werry et al., 1976a; Wong & Cock, 1971).

Some recent studies (Gittelman-Klein et al., 1976b; Greenberg et al., 1972; Saletu et al., 1975b; Werry et al., 1976a) have tried to evaluate the relative efficacy of stimulant and antipsychotic drugs in hyperkinetic children. Greenberg et al. compared CPZ (average dose = 125 mg), dextroamphetamine (average dose = 25 mg), hydroxyzine (Atarax) (average dose = 150 mg), and placebo in outpatient hyperkinetic children. They used a double-blind technique, and the children were randomly assigned to the different groups. It was found that only dextroamphetamine and CPZ produced a significant improvement in hyperactivity at home, and the two drugs were equally effective. However ratings by the staff were not significantly improved by CPZ, and only the pediatrician and the psychologist found a significant improvement with dextroamphetamine. Dextroamphetamine most consistently showed improvement on the performance scale of the WISC and on the Porteus mazes. Contrary to expectations, CPZ did not impair cognitive and motor functioning.

Saletu et al., (1975b), in another double-blind study, compared placebo, dextroamphetamine (mean dose = 12 mg) and thioridazine (mean dose = 51.4 mg). Children improved significantly on all conditions, but only dextroamphetamine produced a statistically significant improvement in the overall clinical symptomatology, as compared with placebo. On the other hand, placebo was superior to thioridazine on the hyperactive-impulsive scale of a parent questionnaire, and more surprisingly, thioridazine led to a significant improvement in inattentive-passive behavior on a teacher questionnaire. These results conflict with many other studies and might be explained by the low doses of medication employed.

Werry et al. (1976a), in a double-blind, placebo controlled, crossover study, compared the effects of methylphenidate (0.3 mg/kg), two doses of haloperidol (0.025 low and 0.05 mg/kg high), and placebo in hyperkinetic children. They found that teachers, parents and psychiatrists each judged all three drugs as superior to placebo on at least one of the measures used. Overall, the drug of choice was haloperidol in both doses for parents, methylphenidate for teachers, and haloperidol in low doses for the psychiatrists.

Some of the haloperidol studies have included evaluation of cognitive functions (Cunningham et al., 1968; Werry & Aman, 1975; Wong & Cock, 1971). Wong and Cock (1971) used 0.05 mg/kg of haloperidol for 6 months and did not find any significant depressant effect on cognitive functions. On the other hand, Cunningham et al. (1968), using doses of about 0.1 mg/kg for 4 weeks, found reduction in the speed of reaction time to a single stimulus, slowing in performance involving eye-hand coordination and fine manual control, and, possibly, reduction in speed of continuously responding to information. Werry and Aman (1975) compared to the effects of placebo, methylphenidate, and low (0.025 mg/kg) and high (0.05 mg/kg) doses of haloperidol on attention, memory and motor activity. They found that the drugs do indeed affect the cognitive functions of vigilance and short-term memory in the laboratory situation. Their data also suggest that methylphenidate and, to a lesser extent, the low dose of haloperidol improve these cognitive functions, while the high dose of haloperidol may possibly deteriorate them. The authors commented that the failure of Wong and Cock (1971) to find cognitive improvement using the same dose might be due to the possible development of tolerance to the depressant effect of the drug, caused by its long-term use.

More definite and highly significant effects were reported in a study of hyperkinetic children by Gittelman-Klein et al. (1976b). They randomly assigned 166 children to 4 different groups (methylphenidate, thioridazine, placebo, and a combination of methylphenidate and thioridazine). The widely-used Teacher Rating Scale (TQ) devised by Conners (1969) (see Chapter 2) served to evaluate the changes of behavior at school. Ratings by the parents, social worker, and psychiatrist were also obtained. At the end of 4 weeks of treatment, they found significant effects across raters for all active treatment ($p < .0001$) with regard to global improvement. In addition, scores on the conduct disorder and hyperactivity factors of the TQ were significantly improved by all active treatments. Methylphenidate and the combination of thioridazine and methylphenidate produced improvement on the TQ inattention factor, while thioridazine alone did not.

The children in the active conditions were treated for an additional 8 weeks to evaluate the relative effectiveness of the different treatments. The behavior ratings and global evaluations by the teachers indicated that improvement from thioridazine decreased over time, while there was increasing improvement with methylphenidate. However ratings of the mothers and psychologist did not shift over time. The authors concluded that although thioridazine seemed to be an effective treatment for hyperactivity it was inferior in this respect to methylphenidate. Furthermore, thioridazine did not improve distractibility, therefore it did not have as broad a scope of action as did methylphenidate. It was also concluded that the initially planned maximum dose of 300 mg of thioridazine was too high, and produced too many side effects. The actual mean doses for this drug were 193 mg. (6 mg/kg) at the end of the fourth week, and 160 mg (4.5 mg/kg) at the end of the twelfth week.

SUMMARY

It would seem that the antipsychotic drugs are less effective in the treatment of hyperkinetic children than are the stimulants. Therefore, as we and others have recommended elsewhere (Wender, 1971; Werry, 1976; Winsberg et al., 1976), they should be used only after a thorough trial of the stimulants and, possibly the antidepressants, has been found ineffective.

Gilles de la Tourette's Syndrome

There are no controlled studies of the use of antipsychotic drugs in this syndrome of multiple tics including vocal ones, but their effectiveness in clinical trials has been repeatedly reported.

Trifluopromazine (Vesprin) and thioridazine (Lucas, 1964) have also been reported as useful in the symptomatic control of this syndrome. However, haloperidol, in doses ranging from 1.5 to 13.0 mg/day has been described as especially effective and appears to have pre-empted the field (Bruun et al., 1976; Chalas & Brauer, 1962; Chapel et al., 1964; Lucas, 1967; Shapiro et al., 1973). In some cases where placebo substitution has been attempted, the symptoms have recurred. In sum, it would seem that haloperidol is the drug of choice in the treatment of this uncommon but distressing disease in adults and children, though controlled and objective data of its efficacy, not too difficult with these easily measurable target symptoms, are desirable.

Anorexia Nervosa

Chlorpromazine has been proposed as useful in the treatment of anorexia nervosa when combined with bedrest and other psychosocial therapies (Dally, 1969).

NONINDICATIONS

Anxiety Disorders (Neurosis)

The single well-controlled study in this area yielded no evidence that antipsychotic drugs are useful in the management of neurotic children. Eisenberg et al. (1961) randomly assigned neurotic children to 3 treatment conditions: psychotherapy without medication, psychotherapy plus placebo, and psychotherapy plus perphenazine (8-16 mg/day). For these children perphenazine appeared to offer no advantage over the other treatments.

It would seem that the lack of demonstrated effectiveness and the potential toxicity of these compounds contraindicate their use in these conditions—which in any case seem to respond to psychosocial therapies.

CLINICAL ADMINISTRATION

When the physician decides that an antipsychotic drug is indicated, he needs to discuss clearly with the parents and the child the advantages and the most common side effects of these drugs. A clear, non-technical explanation of the extrapyramidal effects, with particular emphasis on the dystonic reactions, is very important. It will help the parents to secure rapid treatment for the condition and will decrease the anxiety that this disturbing problem produces in the child and his parents.

Table 2 presents the initial average daily doses of antipsychotic drugs most commonly employed by the present authors. It can be seen that treatment is initiated with small amounts of medication.

TABLE 2

Daily Doses of Antipsychotic Drugs in Children

Name	Initial	Average*
Chlorpromazine	1.5-3.0 mgxkg	3-6 mgxkg (75-150)
Thioridazine	1.5-3.0 mgxkg	3-6 mgxkg (75-150)
Trifluoperazine	0.05-0.1 mgxkg	0.25-0.5 mgxkg (6-15)
Fluphenazine	0.025-0.05 mgxkg	0.15-0.3 mgxkg (3-6)
Haloperidol	0.025-0.05 mgxkg	0.1-0.3 mgxkg (2-5)
Thiothixine	0.025-0.05 mgxkg	0.15-0.3 mg-kg (3-6)

* The numbers in parenthesis are average total daily doses in mg.

For outpatients the total daily amount is administered in 2 or 3 equally divided doses, which are gradually increased until either the target symptoms are controlled or the average daily dose is reached. This usually takes 2 or 3 weeks. During this initial titration of the medication, the patient should be seen once or twice a week. In addition the physician should be available for telephone consultation to reassure the parents regarding mild side effects or to manage more severe reactions, as already outlined in the side effects section of this chapter. On occasion it will be necessary to discontinue the drug and to prescribe another antipsychotic or a different treatment altogether.

The average doses recommended in Table 2 are usually adequate for most children. Nevertheless, in severe cases and especially in the severely disturbed and the mentally retarded child, higher doses, comparable to those used in adults, are necessary. These doses are greater than those recommended by the manufacturers in the package insert; therefore their administration has possible medico-legal complications. The employment of such high doses or of antipsychotic drugs not approved for pediatric use in the Physician's Desk Reference (i.e., fluphenazine, perphenazine, haloperidol, thiothixene, molindone, and loxapine) must be very carefully discussed with the parents, and perhaps signed informed consent should be obtained for the records.

After a stable therapeutic dose is attained, the frequency of visits can be reduced to once a month and the dosage may be translated into once or twice daily administration which is more convenient. Periodic dosage decrements and drug-free periods should be tried in order to find the minimal therapeutic dose to determine if the drug is still necessary and to look for dyskinetic symptoms which may not be apparent on medication. Hopefully, these procedures might minimize or perhaps prevent the appearance or severity of long-term side effects and toxicity.

With inpatients, the regulation of the medication can be achieved more quickly. In cases of severe agitation, parenteral chlorpromazine can be administered intramuscularly in doses of 0.50 to 1.00 mg/kg/dose, which can be repeated every 4 to 6 hours, until the agitation is controlled. However, since the sedative phenothiazines like CPZ and thioridazine are also high dose ones, parenteral administration may be highly irritating and result in aseptic abscesses and tissue necrosis. Thus, high potency drugs such as haloperidol 0.3-0.7 mg/kg may be safer, though EPS are much more likely and, as already noted, most of the high potency drugs are not approved for use in children in the U.S.

The discontinuation of antipsychotics should be a gradual process because their abrupt withdrawal can produce restlessness, insomnia, gastrointestinal distress and vomiting in some patients (Yepes & Winsberg, 1977).

SUMMARY

Antipsychotic drugs constitute a valuable tool for the management of a number of target symptoms, principally psychomotor excitation, occurring among behaviorally disordered children. Their effect seems, however, a quasi-sedative rather than an antipsychotic one, and they also have many short- and long-term side effects not found with other groups of psychotropic drugs. Careful clinical management is the obligation of the pediatric pharmacotherapist who uses these agents. Little information of practical use is available in regard to the pharmacokinetics or mode of action of these drugs among children. Such information might guide the clinician in the more effective clinical use of these compounds.

9

ANTIEPILEPTICS (ANTICONVULSANTS)

GREGORY STORES, M.D.

INTRODUCTION

Antiepileptic Drugs and Psychopharmacology

Antiepileptic drugs, less suitably termed anticonvulsants (many epileptic patients do not convulse), are of psychopharmacological importance in several ways. Not infrequently, epilepsy and psychopathology are closely linked and the control of seizure disorders becomes of considerable importance in the overall management of the child. This is most directly seen in the seizure-related disturbances including *changes of mood* which in some patients portend the occurrence of a seizure, *confusional states* which may follow a generalized convulsion and the diversity of strange, often frightening perceptual and *behavioral* changes sometimes comprising temporal lobe seizures. Absence status (Andermann & Robb, 1972) provides a dramatic example of the influence of seizure activity on behavior, producing a picture of perplexity, intellectual deterioration or psychosis with little motor disturbance, which may escape accurate diagnosis. But, in addition, more enduring inter-seizure disorders frequently occur and psychiatric problems are overrepresented in both children and adults who suffer from recurrent seizures (Werry, in press b). There is no simple explanation for this and organic, psychological and social factors often operate in combination. However, among organic factors, *antiepileptic drugs* themselves appear to figure prominently because of their injudicious or inappropriate use.

Conversely, it has been claimed that certain antiepileptic drugs are capable of improving behavior not only in epileptic patients but in others, including children, with no evidence of organic pathology. Finally, many of the findings arising out of the use of this group of drugs for seizure disorders (including the important pharmacokinetic principles which have come to light in recent years) are relevant to their possible wider use in pediatric psychopharmacology.

For all these reasons, then, it behooves those interested in the use of psychotropic drugs in children to be thoroughly familiar with antiepileptic agents.

Basic Issues

As epilepsy is particularly surrounded by misconceptions and ambiguities, a brief account of the concept will be given in order to establish the approach embodied in this chapter.

First, "epilepsy" is not an adequate diagnosis. The term merely relates to the repeated occurrence of certain clinical events (or seizures), the underlying cause of which may be one of many pathologies. Some are identifiable with precision; others uncertain in the present state of knowledge. Second, clinical observation reveals a wide range of clinical types of seizures. Third, many children and adults have problems, additional to their seizures, of a psychological or social type and these difficult issues must be faced if adequate care is to be provided. A wholly pharmacological approach to treatment is rarely effective. This is highlighted in the considerable number of patients whose seizures are at least partly precipitated by emotional or other psychological factors.

Classification of Seizures

This is essential to any discussion of the use of antiepileptic drugs. This is because a meaningful pharmacotherapy is possible only if traditional crude entities such as *grand mal* and *petit mal* attacks or *major* and *minor* seizures are refined, and if adequate clinical and EEG characteristics of seizures are delineated.

The problems with the traditional terms just mentioned is that they are ambiguous and simplistic. They do not reflect the diversity of forms that seizures can take. This diversity is embodied in the scheme that has been promoted internationally in recent years as a framework in which to place further observations of seizures (Gastaut, 1970). It is clear already that even this extensive scheme is not sufficiently complex to accommodate all the clinical types of seizure that occur. At one extreme, there is the generalized tonic-clonic convulsion popularly associated with epilepsy; at the other extreme, seizures may consist of very brief subjective experiences with little or no external manifestation.

It would be inappropriate to detail the many types of seizures included in the International Classification. Instead, reference will be made to the main seizure types shown in Table 1 which also summarizes the drugs most likely to be effective in each type. Neonatal seizures, infantile spasms and febrile convulsions will not be discussed nor will the emergency treatment of the various forms of status epilepticus or continuous seizures.

TABLE 1

Classification of Seizures and Drugs of Choice

Partial (Focal) Seizures	*Drug*
1. With elementary symptomatology: motor or sensory	Carbamazepine, Diphenylhydantoin Phenobarbital, Primidone
2. With complex symptomatology (temporal lobe or psychomotor)	Carbamazepine, Diphenylhydantoin Primidone
Generalized Seizures	
1. Tonic-clonic convulsions	Diphenylhydantoin, Phenobarbital
2. Myoclonic, atonic or akinetic seizures	Sodium valproate Nitrazepam, Clonazepam
3. Absence seizures	Sodium valproate, Ethosuximide

1) *Partial (or focal) seizures.* These have clinical and, usually, EEG features to indicate that they begin in a circumscribed part of one cerebral hemisphere. The symptomatology may be a) mainly motor or sensory, usually without impairment of consciousness (*elementary symptomatology*), or (b) more complex often with impaired consciousness (*complex symptomatology* or *complex partial seizures* otherwise known as temporal lobe or psychomotor seizures). Daly (1975) has described the very rich diversity of temporal lobe phenomena, the subjective forms of which tend to be underestimated in children because of their inability to describe their experiences.

2) *Generalized seizures.* In these, the clinical features and the accompanying EEG discharge are, from the outset, bilateral and symmetrical and do not include any sign or symptom arising from a *localized* part of one cerebral hemisphere. They are grouped into a) the *tonic-clonic convulsion* (often referred to as *grand mal*) in which body rigidity (tonic) precedes muscle spasms (clonic), b) *other seizures with predominantly motor manifestations such* as the myoclonic seizures of various types and those characterized by a brief loss of postural tone (atonic seizures) or loss of movement without loss of tone (akinetic seizures). Purely clonic and purely tonic seizures are also part of this group. c) *Absence seizure* which is replacing the ambiguous term *petit mal*. Recently, detailed clinical observations (Penry et al., 1975) have

shown that there are several different types within this group. Although impairment of consciousness is the cardinal feature of them all, motor manifestations of one sort or another may predominate and compared with these and the mixed type of absence seizure, simple absences (corresponding to the textbook description of classical petit mal) are unusual.

For various reasons (including treatment) it is important to distinguish between absence seizures and the less dramatic forms of complex partial seizure. The distinguishing features are discussed by Penry et al. (1975). The most important are that complex partial seizures are longer, they are initiated by an aura (preliminary experiential phenomena) and followed by a slow return to full consciousness rather than abrupt recovery, and automatisms are less complex in absence seizures. EEG findings may help distinguish the two types of seizure in difficult cases.

An important group of partial seizures which may well not be recognized as such are those in which the initial focal seizure activity becomes widespread to produce a generalized seizure which is often tonic-clonic in type. The initial features must be known in order to distinguish a partial seizure which has *secondarily generalized* from one which has been generalized from the outset. Sometimes post-ictal focal signs may suggest the former and, occasionally, EEG evidence of the focal origin can be discerned.

It should be emphasized that none of the classificatory systems yet published (and certainly not the truncated account just given) does justice to the variety of seizure manifestations revealed by careful clinical enquiry.

The more behavioral and less motor forms of seizure manifestations may go unrecognized, but quite frequently, the diagnostic error works in the opposite direction, and children are diagnosed as epileptic on inadequate clinical evidence or because of undue reliance on EEG findings. It is of serious consequence to a child to be diagnosed as suffering a seizure disorder, not only because of the social consequences involved, but also because he then runs the risk of being subject to possible harmful effects of antiepileptic treatment. Clinical enquiry about episodes of altered behavior needs to be detailed and directed to *key diagnostic features which tend to characterize seizures in general* (such as paroxysmal and stereotyped quality, brief duration and effect on conscious level) as well as to components of the attack or its aftermath *which might clearly establish the presence of organic dysfunction*. It must be noted, however, that both seizures and psychogenic attacks can occur in the same patient, at least in later childhood and adult life.

Limitations of this Review

A comprehensive account of the use of antiepileptic drugs in seizure disorders is outside the scope of this chapter which will be concerned only with broad principles. For more detailed information the 3 books which have provided the sources for much of the pharmacological data in this review can be consulted. One (Woodbury et al., 1972) gives a detailed account of the pharmacology of the antiepileptic drugs available in the United States at that time; the second (Richens, 1976) brings basic scientific principles to bear on clinical problems; the third (Kutt, 1974) surveys the generally uncertain question of mechanisms of action of antiepileptic drugs.

Useful short reviews of antiepileptic drugs particularly in behavior disorders in children and of effects on intellectual function can be found in Conners & Werry (in press), Reynolds & Trimble (1976) and Stores (1975).

It is worth reflecting on the considerable difficulties involved in attempting a review of antiepileptic drugs in the management of children with seizure disorders or psychiatric problems. Surprisingly in view of their frequency of use, perhaps more than any other group of drugs discussed in this volume, antiepileptic drugs represent a much underresearched area. This is true of their *antiepileptic* properties (hardly any adequately controlled trials have been conducted over the many years that the drugs have been in use) and it is even more the case where *behavior* is concerned.

Most of the evidence about psychological effects (good or bad) consists of clinical impressions or incidental remarks made in the course of reporting on the antiepileptic properties of the drug in question. The result is that opinions differ, sometimes quite remarkably, about even basic considerations. An example of this is the question of how frequently behavior disturbance is a serious complication of the barbiturates. Apparently irreconcilable views are expressed by different people with extensive experience of the drug treatment of childhood seizures (Jeavons, 1976; Livingstone, 1976). The review that follows does not consist, therefore, exclusively of findings from well controlled studies—it would be a very short review indeed if that were so. Instead, an attempt will be made to represent the consensus of opinion derived from studies with various degrees of scientific merit.

Knowledge of the pharmacology of antiepileptic drugs is very incomplete and has generally been derived from adult patients. The information given, therefore, needs to be applied to children more provisionally than usual. This is particularly so with serum half-lives which are likely to be shorter in children because of their generally faster rate of metabolism (see Chapter 1).

Measurement of serum drug levels has become an important part of the management of patients with seizure disorders and *therapeutic ranges* have been published for most antiepileptic drugs. These need to be used with caution, especially in children, and seen as only general guidelines. The relationships between oral dosage and serum level, and between a given serum level and response, vary considerably from one adult patient to another. Much greater variation between children of different ages is therefore likely. The ranges given merely represent the serum levels likely to produce optimum control in most patients. *In individual children, laboratory values are of secondary importance to clinical condition.*

General Comments and Organization

1) *Clinical effects* of each group of drugs will be discussed in relation to the treatment of seizure disorders and then, separately, in relation to non-epileptic conditions.

2) *Treatment emergent or side effects* will be divided into physical and behavioral complications with emphasis on the latter. As far as possible general disturbances of behavior will be presented before cognitive deficits are discussed. Ideally, a distinction would be made between three types of adverse drug effect (Kutt & Louis, 1972), the treatment of each of which is quite different. These three types are: a) symptoms and signs of intoxication occurring predictably at high dosage or high blood levels; b) side effects which are seen quite commonly and are produced by usual therapeutic doses of a drug; c) idiosyncratic responses which are unusual, unpredictable and not related to dosage or drug concentration. Unfortunately, it is often impossible to classify complications in this way because in many reports little or no information is given about dosage or serum levels. Perhaps because the main types of antiepileptic drugs are all basically cyclic compounds, many of their adverse effects on behavior consist of sedation, confusional states, mood changes or other non-specific disturbance without distinctive features. Occasionally, however, a reaction characteristic of a particular drug or group of drugs is encountered, such as the frequently intolerable irritability, depression or increased activity which barbiturates seem to produce in many children.

The generally neglected subject of the adverse physical effects of antiepileptic drugs is comprehensively reviewed in three recent articles which look at the problem from the points of view of idiosyncratic reactions (Booker, 1975), acute toxicity (Plaa, 1975) and chronic toxicity (Reynolds, 1975).

3) *Drug interactions.* Those more likely to be encountered in children will be emphasized particularly.

4) *Clinical indications* are necessarily presented tentatively; contraindications are principally a history of previous idiosyncratic response or severe and persistent adverse side effect.

5) *Interactions with other treatments.* The interactions between drug treatment and other forms of therapy, including non-pharmacological approaches to seizure disorders (such as behavior modification or biofeedback), have apparently not been investigated at all.

6) *Clinical administration, dosage and precautions.* To locate these as they apply in the treatment of seizure disorders, reference should be made to the appropriate manufacturer's data sheets or to Richens (1976). The International Glossary of Anticonvulsants (1977) published by the International Bureau for Epilepsy is useful for identifying antiepileptic drugs used in different countries from their proprietary names.

7) *General issues* not dealt with in relation to individual drugs will be discussed at the end of the chapter.

8) *Classification of anticonvulsant drugs.* The following subgroups will be distinguished on the basis of *chemical composition.* However, in many cases, these chemical differences are more apparent than real, since the drugs often have a structural or steric common denominator (see Figure 1.).

1. Hydantoins
2. Barbiturates
3. Carbamazepine
4. Succinimides
5. Benzodiazepines
6. Sodium Valproate
7. Miscellaneous

Fig. 1

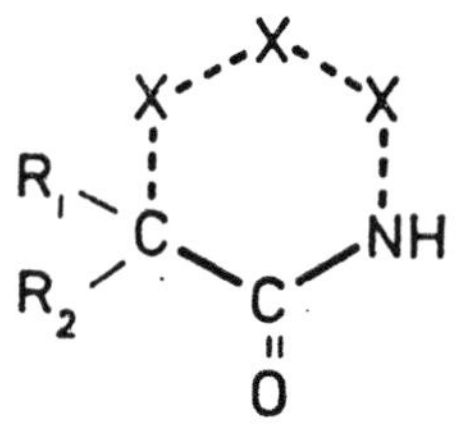

ANTIEPILEPTIC
COMMON DENOMINATOR

Fig. 2

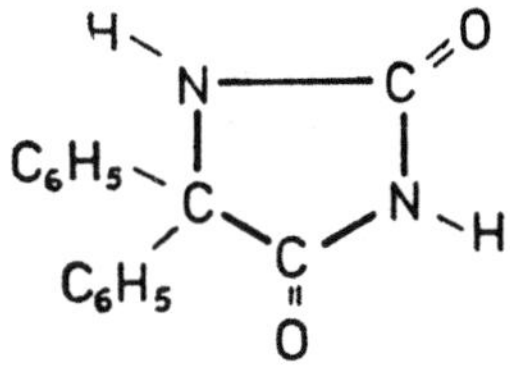

DIPHENYLHYDANTOIN
(Dilantin)

HYDANTOINS

Introduction

This group of drugs which forms one of the cornerstones of the treatment of epilepsy was introduced in 1938 after a widespread search in laboratory animals for drugs which would lower electroshock convulsive thresholds.

Diphenylhydantoin (DPH) will be discussed in some detail as the principal and very widely used member of this group. Methoin, ethotoin and albutoin have been used less extensively and will be referred to only briefly at the end of this section.

Diphenylhydantoin (Dilantin, Epanutin)

CHEMICAL STRUCTURE

By comparing Figure 2 with Figure 1, it can be seen that DPH has the typical structural common denominator of antiepileptic drugs.

PHARMACOLOGY

1) *Absorption and Distribution.* DPH is relatively insoluble in aqueous media, but this can be improved by administering microcrystalline preparations (which are very well absorbed because they present a much greater surface area for dissolution to take place) or the sodium salt of phenytoin which forms a microcrystalline suspension in the stomach and is therefore also well absorbed. Richens (1976) has emphasized that, because different DPH preparations may contain different forms of the drug which are absorbed at unequal rates, there is a risk of intoxication if these preparations are interchanged. *Prescriptions for children should therefore specify the particular type of preparation as well as dosage.*

Whereas the activity of most enzyme systems is proportionate to the serum concentration of the drug, this is not so with DPH, the enzyme system of which becomes heavily saturated, to a point within the therapeutic range at which its action stops increasing no matter how much more the serum concentration rises. As the elimination phase is not exponential, it is not appropriate to calculate an overall half-life value which varies with the serum level of the drug, being longest at toxic levels.

After absorption about 90% of DPH in the bloodstream binds reversibly to plasma proteins, especially albumin. Diffusion of the drug into brain and other tissues is determined by the free drug in the plasma. General medical conditions which lower serum albumin increase the risk of adverse effects. High concentrations are produced in brain as well as in other tissues.

2) *Metabolism/Excretion.* DPH is extensively metabolised by the liver mainly to a parahydroxylate derivative which is excreted in the urine. In keeping with other drugs, the rate of metabolism of DPH increases with decreasing age in children.

3) *Site and Mode of Action.* The important active principle is DPH itself. Particular anatomical sites of action have not been established. The mode of cellular action most clearly understood is the depression at relatively low doses—probably by membrane ionic stabilization rather than depression of cell function—of post-tetanic potentiation which occurs excessively in association with seizure activity. The effect, then, seems to be that seizure threshold is stabilized and spread of seizure activity is limited rather than that the source of seizure activity is abolished.

4) *Dose/Response Data.* Wide differences exist between individuals in the serum levels produced by a given dose of DPH even where adjustment for body weight or surface area is made and only general guidelines can be provided about the weight-related starting doses required to produce average serum concentrations within the *therapeutic range* (see Richens, 1976).

5) *Clinical Administration.* Initial dosage is 5-10 mg/kg depending on body weight (Richens, 1976). It is commonly stated that serum concentrations in the range of 10 to 29 μg/ml give maximum control of seizures in most patients. However this can only be taken as a general guide because of considerable individual differences. Some patients appear to be controlled at serum levels generally considered subtherapeutic. Because of individual variations in serum enzyme saturation point, the relationship

between dose of DPH and serum level is not linear, and a small increase in dose can produce a disproportionate rise in serum levels within the therapeutic range. Therefore increments given to achieve better control should become progressively smaller and more spaced as the serum concentration increases, and this may mean changes by as little as 25 mgm and as long as at two weekly intervals. There is recent evidence to suggest that, in spite of the accelerated rate of metabolism in children, a once-daily dosage of DPH can control seizures as well as divided doses.

CLINICAL EFFECTS

1) *Antiepileptic.* DPH can be expected to be effective in a variety of seizure disorders, excluding absence seizures and probably myoclonic, atonic and akinetic attacks, which have tended to be resistant to most traditional forms of treatment. In contrast to phenobarbital, its antiepileptic action is achieved without depression of the central nervous system (CNS).

2) *Psychotropic.* The place of DPH in the treatment of non-epileptic disorders of behavior is difficult to judge, in spite of the many reports since the 1940's of its use for different types of disturbance in children and adults. These reports have been catalogued (without critical appraisal) by Bogoch and Dreyfus (1970, 1975) and range from personal testimonies as to its efficacy, to more scientific and controlled evaluations. At present, the picture is unclear though it is significant that in the U.S. the only FDA approved indication for the use of DPH is epilepsy.

However, there have been some interesting reports that DPH can have selectively beneficial effects on certain aspects of *cognitive function.* Haward's (1970, 1973) double-blind cross-over studies of normal subjects carrying out perceptual accuracy and vigilance tests suggest that single modest doses of DPH can improve performance. Smith and Lowry (1972, 1975), also using double blind cross-over design, report improvements especially of verbal skills in normal adult subjects (including elderly people) after short-term continuous DPH medication. These careful investigations contrast with other studies of DPH in child and adult psychiatry which have usually been concerned with ill-defined and heterogeneous patient groups and impressionistic evaluation rather than measurement of change in particular aspects of behavior. The paper by Uhlenhuth et al. (1972) contained a review of most of the literature up to that time which highlighted the paucity of controlled studies in this area. The same is still true. Several important points arise from the many reports available: a) Beneficial effects of DPH are claimed for a very wide range of conditions, although at any age, *antisocial behavior*, *impulsiveness* and *restlessness* feature prominently in most reports. However, most of these positive claims are from uncontrolled studies and where controlled procedures have been attempted the findings are less convincing, with good results being described in some (Boelhouwer et al., 1968; Resnick, 1967; Stephens & Shaffer, 1970) and poor results in others (Case et al., 1969; Conners et al., 1971; Lefkowitz, 1969; Looker & Conners, 1970; Malitz & Kanzler, 1971). b) dosage of DPH varies greatly from one study to another and sometimes the drug has been given alone, at other times in combination with other drugs. There is no mention in these studies of *serum levels* which, from epilepsy research, might be expected to be crucial. This seems to have been the case in Malitz and Kanzler's (1971) study in which the response of patients taking up to 600 mgs a day of DPH was significantly worse than those on placebo, a result which could well have reflected toxic effects. c) In several reports, children are described as having "epileptic" or "convulsive equivalents" (Chao et al., 1964; Zimmerman, 1956) or significance has been attached to the presence of "abnormal EEGs" in children without clinical seizures who have responded to DPH. Both these dubious concepts will be discussed later.

It seems that, on the present evidence, DPH does not deserve the wide acclaim as a psychotropic agent that it has been given in the past. However, there are indications that certain types of patient with impulsive or aggressive tendencies or attention deficits may benefit and further, more precise and properly controlled evaluation needs to be carried out. The undesirable psychotropic effects are discussed in the next section.

TREATMENT EMERGENT (SIDE) EFFECTS

1) *Idiosyncratic reactions* to DPH include skin lesions of varying severity, immunological disorders, hepatic dysfunction and bone marrow depression. These are rare.

2) *Skin and Mouth*. DPH commonly causes cosmetic problems, especially gum hyperplasia which, if a problem, calls for discontinuation of the drug. Acne, hirsutism, and coarsening of the skin and facial features (Falconer & Davidson, 1973) are also seen frequently and are likely to produce self-consciousness and social disadvantage to the child. For this reason alone, DPH needs using with great caution in childhood, especially for girls.

3) *Nervous System* (*including behavior and cognitive function*): Mild peripheral neuropathies have followed on prolonged ingestion of DPH.

The question of whether persistent cerebellar damage can result remains uncertain. The characteristic picture of *reversible* DPH toxicity, usually occurring above serum levels of 20 µg/ml, includes the development of cerebellar signs—nystagmus (oscillatory eye movement), ataxia (staggering gait), dysarthria (slurred speech), and lethargy, often in a predictable sequence. Above 40 µg/ml, very obvious mental changes, including acute confusional states, usually occur. There are reasons to suppose, however, that this classical picture of DPH intoxication is only one of several possible syndromes associated with raised serum levels. Glaser (1972) has described a serious condition of *diphenylhydantoin encephalopathy* associated with overdosage, or average oral dosage but with high serum levels, sometimes occurring abruptly in patients who have not had any recent change of medication. The picture includes an increase in seizures (often with a change of seizure pattern towards more tonic or opisthotonic attacks), slowing of basic EEG rhythms, the development of altered mood or other behavioral change, and, in some instances, the development of focal neurological signs. Nystagmus may not be evident at any stage. Similar reactions to DPH have been described more recently, with the additional clinical features of choreoathetosis (spontaneous movements) and dystonia (isolated muscle spasms) (Ahmad et al., 1975; McLellan & Swash, 1974).

Chronic DPH intoxication, producing a picture of *degenerative disorder,* has also been described by Vallarta et al. (1974) and, in children, by Crichton and Patel (1968), Logan and Freeman (1969), Weiss et al. (1969), and Prensky et al. (1971). Points of particular emphasis in these reports are that toxicity may occur with conventional or previously well tolerated dosage, and the usual premonitory classical cerebellar signs may not be seen, especially in young children. Disturbed behavior may therefore not be recognized as a symptom of intoxication. Judging from some of these reports, although discontinuation of treatment with DPH may halt intellectual deterioration in many cases, complete recovery may not always occur.

Although DPH has been said to produce a wide range of other *psychiatric conditions,* including conversion symptoms (*Bulletin of the Johns Hopkins Hospital,* 1964; Niedermeyer et al., 1970), tactile and visual hallucinatory states with somatic delusions (Hoaken & Kane, 1963) and schizophrenic psychoses (Peters, 1962), the precise nature of the relationship is obscure, and is dubious in some cases. Interpretation of some of these claims is made difficult by international differences in psychiatric terminology.

The possibility that serum levels of antiepileptic drugs within the commonly accepted therapeutic range may be associated with *behavioral change* is suggested by Reynolds and Travers (1974) who found that (independently of seizure frequency) epileptic patients with psychomotor slowing, intellectual deterioration, psychiatric illness or personality change generally had higher serum concentrations of DPH and phenobarbital than patients without such characteristics.

A similarly insidious *impairment of intellectual ability* was reported by Rosen (1968) in a small number of patients on long-term treatment with DPH in whom there was otherwise no evidence of intoxication. Although details are not provided in this report, it is stated that "remarkable improvement" in overall intelligence, perceptual and other specific abilities followed discontinuation of DPH and (surprisingly) substitution of phenobarbital or primidone (Mysoline) in many of the cases. Dodrill (1975a) describes selective impairment of motor skills in patients taking DPH alone. In a recent study of factors associated with poor school progress of children with epilepsy attending ordinary school (Stores & Hart, 1976), it was found that the reading skills of those children who had taken DPH for at least 2 years was significantly inferior to those who had taken other antiepileptic drugs over a similar period. Ideström et al. (1972) have reported marginally adverse effects on some aspects of attention following the acute administration of DPH to healthy adults in doses sufficient to produce low serum levels, but it is difficult to assess the relevance of these findings to long-term ingestion of the drug.

DRUG INTERACTIONS

Many interactions between antiepileptic drugs themselves and between them and other drugs have been described and DPH figures prominently in both types of interaction. The effects vary considerably depending on the clinical management and only those of particular importance will be mentioned here.

Of the interactions between antiepileptic drugs themselves, that between DPH and sulthiame (Ospolot) needs emphasis because the combination is quite commonly prescribed. Sulthiame inhibits the metabolism of DPH, phenobarbital and primidone (Mysoline). The addition of sulthiame, therefore, can cause a rise in the serum concentration of these drugs which, in the case of DPH, may easily reach toxic levels. Of the other antiepileptic drugs, pheneturide (Benuride) (and possibly phenobarbital and ethosuximide) may have a similar but clinically less important effect. Different types of drugs implicated in this way include methylphenidate (Ritalin) although the evidence is conflicting. In contrast, benzodiazepines and carbamazepine (Tegretol) appear to *reduce* serum levels of DPH by inducing its metabolism.

Antiepileptic drugs may accelerate the metabolism of other drugs and exogenous substances by inducing liver enzymes. These effects, which occur with phenobarbital, primidone, pheneturide and carbamazepine, as well as DPH, affect antidepressants, anticoagulants, folic acid, vitamin D, steroids, sex hormones and various other drugs. The clinical significance of the much publicized folate deficiency which might result in this way is still unclear (Reynolds, 1975).

CLINICAL INDICATIONS AND CONTRAINDICATIONS

DPH is a satisfactory drug for the control of generalized tonic-clonic convulsions, and partial seizures with elementary symptomatology including those which secondarily generalize. It is of no value in absence seizures and alternative treatments for complex partial seizures and for myoclonic, akinetic and atonic seizures are probably more effective. *There are no established indications, as yet, for the use of DPH in non-epileptic disorders.*

SUMMARY AND CONCLUSIONS

DPH is a useful antiepileptic drug with a wide range of applicability in the treatment of seizure disorders.

Despite not uncommon use, the place of DPH in non-epileptic psychopathological disorders of childhood, even those with abnormal EEGs, remains uncertain. Although there are suggestions in the literature that children with impulsive or aggressive tendencies might benefit, administration of DPH for these broad categories of disturbance outside properly controlled clinical trials is not justified on the available evidence, particularly in view of the drug's toxicity.

Because of the unusual nature of its pharmacokinetics, particular care needs to be taken with dosage of DPH and its combined use with other drugs. Caution is also necessary in view of its widespread effects on physical systems and the potentially serious and irreversible effects on behavior and intellectual function of its long-term use.

Other Hydantoins

Methoin (Mesantoin) appears to be effective in generalized tonic-clonic convulsions and partial seizures with elementary symptomatology but it is of less certain value in complex partial seizures and is ineffective for absence seizures. It is generally more toxic than DPH especially in its effect on bone marrow and as a result has found a very limited place in treatment. Ethotoin (Peganone), although safer, is much less potent than the other hydantoins. The place of albutoin remains uncertain. None of these other hydantoins appears to have been used for behavior disorders.

BARBITURATES

Introduction

After bromides, these are historically the oldest antiepileptic agents (since 1912).

All members of this group are derivatives of barbituric acid and are closely related structurally to each other as well as to the hydantoins and other antiepileptic drugs sharing the chemical or steric common denominator (see Figure 1). The most commonly used for seizure disorders are phenobarbital (Luminal) and primidone (Mysoline) which is a desoxy-barbiturate.

Fig. 3.

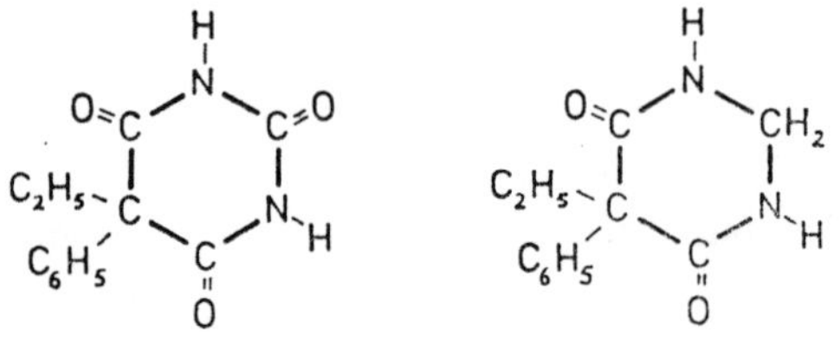

PHENOBARBITAL   PRIMIDONE
                     (Mysoline)

Methobarbital (Prominal) and metharbital (Gemonil) are little used and will not be discussed further.

Phenobarbital (Luminal)

CHEMICAL STRUCTURE

See Figure 3 and compare with Figure 1.

PHARMACOLOGY

1) *Absorption and Distribution.* Phenobarbital is rapidly absorbed, but its serum half-life in children is long—from 37 to 73 hours. Only about 60% is bound to plasma albumin, making reduction of plasma albumin

levels less clinically important than in the case of DPH. Phenobarbital appears to enter the brain slowly, but eventually it is distributed in equal concentrations in all tissues and body fluids.

2) *Metabolism/Excretion.* Phenobarbital is parahydroxylated in the liver with 10% to 40% excreted unchanged in the urine. Both metabolism and excretion are slow but less so in children than adults. The parahydroxylate derivative, which appears to be the major metabolite, has no antiepileptic action itself.

3) *Site and Mode of Action.* The anatomical site of action has not yet been determined. Phenobarbital has a widespread depressive effect on all excitable tissue but especially in the CNS and on polysynaptic pathways. Both the initiation and the spread of seizure discharge are prevented or modified. The cellular basis of this depression is unknown but it is thought to involve synaptic transmission in some way.

4) *Dose-Response Data.* Unlike DPH, the enzyme system by which phenobarbital is metabolized does not become saturated within the therapeutic range, and serum concentrations in children correspond in a relatively simple way to dosage on a body weight or similar basis.

5) *Clinical Administration.* Ordinarily, initial dosage is 2-4.5 mg/kg/day depending on body weight (Richens, 1976). The usual therapeutic range for phenobarbital in serum is 15-40 μg/ml. Although phenobarbital is usually administered twice daily, because of its slow metabolism and excretion, a once daily dosage will probably give stable serum levels.

CLINICAL EFFECTS

1) *Seizure Disorders.* Phenobarbital is effective in tonic-clonic convulsions and partial seizures with elementary symptomatology. Much less success is reported in complex partial seizures and no effect in absence seizures. In contrast to DPH, phenobarbital produces its antiepileptic effect by depression of CNS function. In the types of seizure disorder for which it is effective, there seems to be little to choose between phenobarbital, DPH and primidone (Mysoline) as far as antiepileptic action is concerned, although their adverse behavioral effects may be quite different in individual children.

2) *Nonepileptic Disorders.* Very little can be said about the psychotropic value of the barbiturates in nonepileptic psychopathological states in children, since controlled trials are almost nonexistent (Conners & Werry, in press) and they have been largely superseded. Because of their

toxicity in overdose there is an increasing reluctance in medicine in general to use this group of drugs as sedatives or hypnotics. A common problem with barbiturates in children, whatever the cause of their disorder, seems to be that they are prone to cause behavioral deterioration, sometimes quite dramatically (see below). It is also felt inappropriate ordinarily to adopt a wholly pharmacological approach to anxious children whose problems usually require psychological attention. As adjuvant therapy for anxiety states, because of their greater safety, the benzodiazepines or antihistamines are preferable (see Chapter 10).

TREATMENT EMERGENT (SIDE) EFFECTS

1) *Physical (other than CNS).* Compared with DPH, phenobarbital produces few adverse *physical* effects in normal clinical dosage. Occasionally, severe, idiosyncratic skin reactions may occur although, more usually, the various rashes caused or aggravated are benign. Neonatal coagulation defects due to vitamin K deficiency have been reported in infants born to mothers treated with phenobarbital (or DPH). Folate deficiency and disorders of calcium metabolism have been attributed to phenobarbital (as well as to DPH and primidone) although the overall clinical significance of these effects remains unclear.

2) *Nervous System (including behavior or cognition).* As noted above, phenobarbital acts by a widespread dose dependent depression of CNS function. Drowsiness appears to be a common initial effect of phenobarbital. It usually lasts only for several days but, in a few patients, the reaction is protracted. An effect seemingly common with phenobarbital or other barbiturates is the excitement, irritability, tearfulness or aggression often reported in children taking these drugs. Surprisingly, this phenomenon has not been studied objectively. There is no clear indication what proportion of children suffer these complications or the ways in which they might be predicted except that a child who is already disturbed, particularly if hyperactive, is said to be more likely to be made much worse by the introduction of barbiturates (Conners et al., 1965). Some pediatricians feel that the risk of these unpleasant effects is so great that they avoid prescribing phenobarbital for children with epilepsy. Fortunately, only few epileptic children develop the severe hyperkinetic reaction described by Ounsted (1955) (gross overactivity, short attention span, distractibility and destructiveness or aggression) with phenobarbital. Blood levels of phenobarbital above 60 $\mu g/ml$ predictably result in acute or subacute confusional states often with ataxia, dysarthria and nystagmus, as well as clear evidence of intellectual deterioration. Severe

developmental delay in childhood, misinterpreted as permanent handicap, has been attributed to such chronic intoxication with phenobarbital (Cordes, 1973).

The study by Mirsky and Kornetsky (1964), showing how barbiturates impair performance on vigilance tests, and, even more, cognitive processes involving cortical rather than subcortical mechanisms, might be taken to suggest that barbiturates can indeed be incriminated in learning difficulties of children with epilepsy. However, these investigations are not strictly relevant to the child who has been on continuous barbiturate medication because tolerance develops in a matter of days and these acute effects can be expected to diminish. The study by Hutt et al. (1968) is, on the face of it, more relevant. In this study normal adults were given phenobarbital sufficient to produce what would normally be considered therapeutic serum levels. After a period of 12 days delay to allow initial tolerance to develop, performance on a variety of tests was measured over a 4-week period. The main finding in this preliminary study was that phenobarbital appeared to have no effect on simple and brief tests but those requiring sustained effort were affected adversely, although these deficits were not absolute and could be corrected by social stimulation. The selective adverse effects in healthy subjects of amylobarbitone sodium and diazepam, given in commonly prescribed dosage, on prolonged and monotonous tasks and on those involving short-term memory have been demonstrated by Hart et al. (1976).

Clinical investigations, on the other hand, seem to have provided little support for the view that phenobarbital (or other antiepileptic drugs) is a particular cause of poor performance on tests of intellectual abilities. At least one early study (Somerfeld-Ziskind & Ziskind, 1940) suggested that such effects are more than outweighed by the reduction in seizure frequency that the phenobarbital may produce. The design of this study can be criticized, but Wapner et al. (1962), in a better controlled investigation, also found no evidence of deterioration of intelligence or learning ability in a group of epileptic children who had taken phenobarbital for 6 weeks. Seizure frequency, rather than amount or duration of drug treatment, appeared to be of particular importance in the study of intellectual deterioration in epileptic children by Chaundry and Pond (1961). At variance with these findings, is the report by Tchicaloff and Gaillard (1970) that dosage of phenobarbital and impairment on some of the Wechsler Intelligence Scale subtests are correlated.

The apparent conflict between positive laboratory findings and the negative results of clinical studies may seem surprising, especially in view of the frequency in which other aspects of behavior are said to be upset by phenobarbital. They are, however, consistent with findings in pediatric psychopharmacology in general, whatever the drug, and raise the issue of the validity of laboratory type tests for the naturalistic situation. This issue is discussed in detail in Chapter 3.

DRUG INTERACTIONS

Both sulthiame and pheneturide (Benuride) can increase serum concentrations of phenobarbital although their effect is less than on DPH levels. The effects of interactions between phenobarbital and DPH are variable. Substances which make urine acid decrease the urinary excretion of phenobarbital and, therefore, increase serum levels; agents which make the urine alkaline have the opposite effect. The liver enzyme-inducing properties of phenobarbital, affecting other drugs such as antidepressants and vitamins, were mentioned earlier.

CLINICAL INDICATIONS AND CONTRAINDICATIONS

Phenobarbital can be expected to be effective in controlling generalized tonic-clonic convulsions and partial seizures with elementary symptomatology but because of its tendency to cause behavioral deterioration, its place in the management of children is more limited than in adults. It should be used with particular caution in any epileptic child already behaviorally disturbed, and has no established place as an anxiolytic or sedative in pediatric psychopharmacology.

SUMMARY AND CONCLUSIONS

Phenobarbital and other barbiturates have only a limited place in the treatment of seizure disorders in children because of apparently common adverse behavioral effects. Alternative drugs, free of these adverse effects, are readily available. There is no convincing evidence to suggest that phenobarbital is of value in non-epileptic child psychiatric disorders (see Chapter 10).

Primidone (Mysoline)

CHEMICAL STRUCTURE

See Figures 1 and 3.

PHARMACOLOGY

As the main active metabolite of primidone is phenobarbital, the latter's pharmacology (see above), is really more relevant than that of primidone itself and other derivatives.

Absorption of primidone is relatively rapid and it is metabolized, probably incompletely, by the liver into 2 active compounds, phenobarbital and phenylethylmalonamide (PEMA). The conversion to phenobarbital is slow. Very little primidone and PEMA are protein-bound and both are distributed more readily to brain than is phenobarbital. Little is known about excretion and detoxication of primidone or PEMA in man. Although the main active principal is phenobarbital, there is some evidence in animals, that both unchanged primidone and PEMA have anti-epileptic activity. However, the site and mechanism of this action are not yet known.

As administration of primidone provides much higher serum concentrations of phenobarbital than of primidone and as the anti-epileptic contribution of primidone itself is not yet known, dose-response and time-response data are best judged in terms of phenobarbital concentrations. As noted, a therapeutic range of 15-40 μg/ml is usually used for phenobarbital whether administered directly or derived from primidone.

CLINICAL EFFECTS

Primidone appears to have the same range of effectiveness as phenobarbital in the control of seizures, but in addition it is likely to be effective in the control of complex partial seizures. It is of no value for absence seizures. Primidone has not been used as a psychotropic agent, no doubt because its psychotropic effects are mostly undesirable (see next section).

TREATMENT EMERGENT (SIDE) EFFECTS

These are similar to those with phenobarbital, but with the important addition of an idiosyncratic response, possibly due to the unmetabolized form of primidone. This consists of pronounced sedation or acute confusional state often accompanied by ataxia, nausea and vomiting. The effect often comes on within the first hour or two of a single dose and persists after discontinuation for periods between a few hours and a few days. Some physicians feel it necessary to give patients a small test dose before instituting treatment. A few cases in which primidone has been successfully introduced appear later to develop a florid confusional state, sometimes with paranoid features, at doses normally considered to be within the therapeutic range. The effects of long-term administration are difficult to determine. Reports from Europe have for some time now remarked on "personality deterioration," mood swings and what appear to be confusional states, as well as paranoid psychoses associated with ingestion of the drug, but it is difficult to evaluate these reports as serum level estimations or other details of dosage have not been included.

DRUG INTERACTIONS

See phenobarbital and DPH.

CLINICAL INDICATIONS

Indications are as for phenobarbital with the addition of complex partial seizures. Behaviorally disturbed children may well become worse on primidone. A previous history of idiosyncracy should be sought.

SUMMARY AND CONCLUSIONS

Primidone is a widely effective anti-epileptic drug but its behavioral effects may limit its usefulness perhaps as much as with phenobarbital. There is no evidence that it has any place in the treatment of non-epileptic conditions.

CARBAMAZEPINE (TEGRETOL)

CHEMICAL STRUCTURE

Carbamazepine is chemically related to the tricyclic antidepressant drugs, differing in having a single rather than three carbon (propyl) side chain. As with the chemically related phenothiazines (see Chapter 8), this shortening of the side chain radically alters its neuropharmacological properties.

Fig. 4

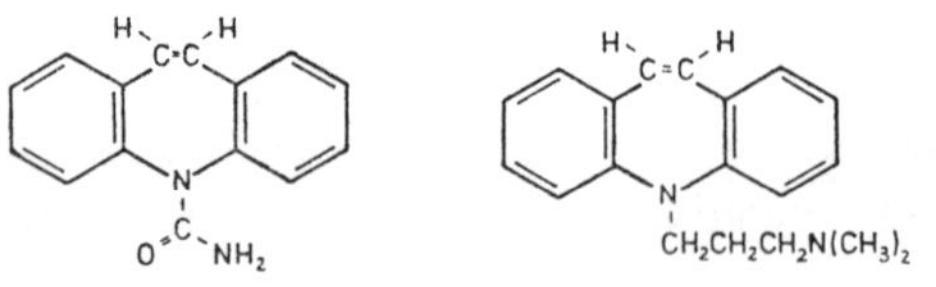

CARBAMAZEPINE
(Tegretol)

IMIPRAMINE
(Tofranil)

PHARMACOLOGY

In contrast to other antiepileptic drugs and its tricyclic antidepressant relatives, the pharmacology of carbamazepine is not well worked out. Absorption appears to be quite rapid. Carbamazepine's metabolism is autoinducible. Following single dosing in adults, the half-life is around 36-72 hours but following chronic dosing it falls to 12-24 hours. The same effect is to be expected in children although the details have not been studied. Average half-life in children is probably about 12 hours. Distribution into CSF (cerebrospinal fluid) occurs quickly. Carbamazepine is metabolised mainly to the 10, 11-epoxide which is pharmacologically active. In fast metabolisers such as children (see Chapter 1), the serum level of this metabolite can be as great as or even exceed that of the parent drug and therefore makes a significant contribution to the total antiepileptic effect. Anatomical sites of action are not known. The drug may limit the spread of seizure activity by depressing post-tetanic potentiation. Although the exact mechanism is unclear, it seems to resemble that of DPH. Like the tricyclic antidepressants, the relationship between oral dose and blood concentration is quite irregular, making estimation of serum concentrates important (therapeutic range about 4-8 µg/ml). Time response relationships have not yet been established but it is usual to follow medical custom and administer carbamazepine twice a day.

CLINICAL EFFECTS

1) *Antiepileptic.* The very comprehensive review of the antiepileptic properties of carbamazepine by Cereghino et al. (1974) suggests that the best results are obtained in generalized tonic-clonic seizures and complex partial seizures. Little effect is seen with absence seizures. With carbamazepine, clinical improvement and EEG changes appear to be unassociated; indeed, clinical improvement may be accompanied by an increase in EEG discharges (Jeavons, 1973). From the results of uncontrolled studies, there seems to be little to choose between the antiepileptic effects of carbamazepine and of DPH, phenobarbital or primidone, although a distinct preference for carbamazepine is stated by some authors for the treatment of complex partial seizures in adults (Parsonage, 1975) and children (Gamstorp, 1975).

2) *Psychotropic—Epileptic Conditions.* Several reports of the effectiveness of carbamazepine as an antiepileptic medication have noted associated improvement in the mental state of patients and this is of particular interest in view of the structural relationships bewteen carbamazepine and the tricyclic antidepressants. A wide range of abnormal mental states are said to have improved, but perhaps especially antisocial and apathetic behavior and psychomotor retardation.

There are suggestions in some reviews of its use in seizure disorders that this psychotropic effect is independent of its antiepileptic action but this is not clearly supported by the available evidence. A frequently quoted paper on the subject is that by Dalby (1971) in which 93 patients with complex partial seizures were treated with carbamazepine and observed for up to 6 years. Over half of these patients were psychiatrically abnormal at the outset and a substantial number of them improved during the period of observation, particularly those with episodic disorders (especially depression). As Dalby himself points out, however, *these improvements in mental state were significantly related to better control of seizures and to the withdrawal of previous medication with socially disabling side effects.* Far from there being evidence of direct psychotropic action, the administration of carbamazepine was convincingly associated with the onset of severe mental disorder in 5 patients in this series. One developed a schizophrenia-like psychosis, another suffered an increase in the frequency of his attacks (which took on new psychotic proportions) and 3 other patients are said to have become emotionally explosive and confused. That all 5 of the patients had objectively demonstrated cerebral atrophy raises the interesting possibility that carbamazepine may actually be contraindicated in similarly brain damaged patients.

Rajotte et al. (1967) and Marjerrison et al. (1968) conducted controlled studies in which improvements in behavior occurred when carbamazepine was substituted for DPH and phenobarbital respectively in chronically institutionalized patients. Again it is difficult to apportion this improvement to carbamazepine itself or to relief from the adverse effects of other drugs. Less certain beneficial effects were seen when carbamazepine was compared in a controlled manner with placebo by Pryce-Phillips and Jeavons (1970) and Rodin et al. (1974).

3) *Psychotropic—Non-epileptic Conditions.* The reported beneficial effects of carbamazepine on the behavior of patients with epilepsy led many clinicians, especially in Europe, to prescribe the drug for nonepileptic children and adults with a variety of types of disturbed behavior. The difficulties of evaluating the resulting claims for its efficacy exactly parallel those already discussed in connection with DPH. Most favorable reports are based on uncontrolled studies of heterogeneous clinical groups with little effort made to measure particular aspects of behavior. Nissen (1976), for example, on the basis of clinical experience recommends the use of carbamazepine in the anxious and hyperkinetic groups of children which constitute 2 of his 3 broad categories of behavioral disorders of childhood (the other being children with inhibition of drive) *in spite of his own negative findings in a controlled study.*

Remschmidt (1976) provides a thoughtful review of the evidence, particularly as it relates to children. Of the 7, double-blind, placebo-controlled trials which he quotes, 3 (Groh et al., 1971; Puente, 1976; Puente et al., 1973) suggested that carbamazepine was significantly better in enhancing drive, purposeful activity, mood and social adaptation. In the other 4 (Bettschart et al., 1969; Kivalo et al., 1968; Nissen, 1976; Schifino et al., 1976), no significant differences were found, though a trend in favor of carbamazepine was seen in the first 2 of these studies for behavioral disorders. In the many other uncontrolled studies there is a tendency to report that overactivity and aggressiveness are particularly helped by carbamazepine and usually the presence of nonspecific "EEG abnormalities" is seen as a good prognostic sign, though the latter is a recurrent yet quite unestablished theme in pediatric psychopharmacology (see Chapters 2 and 6).

The findings taken as a whole do not permit more than the tentative conclusion that there is some evidence to suggest that carbamazepine *may* benefit disturbed children, perhaps particularly those whose problems show themselves as motor overactivity or aggression. It is of interest that this is the diagnostic group which responds to antidepressants and it is possible that this is simply a weak residual antidepressant-like effect. If so it would have to be shown that carbamazepine was safer, more effective or had different indications. However, it is not yet possible to say really how many children profit in this way from the psychotropic effects of carbamazepine or what characterizes the responders in terms of precise psychopathological or physiological variables. Rett (1976) has suggested that girls and older children generally respond more favorably, but this too awaits confirmation.

TREATMENT EMERGENT (SIDE) EFFECTS

These appear to be relatively infrequent. Initial dizziness, drowsiness, restlessness, gastro-intestinal upset or skin reactions may occur at low serum levels. Drowsiness, ataxia or diplopia often develop above serum levels of 8 μg/ml. A number of serious idiosyncratic effects, such as depression of bone marrow function and liver toxicity, have been reported but appear rare.

DRUG INTERACTIONS

The ability of carbamazepine to induce liver enzymes and the consequent effects on the metabolism of other drugs were mentioned earlier (see DPH).

CLINICAL INDICATIONS

The best established indication for the use of carbamazepine is the repeated occurrence of generalized tonic-clonic convulsions or partial seizures including those with complex symptomatology. It is not effective in absence seizures. In children in particular, carbamazepine may be preferable to other major antiepileptic drugs because of its apparently low incidence of adverse behavioral effects or other unwanted actions.

There are not yet any well-established indications for the use of carbamazepine in nonepileptic behavioral disorders of childhood, but this area deserves further study.

SUMMARY AND CONCLUSIONS

Because of its efficacy as an antiepileptic and relative freedom from adverse effects, carbamazepine is considered by some the drug of first choice in the generalized tonic-clonic convulsions and partial seizures of childhood. Its place in the management of other child psychiatric disorders is uncertain.

SUCCINIMIDES

Introduction

This group of drugs was derived from a systematic search, based on known chemical properties of antiepileptic drugs, for safer drugs effective in absence seizures, which it will be noted are not helped by any of the preceding drugs.

Ethosuximide (Zarontin) is the most commonly used member of this group which also includes methsuximide (Celontin) and phensuximide (Milontin).

Fig. 5

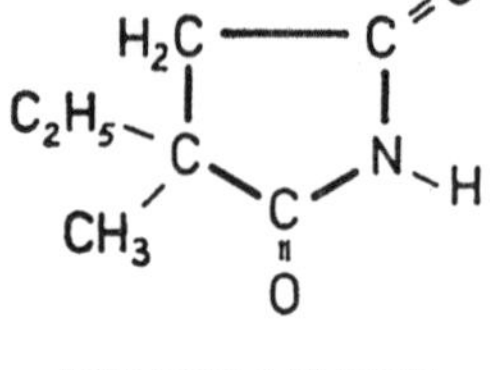

ETHOSUXIMIDE
(Zarontin)

CHEMICAL STRUCTURE

As can be seen in Figure 5, this contains the typical common denominator illustrated in Figure 1.

Ethosuximide (Zarontin)

PHARMACOLOGY

Absorption is rapid, and the serum half-life in children is about 30 hours. Protein-binding is negligible, but little is known of distribution except in animals where it is evenly distributed in most tissues. About 10 to 20% is excreted in the urine unchanged; the remainder is metabolized in the liver. At least two metabolites are produced, one of which has no antiepileptic action. Sites and mechanism of the action of ethosuximide are not well understood, though the end result in animals is to raise seizure threshold. Serum levels are reasonably well related to dosage but with variability between patients, and there is good evidence that seizure control is closely related to concentration of ethosuximide in serum.

CLINICAL ADMINISTRATION

Ethosuximide is usually given twice a day though once may be sufficient in view of the steady serum levels achieved after treatment has been established. Onset of antiepileptic action is rapid and maximal within a few days. Most patients require serum levels between 40 and 100 μg/ml for optimum control.

CLINICAL EFFECTS

1) *Seizure Disorders.* One of the few generalizations possible from Coatsworth's review (1971) was that ethosuximide consistently showed good results in the treatment of absence seizures. This has been borne out in later studies. Despite its action in animals there is little evidence of efficacy in other types of seizure disorders and it has been claimed that generalized tonic-clonic convulsions can be induced in patients who previously had only absence seizures.

2) *Nonepileptic Disorders.* Ethosuximide has been used in nonepileptic children with learning difficulties and the 14 and 6 per second spike and wave phenomenon (the psychiatric significance of which remains contentious—see Werry, in press b). Smith et al. (1968) carried out a double-blind cross-over trial on such children using very small amounts of ethosuximide compared with the usual antiepileptic dosage. They reported a

general improvement in behavior as well as significant and selective improvement in verbal skills as measured by the Wechsler Intelligence Scale for Children (see below).

TREATMENT EMERGENT (SIDE) EFFECTS

1) *Physical (other than CNS)*. Ethosuximide is relatively safe with few physical complications. Mild transient side effects include gastric upset, drowsiness and dizziness. Serious skin reactions or hematological change are rare.

2) *Nervous (including Behavior and Cognition)*. Mood changes such as lethargy and euphoria are said to be possible side effects of ethosuximide and more dramatic psychotic illnesses have also been attributed to this drug (Roger et al., 1968). Descriptions of these disorders suggest that they were actually acute organic confusional states rather than psychoses in clear consciousness.

Ethosuximide has also been linked with effects on learning in children though contradictorily. Alarming consequences were reported in some children from the addition of ethosuximide to phenobarbital (Guey et al., 1967). Global intellectual impairment and speech difficulties appeared to follow, as well as confusional states and possibly other psychotic disorders. It is difficult to know from this uncontrolled study how these effects might have been produced. In contrast, a multi-center control trial of ethosuximide given to therapeutic serum levels for absence attacks in previously untreated children produced no evidence of intellectual deterioration or any other behavioral disturbances after eight weeks of treatment (Browne et al., 1975). Indeed, there was some evidence of improvement in psychological function, as might be expected from seizure control.

DRUG INTERACTIONS

There appear to be none of clinical significance.

CLINICAL INDICATIONS AND CONTRAINDICATIONS

Ethosuximide is indicated in absence seizures associated with the three per second spike and wave discharge. However, sodium valproate (either alone or combined with ethosuximide) may be preferable, especially when the absence takes a clinically more complicated form although accompanied by generalized discharge. There is no convincing evidence of its value in other seizure disorders and there is little to commend the practice of routinely combining other drugs with ethosuximide with the intention of preventing the development of generalized tonic-clonic convulsions on the grounds that this happens in a proportion of children who initially have only absence seizures.

Although the possibility of an independent psychotropic action has been raised, this requires much more confirmation.

SUMMARY AND CONCLUSIONS

Ethosuximide remains an effective and safe treatment for the control of absence seizures, but may be superseded by sodium valproate for this purpose. Any use in nonepileptic conditions is yet to be established.

Other Succinimides

Phensuximide, the first succinimide to be introduced for the treatment of absence seizures, is as safe as but less effective than ethosuximide. Methsuximide appears to be effective in this type of seizure disorder (though to a less extent than phensuximide) but may also control complex partial seizures.

BENZODIAZEPINES

Introduction

Though most mental health professionals probably think of this group of drugs as anxiolytics and this no doubt accounts for most of their dispensing, some of them have useful, indeed lifesaving, antiepileptic properties. Their pharmacology and psychotropic use are discussed in Chapter 10.

The structure of diazepam is presented in Fig. 1, Chapter 10 (p. 336). Variations within the group are minor. Though the two-dimensional structure looks different from that of the antiepileptic common denominator in Figure 1 of this chapter, it is said to be similar sterically.

While the members of this group of drugs have increased steadily in recent years, only 3 have found a regular place in the treatment of seizure disorders to date. Diazepam (Valium) is of particular value in the treatment of status epilepticus (continuous seizures) of both the convulsive and absence types, and nitrazepam (Mogadon) and clonazepam (Rivotril) have some value as maintenance therapy for certain types of seizure disorder. Chlordiazepoxide (Librium) is thought to have less direct antiepileptic value in clinical practice than these other benzodiazepines although it may be the most effective member of this group in suppressing generalized seizure discharge in the EEG (Jeavons, 1962).

The mode of action of diazepam is thought to be mainly depression of synaptic transmission with limitation of spread of seizure discharge especially in the hippocampal formation, amygdaloid complex and the septal area. After intravenous injection, penetration into the CNS is very rapid, but concentrations there decline quickly as distribution occurs into non-lipoid tissues. This may result in a recurrence of seizures after 30-60 minutes.

Clinical Effects in Seizure Disorders

In contrast to the emergency use of diazepam in status epilepticus, there is little evidence that the benzodiazepines are effective in the long-term treatment of generalized tonic-clonic convulsions or partial sizures, except in those cases where emotional factors such as anxiety may act as a consistent precipitant of seizures. In such cases, the psychotropic properties of diazepam or chlordiazepoxide, rather than their antiepileptic properties, may aid satisfactory seizure control. Because of inadequate evaluation (including the tendency to use them as adjuvant therapy), it is not possible to know whether benzodiazepines have a direct antiepileptic action in the case of absence seizures, although clonazepam has been reported to be promising in this respect. In contrast, benzodiazepines (especially nitrazepam and clonazepam) appear to be effective in *myoclonic, atonic* and *akinetic* seizures which are otherwise very difficult to treat.

The benzodiazepines appear to be relatively non-toxic. Drowsiness quite often occurs initially but this is transient. Indeed, one of the limitations of this group of drugs is the tendency for tolerance to develop at the expense of their antiepileptic action. Over-sedation may be a particular problem with clonazepam. The long-term administration of benzodiazepines has not usually been associated with harmful direct effects on mental state, but recent evidence suggests that in certain circumstances benzodiazepines may provoke hostile or otherwise disinhibited behavior (*British Medical Journal*, 1975). This could be important in epileptic children exhibiting irritable or aggresssive behavior. Disinhibition is discussed in detail in Chapter 10.

Interactions

The sedative properties of benzodiazepines are likely to be potentiated by sodium valproate. Apparently, clonazepam may lower levels of DPH by induction of its metabolism despite the low capacity of benzodiazepines for induction.

Clinical Indications

Because of its safety and rapid penetration of the CNS, diazepam is particularly useful for the treatment of the serious condition of status epilepticus or continuous seizures. On the present evidence, the place of long-term treatment with nitrazepam and, possibly, clonazepam is confined to the myoclonic, atonic and akinetic seizures where these drugs probably represent a significant advance over other antiepileptic drugs with the possible exception of sodium valproate.

The benzodiazepines are an important and relatively safe group of antiepileptic drugs especially valuable acutely in status epilepticus and in long-term treatment of the otherwise difficult myoclonic, atonic and akinetic seizures.

Fig. 6.

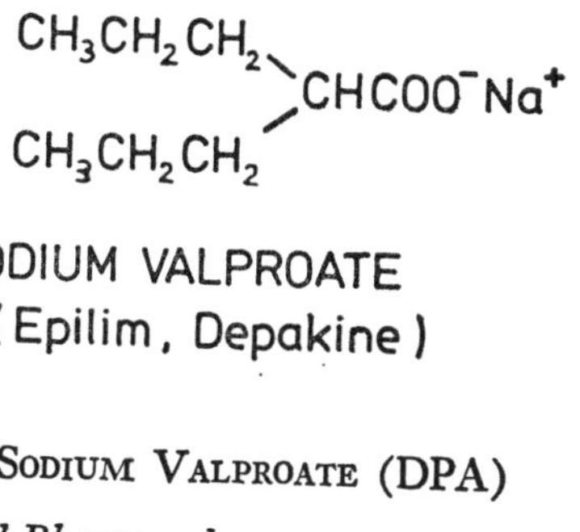

$$\begin{array}{c} CH_3CH_2CH_2 \\ CH_3CH_2CH_2 \end{array}\!\!\!>\!CHCOO^-Na^+$$

SODIUM VALPROATE
(Epilim, Depakine)

Sodium Valproate (DPA)

Chemical Structure and Pharmacology

Sodium valproate (Epilim, Depakine) is the sodium salt of valproic acid, or dipropyl-acetic acid, often abbreviated to DPA. It has been used in the treatment of seizures since 1963 but only became generally available in Britain in 1972 and is still undergoing evaluation in the United States. Sodium valproate is a branched chain carboxylic acid salt and is structurally quite unlike other antiepileptic drugs. Pinder et al. (1977) have published a comprehensive review of this drug.

Sodium valproate is rapidly absorbed and its half-life in children is probably less than 7 to 9 hours. It is about 90% bound to serum albumin and rapidly distributed, mainly in the extracellular fluid. It is omega oxidised to a variety of pharmacologically inactive metabolites which are excreted mainly through the kidneys. Its site of action has not been established. The mechanisms of action involved are uncertain, but there are suggestions that DPA may partially be effective by raising brain levels of the inhibitory neurotransmittor gamma-amino butyric acid (GABA). There seems to be a poor correlation between body-weight related dose and serum levels.

Clinical Administration

A therapeutic range of 50-100 µg/ml can be accepted provisionally although doubts have been expressed about the value of serum levels in clinical practice (Jeavons et al., 1977). It appears that DPA needs to be given at least twice a day. It has been suggested that the most responsive type of seizure disorder, namely absence seizures, begin to improve within one to three weeks (Jeavons et al., 1977).

Clinical Effects

1) *Seizure Disorders.* There are difficulties in the evaluation of DPA because of the usual lack of controlled studies and the fact that it is usually used in combination with other drugs. However, there is general agreement that DPA is most effective in the generalized seizure disorders, especially absence seizures associated with three per second spike and wave discharge. Many investigators have been impressed by improvement in myoclonic seizures, which are often resistant to other forms of treatment (Jeavons et al., 1977), as well as in generalized tonic-clonic convulsions. Partial seizures with elementary symptomatology may also respond (possibly only at higher dosage than that required for absence seizures) but the evidence for complex partial seizures is less convincing.

Several authors have emphasized the improvement in mental state of patients with epilepsy following the introduction of DPA. Jeavons et al. (1977) feel that its alerting effect makes it particularly valuable in the treatment of school children. As always with antiepileptic drugs, it is difficult to tell, however, how far such changes are the results of improved seizure control and/or the concomitant withdrawal of other drugs which have adversely affected behavior.

2) *Psychotropic Effects.* In a very preliminary double-blind study of largely subnormal patients, aged 6 to 35, with mainly aggressive behavior (Sonnen et al., 1975), no significant difference was seen between the psychotropic effects of DPA administered over a 3-week period and placebo. Nevertheless, the possibility exists that DPA has independent psychotropic

action of other types (including an alerting effect) perhaps after longer administration or in certain groups of patients. This is suggested by the findings of Linnoila et al. (1976). In their double-blind cross-over study on elderly chronic psychiatric patients who had been on heavy neuroleptic medication for several years, DPA produced a significant improvement in tardive dyskinesia and, independently, in psychiatric symptoms, especially poor cooperation and emotional withdrawal. In contrast, single modest doses of DPA administered alone can have an hypnotic effect on healthy subjects (Boxer et al., 1976). This area, however, needs further study.

Treatment Emergent (Side) Effects and Interactions

The adverse effects associated with DPA are relatively few and not serious, the most common being gastro-intestinal disturbance which can usually be prevented by taking it with or after food. Other unwanted physical effects include temporary hair loss and tremor (in high dosage). Platelet deficiencies may occur at very high serum levels and DPA may potentiate the sedative effects of other drugs, especially phenobarbital (the serum levels of which may be increased) and clonazepam. The effects of antidepressant drugs may also be potentiated. Overactivity and other troublesome behavior have occasionally been reported but, again, it is difficult to assess the possibility in most cases of interaction of DPA with other drugs or the role of serum levels as they are rarely reported.

Potentiation of sedating and antidepressant drugs has already been mentioned.

Clinical Indications and Contraindications

DPA appears to be effective over a wide range of seizure disorders, especially the generalized epilepsies and, in particular, absence seizures associated with three per second spike and wave discharge. At least as adjuvant therapy, it appears to have been very helpful in many cases previously resistant to other forms of antiepileptic treatment including the myoclonic seizures. There are no known absolute contraindications to its use. DPA should be withdrawn in the event of spontaneous bruising or bleeding and the cause investigated.

DPA appears to be a significant advance in the treatment of seizures. It has the advantage of a wide range of effectiveness including some otherwise refractory seizure states. It also appears to have relatively few adverse effects. It is potentially the drug of choice in absence seizures and at least the equal of ethosuximide. Occasionally the combination of these two drugs appears to be helpful for otherwise resistant absence seizures. DPA has the advantage over phenobarbital and DPH in terms of adverse effects but direct comparisons of the antiepileptic properties of these drugs have yet to be made. The full extent of its place in the treatment of seizure disorders will only be clear when further studies of its use as a single agent in comparison with the more established drugs have been carried out.

Its psychotropic properties, both direct and indirect, deserve further study.

Miscellaneous Antiepileptic Drugs

Sulthiame (Ospolot)

This is a sulphonamide derivative which weakly inhibits carbonic anhydrase. Its antiepileptic properties have been demonstrated in animals for some years and it has been considered useful (usually in combination with other drugs) in a variety of types of seizure disorder, perhaps especially complex partial seizures. It has also been promoted as having psychotropic properties. More recently, the results of controlled studies (Green et al., 1974) have raised doubts whether it has independent antiepileptic action or whether it works by raising the serum levels of phenobarbital, primidone and especially DPH, by inhibiting the metabolism of these drugs. As well as carrying the risk of intoxication because of these interactions (which become apparent 10 to 20 days after the introduction of sulthiame), sulthiame has adverse physical effects of its own, especially headache, drowsiness, hypernea, paresthesiae of the extremities, anorexia and weight loss. Sulthiame has also been thought to produce depression and psychotic states.

Its reported effects on cognitive function are conflicting. Hutt et al. (1966) claim a selectively beneficial effect on sustained attention but a more recent report of a double-blind comparison of DPH and sulthiame taken singly (Dodrill, 1975b) suggests that, although patients may feel more alert when on sulthiame, they show widespread intellectual and social deficits on testing, with significantly less impairment when taking DPH. Sulthiame treatment was particularly associated in this study with general intellectual impairment, poor performance in complex tasks requiring sustained attention and complex psychomotor tasks. Social functioning was also said to be adversely affected. This is an important study but it leaves open the question of how far these deficits are ascribable directly to sulthiame or whether they are not the result of less satisfactory control of seizure activity with sulthiame compared to DPH. Ingram and Ratcliffe

(1963), reporting the value of sulthiame (often combined with other drugs) in children with seizures and, in most cases, other neurological and intellectual handicap, claimed that "hyperkinetic behavior" (undefined) was much improved in half the cases. Kneebone (1965) in a comparable study reported similar but more consistent effects and claimed that hyperkinetic behavior increased when sulthiame was withdrawn and improved again when it was reintroduced. Sulthiame was assessed by Liu (1966) over periods from 6 months to 4½ years in mentally handicapped and disturbed adult patients most of whom had seizures. Liu concluded that sulthiame was a valuable drug both in terms of controlling seizures and improving behavior but, even more than in the 2 previous studies, the information provided does not allow the behavioral changes claimed to be assessed precisely, still less can any such change be attributed directly to sulthiame itself. None of these 3 studies was adequately controlled.

However, in the last few years, 2 reports have been published which are more convincing. The studies by Moffatt et al. (1970) and Al-Kaisi and McGuire (1974) have been quite large, well controlled investigations in which standardized measurements have been made of different aspects of behavior in both epileptic and nonepileptic patients suffering severe subnormality and serious behavioral disturbance. From these reports, it seems that sulthiame may produce a significant and genuine reduction of disturbed behavior in such patients, perhaps especially in motor excitement and aggressiveness, which is not simply attributable to a reduction in seizure frequency or to improved standards of care and attention.

At the present time it seems that there is little support for the view that sulthiame has independent properties as an antiepileptic and its psychotropic properties require further study. As will be discussed later, the physical and behavioral risks of adding it to other antiepileptic treatment (especially DPH) are considerable.

Acetazolamide (Diamox)

Like sulthiame, acetazolamide is also a sulphonamide derivative and a carbonic anhydrase inhibitor. It was introduced in the 1950's as an alternative to a ketogenic diet for the treatment of absence seizures. Its value in the treatment of seizure disorders is uncertain and it appears to have no particular psychotropic indications.

Pheneturide (Benuride)

Pheneturide, like its highly toxic predecessor phenacemide, is an acetylurea. It has been claimed to be effective in complex partial seizures but has been the subject of very little satisfactory evaluation. Its place in the treatment of seizures is further limited by its high rate of adverse effects. It can inhibit the metabolism of DPH and is a potent inducer of liver enzymes. Pheneturide is undoubtedly safer than its predecessor, but it is thought to produce confusional states, other psychotic disorders and depression in a proportion of patients although it is again impossible to ascertain the particular circumstances in which these complications might occur.

Beclamide (Nydrane)

This is a chlorpropamide derivative with an uncertain place in the treatment of seizure disorders. If it has an antiepileptic action, it is weak. Its interest lies in the fact that of all the antiepileptic drugs perhaps the greatest claims of psychopharmacological benefit have been made for it. It is publicized as having a beneficial effect on a very wide range of disturbed behavior as well as on learning difficulties and involuntary movements, especially in children whether suffering from epilepsy or not. There is even more than the usual disparity (characteristic of the antiepileptic drugs) between these claims and the supporting evidence for psychotropic action and there is only one investigation which provides any suspicion of a real reason to believe that this drug may be of psychiatric value. This was a double-blind cross-over trial of beclamide given to very seriously disturbed and severely subnormal patients ranging from 7 to 30 years of age (Price & Spencer, 1967). The precise results are not given in this report but it is stated by the authors that a statistically significant improvement of behavior was obtained in the vast majority of patients. There is no mention of the particular behaviors that improved nor of the practical significance of the improvements so that this report is hardly substantial evidence in favor of a psychopharmacological role for beclamide.

Troxidone (Tridione)

This is a member of the oxazolidinedione group of drugs of which other less effective members have been produced for the treatment of absence seizures. It can cause a range of adverse effects including the so-called glare phenomenon, skin reactions and bone marrow depression. There have been reports that it can precipitate generalized tonic-clonic convulsions in patients who previously had only absence seizures (the same has been said for ethosuximide). Coatsworth's review (1971) accorded with general experience that ethosuximide is more effective for absences and less toxic than troxidone which is therefore not often used now. There seem to be no particular psychotropic aspects to this drug.

Overview and Conclusions

In reflecting the place of antiepileptic drugs in present-day pediatric practice, this chapter has naturally been very largely concerned with their use in children with seizures although many of the points discussed are directly relevant to their use in any context, including as primarily psychopharmacological agents.

Basic Principles

Certain basic principles arise concerning the use of these drugs as antiepileptic agents.

CHOICE OF DRUGS

This should be appropriate for the type of seizure disorder in question. Some drugs are likely to be more effective than others for a given type of epilepsy. Some drugs are not effective at all in certain circumstances and can even increase the severity of certain seizures. Rational therapy is only partly possible in the present state of knowledge, but it should be attempted initially. This presupposes, however, a much more precise description of each patient's seizure disorder than is often the case at present.

DRUG REGIMENS

1) *Treatment should be simple wherever possible.* It should be dictated largely by practical considerations and by pharmacological properties of the drug rather than by medical folklore. Depending on the serum half-life of the drug, the *minimum number of daily doses* needed to maintain the serum concentration within the optimum range for the child should be prescribed. Once daily doses of DPH have been recommended for adults (Reynolds et al., 1976) and children (Buchanan et al., 1973) as adequate for maintaining satisfactory serum levels over 24 hours. There may be problems, however, in giving a large dose (especially if more than one drug is required) rapidly and absorbed drugs might produce toxic serum levels if only transiently. If a single daily dose is preferred, it is probably best taken last thing at night. Avoiding an unnecessary midday dose at school is important because such a dose may be forgotten

and because the risk of the child being stigmatized as someone different and in need of drugs is lessened. Treatment should also be simple in the sense of *minimizing the number of drugs* prescribed. Reynolds et al. (1976) have demonstrated that many patients' seizures can be controlled with DPH alone if adequate blood levels are achieved. Small doses of more than one drug (sometimes combined in proprietary preparations), given to minimize the risk of adverse effects from any one, may well result in generally sub-therapeutic serum concentrations. Interactions have been stressed at various points in the preceding account and have been well reviewed by Richens (1975). Among the most troublesome are DPH with sulthiame, and barbiturates or benzodiazepines with sodium valproate. *Toxic levels of DPH (however produced) or over-sedation may increase seizure frequency.*

2) *Drugs need an adequate trial before their value can be realistically assessed.* Serum levels take time to stabilize from several days to 2 or 3 weeks depending on the drug (Kutt & Penry, 1974), and failure to respond immediately is not a reason for change of treatment. Parents often need to be reassured about this. Because of the slow rise of the serum level to therapeutic concentrations, a drug can generally be introduced at average dosage or above. Exceptions to this rule are primidone (because of the possibility of an idiosyncratic response) and carbamazepine which may well cause drowsiness if not introduced gradually. The potential effectiveness of a drug can be assessed by increasing the dosage up to the point at which toxic signs first appear. It should be then reduced until such signs disappear, or substituted if it has not produced satisfactory control of seizures.

3) *Changes of treatment should be carried out with care.* The risk of serious seizures on abrupt withdrawal of treatment is generally well-known, but even gradual discontinuation of a drug with a view to introducing a substitute may leave the child inadequately treated in the interim period. It is generally advisable to introduce the new treatment quite quickly to an average level and maintain that for about a week (being vigilant for adverse effects) before withdrawing the old treatment. In general, antiepileptic drugs should not (indeed do not need to be) withdrawn for the purposes of EEG investigations.

SERUM LEVELS AND TREATMENT

Measurement of serum levels of antiepileptic drugs has clearly become an important part of this management of patients with seizure disorders and has already given insights into some of the apparent anomalies of treatment in the past. Kutt & Penry (1974) and Richens (1976) have concisely discussed the clinical value of drug levels. The value probably varies with each drug depending on the complexity of its metabolism, the ease with which adverse effects may be produced by a slight increase in serum level, and the diversity of ways in which toxicity may show itself. On these counts, DPH estimations are particularly important, but it is possible to state general indications for the measurement of any antiepileptic drug. These include: a) *poor seizure control*, which might be due to inadequate or excessive treatment (although psychological precipitants should not be forgotten); b) serious *adverse effects* in a child on several drugs (to assess their relative contributions to the problem); c) *alteration in learning, general behavior or neurological state* in a child on antiepileptic medication as drug effects feature prominently in the differential diagnosis of all such cases. The introduction of *additional* treatment and the presence of other *diseases* which might affect drug metabolism or excretion are other indications. Serum levels should also be checked routinely every 6 months or so, especially in growing children whose dosage may well need adjustment. Serum level estimation should be standardized. Fasting samples taken early in the day are probably the most generally acceptable. Because of the technical difficulties involved, laboratory methods must be demonstrably reliable and the results comparable from one centre to another.

NON-PHARMACOLOGIC MANAGEMENT

Repeated explanations about the nature of the seizure disorder and its management are usually needed by parents and older children in order to ensure their acceptance and cooperation. The uncertainties of the response in many cases is worth admitting in order to avoid loss of confidence. Failure to secure active cooperation of parents and patients probably contributes significantly to the high rates of noncompliance reported in patients with epilepsy. Ley (1977) has summarized in a very persuasive way the reasons for patients' poor compliance and the ways in which physicians can raise their standards of care by improving communication. The points made by Ley apply to any area of clinical practice but they are likely to be particularly relevant to the management of childhood epilepsy which is fraught with anxieties and misconceptions (Voeller & Rothenberg, 1973).

Although the emphasis so far has been on drugs, a wholly pharmacological approach to the management of children with seizures is mistaken.

Many children with seizure disorders have additional complications to their lives of a psychological or social nature and adequate care must include attention to these problems. But, that apart, psychological factors can act as potent precipitants of seizures whatever their basic etiology, and modification of such factors can often be at least as important as drugs in obtaining satisfactory control. The need to explore and modify harmful parent-child relationships and other emotional precipitants, or investigate the influence of certain types of school work or levels of interest or arousal (Stores, 1973), illustrates how intimately related are physical and psychological processes in this particular area of medical practice. Although there has been some demonstration of the importance of psychological precipitants and their inhibiting factors in some seizure disorders, as is to true of pediatric psychopharmacology in general (see Chapter 3), very little systematic study of their therapeutic relevance and interrelations with drug treatment has been carried out.

Evaluating Antiepileptic Drugs (See Also Chapters 2, 3 and 4)

Generalizations about "epileptics" and heterogeneous groupings bedevil the subject of epilepsy. Failure to specify the types of patients studied, their circumstances or their treatment may well explain some of the conflicting reports and the negative findings in some studies on the behavioral effects of antiepileptic drugs such as those by Loveland et al. (1957).

Studies of various behavioral aspects of childhood epilepsy, including reading skills (Stores & Hart, 1976), attentiveness (Stores et al., 1977), different types of disturbed behavior at school (Stores, 1977) and dependency (Stores & Piran, 1977), suggest that EEG type of epilepsy and sex may be crucial variables, boys being consistently more affected than girls. Some behavioral effects of treatments may be age dependent. The serious disturbances of learning attributed to ethosuximide by Guey et al. (1967) were predominantly in adolescents rather than in younger children. Intellectual level and the presence of gross structural brain pathology could also be important. Is carbamazepine particularly troublesome behaviorally in patients with cerebral atrophy as Dalby's (1971) findings might suggest? Are the severely subnormal at special risk of DPH intoxication (Logan & Freeman 1969)? Drug toxicity, especially as it affects behavior, may be easily overlooked in patients whose behavior is already severely disturbed. On the other hand, does sulthiame improve disturbed behavior only in severely subnormal populations? Studies of the antiepileptic properties and behavioral effects of drugs must aim at more precise definition of the *condition* in question and also the *circum-*

stances of the patient at the time of assessment. The social environmental circumstances of the patients studied are rarely documented and yet reports of benezodiazepine-induced hostility suggest that this may be another important factor.

An aspect of the psychopharmacology of antiepileptic drugs, which requires much more attention than it has so far received, is the way in which behavior is assessed. Reference has already been made to the unsophisticated ways in which behavioral complications are reported in studies of the antiepileptic properties of drugs. Impressions and global judgments about "improvement" or "deterioration" are common but give no clear idea of what particular behavioral change has come about. Behavior should be measured whenever possible, not by means of multifactorial tests which use gross measures such as IQ (or even subtests on the Weschler scales which themselves are multifactorial and unreliable), but by relatively specific measures which allow functional analysis of the impaired performance (see Chapters 2 and 3).

It has not been clear which are the more fundamental functions and most discriminating test used in epilepsy research. This is reflected in the diversity of tests employed to study the behavioral effects of seizure activity (Penry, 1973). But sensitive tests for drug research with antiepileptics can be identified. Hart et al. (1976) have demonstrated the sensitivity of auditory vigilance tests to low doses of amylobarbitone and diazepam; McNair (1973), reviewing the many different measures used in studies of anxiolytic drugs such as diazepam, highlights the more useful of these for future research. The Werry-Weiss-Peters activity rating scale (Werry & Sprague, 1970) and simple performance measures of vigilance, visual search and auditory distractibility have been shown to distinguish between epileptic and normal boys (Stores et al., 1977) although the contribution of drugs to this difference has not yet been ascertained. Where only descriptive accounts are feasible, international differences in terminology should be acknowledged and precise operational definitions given. At the moment, a serious imbalance exists between the increasingly sophisticated pharmacological accounts of antiepileptic drugs and the relatively amateurish reporting of their behavioral effects. The general question of measurement in pediatric psychopharmacology is discussed in detail in Chapters 2 and 3.

Dangers of Antiepileptic Drugs

It is clear from this brief review that there is enough known or suspected to make the administration of antiepileptic drugs to patients a serious matter. Drug treatment of seizures is of great importance in most cases but it has to be recognized that adverse effects are common and sometimes very serious. For the most part, fortunately, harmful behavioral effects seem to remit on reduction or discontinuation of the drug in question, although fears have been expressed that the deterioration sometimes associated with chronic DPH intoxication may be irreversible (Vallarta et al., 1974). As implied earlier, very few follow-up studies have been carried out to explore the possible long-term effects on learning or other aspects of behavior of antiepileptic drug administration. Apart from the direct behavioral effects of drugs taken over long periods, there may be serious psychological consequences of the unpleasant cosmetic effects of certain drugs, particularly DPH as mentioned earlier.

There needs to be good reason to believe at the outset (with periodic reassessments afterwards) that the child will on balance benefit from taking antiepileptic drugs. Not all seizures need to be treated this way. A reasonable general principle is that a first seizure needs investigation but no treatment. However, on recurrence (if the seizures are likely to be detrimental to the child's progress), appropriate treatment should be started. Thus, mild, infrequent, non-convulsive seizures might be best left untreated. Uncomplicated television-induced epilepsy is an example of where drug treatment may well not be required at all (Jeavons & Harding, 1975).

Epilepsy, Behavior Disorders and the EEG

A numerically more serious cause of unnecessary treatment is *misdiagnosis*. Jeavons (1975) reports that 20% of children attending an epilepsy clinic had been diagnosed as epileptic when, in reality, they had suffered syncope, attacks of a psychological nature or other non-epileptic conditions. Another source of diagnostic error is the injudicious use of the EEG which is still sometimes erroneously seen as a substitute for close medical enquiry. Apart from very special circumstances, it is not the purpose of the EEG to diagnose a seizure disorder *which is essentially a clinical procedure*.

Diagnostic indeterminacy appears to underlie some of the wider uses of antiepileptic drugs in child psychiatry. Particularly in some of the claims for DPH in this context, significance is attributed to the presence of EEG abnormalities as part of a syndrome, which (it is thought) has such features in common with undoubted seizure disorders that the use of antiepileptic drugs is appropriate. Thus Chao et al. (1964) wrote about the *convulsive equivalent syndrome of childhood*. Other writers refer to *epileptic equivalents* (an ambiguous term which has also been used for non-convulsive seizures in patients who undoubtedly have epilepsy). The behavioral features emphasized in these conditions have been their paroxysmal character and signs of autonomic disturbance. EEG "abnormalities" (including the 14 and 6 cycles per second positive spike phenomenon) and supposed response to antiepileptic drugs have reinforced the view that organic pathology underlies these conditions.

In fact, none of these features constitutes adequate evidence of an epileptic basis. Many nonepileptic behaviors are intermittent or paroxysmal. Paroxysmal behavioral disturbance and autonomic changes are in no way specific to seizures. In the conditions in question, a close association in time between either type of change and the occurrence of seizure activity has not usually been demonstrated. Lack of normative data makes the definition of EEG abnormality itself in children very difficult and features judged "unusual" not infrequently occur in perfectly healthy children. The 14 and 6 cycles per second positive spike phenomenon (to which much psychopathological significance has been attached in the past) is of this type as Eeg-Olofsson (1971) has shown. It seems likely to represent a normal developmental process; at worst it is "a signal in a search for significance" (Walter & Grossman, 1963). The presence of abnormal slowing of basic EEG rhythms and other unusual electrographic features, have, in fact, *not* been consistently associated with behavioral response to DPH. Freeman (1967) has emphasized the general problem of the reliability and interpretation of EEG findings in child psychiatry. Especially where the total clinical context is ignored, importance is often still attached to non-specific EEG abnormalities the true significance of which is quite unknown. Finally, as far as response to anti-epileptic drugs is concerned, the possibility of placebo response must constantly be borne in mind (see Chapter 4).

Summary

More than ordinary caution is required in the use of antiepileptic drugs for children, not only because of their potentially hazardous effects but because, by their injudicious prescription, the implied diagnosis of epilepsy or some quasi-epileptic disorder puts the child at risk of social stigmatization, and lifelong disadvantage. At the moment, while some of the antiepileptic drugs show possibilities as psychotropic agents, their use in children with nonepileptic conditions such as behavior or learning disorders of childhood cannot be justified except as a carefully controlled research exercise.

10

ANTIMANIC, ANTIANXIETY, HALLUCINOGENIC AND MISCELLANEOUS DRUGS

JUDITH L. RAPOPORT, M.D.,
EDWIN J. MIKKELSEN, M.D., and
JOHN S. WERRY, M.D.

ANTIMANICS*

Definition

Antimanic drugs are those which *specifically* inhibit or prevent the manic or excited phase of manic-depressive illness. This specific action stands in sharp contrast to the symptomatic suppression of manic excitement by sedatives or antipsychotic drugs in which *sedation* is clinically conspicuous and the source of the therapeutic effect. Once again, the term is unsuitable for children since, as was seen in Chapter 5, manic-depressive illness does not appear in the proposed American and International classifications of children's psychiatric disorders, beginning only in adolescence; further, if antimanics prove to have a place in pediatric psychopharmacology, it will be, most probably, in other than true manic states. However, in keeping with the functional classification derived from adult psychopharmacology reluctantly accepted in this book, the term antimanic will be used, again without implying any therapeutic indication. Fortunately, the fact that there is only one antimanic drug, lithium, at present, means the problem can be obviated to a certain extent by referring to it in this review by name rather than by class.

---

* This section was written by J. Rapoport and E. Mikkelsen who would like to thank William E. Bunney, Jr., M.D. for helpful discussion and advice.

Introduction

The use of lithium carbonate is a major advance in the treatment of manic-depressive disorders. First described by Cade (1949), who reported that lithium salts seemed efficacious in *treating* acute affective disorders of manic-depressive type, lithium now appears effective as a *prophylactic* agent in preventing or minimizing recurrences (Basstrup and Schou, 1967; Schou, 1976). Though lithium has not played a significant role in child psychiatry to date, its actions and the few clinical studies with children are reported here in some detail, as greater use of lithium salts with pediatric patients seems certain to occur, not only by a sort of osmosis of clinical practices from adult psychopharmacology but because of its interesting and powerful effects on brain function.

Chemical Structure and Pharmacology

Lithium is an hydrophilic alkali metal found in many minerals in the earth's crust and in sea water. It is the lightest of all the solid elements, with an atomic weight of 6.9M., and is the least lipid-soluble of the alkali metals.

ABSORPTION AND DISTRIBUTION

Lithium is rapidly absorbed via the gastrointestinal tract, with blood levels peaking in 2-4 hours after a single oral dose (Amdisen, 1969). The serum half-life is quite long, approximately 24 hours.

As lithium is not protein bound, it distributes throughout intra- and extracellular body water (Foulks et al., 1952; Schou, 1958). It cannot be pumped out of cells as efficiently as sodium, though it can be actively transported across cell membranes (Maizels, 1961; Zerahn, 1955). Because of these properties, tissue lithium concentration depends on at least 4 factors: serum lithium concentration, tissue water content, rate of penetrance into intracellular fluid, and rate of removal from intracellular fluid (Baer, 1973).

Autopsy studies in patients dying of lithium overdose have shown no major differences between concentrations in heart, liver, muscle, kidney or brain (Trautner et al., 1955). However, other studies in man have shown that lithium is not uniformly distributed between serum and cerebrospinal fluid with a mean serum to CSF ratio of 3:1 to 4:1 during chronic administration (Baker & Winokur, 1966; Platman & Fieve, 1968). There is a similar differential distribution of approximately 3:1 between serum and red blood cell (Baer, 1973).

METABOLISM, EXCRETION AND ACTIVE PRINCIPLES

Being an ion, lithium is not metabolized in any way. It is excreted almost entirely by the kidneys (Talso & Clarke, 1951). This is somewhat slow with average rates of 50% in the first 24 hours, 90% within 48 hours and trace amounts still detectable in urine for weeks after ingestion of even a single dose. As lithium is not protein-bound, it is freely filtered by the glomerulus, with lithium to creatinine clearance rations averaging 0.2 to 0.3 in man. Clearance seems independent of serum concentration and is not significantly influenced by water-loading or potassium-loading (Thomsen & Schou, 1968). The proximal renal tubule appears to be the primary site of reabsorption (Baer et al., 1971; Thomsen & Schou, 1968) and thus diuretics which act on the proximal tubule should only be used with great caution. Lithium excretion is tied to that of sodium. Increased proximal tubular reabsorption of sodium is generally accompanied by decreased reabsorption of lithium leading to increased excretion and vice versa (Shopsin & Gershon, 1973). This major regulatory role of sodium in controlling renal lithium excretion is of utmost clinical importance.

SITE AND MODE OF ACTION

Lithium has important effects on body electrolytes, biogenic amines, and cellular transport mechanisms.

1) *Electrolytes.* There is an initial increased loss of *sodium* and *potassium* following the onset of lithium treatment which is thought to be due to displacement of these ions by lithium in intra- and extracellular fluid compartments. After appproximately one week of lithium administration, sodium and potassium excretion return to normal (Baer, 1973). Studies of its effect on *magnesium* have shown conflicting results (Aronoff et al., 1971) *Calcium* excretion has been shown to decrease (Tupin et al., 1968) and serum levels have increased in animal studies (Mellerup et al., 1970). Shopsin and Gershon (1973) have speculated that the action of lithium in the central nervous system may parallel its inability to substitute for sodium in renal transport systems; thus, its inefficient pumping out of neurons could alter electrical transmission.

2) *Monoamines.* Acute and short-term administration of lithium has been shown to increase the turnover of *norepinephrine* (noradrenalin) (Stern et al., 1969) though no such change is found when administration exceeds 2 weeks (Corrodi et al., 1969). Data showing a transient increase in urinary excretion in man of MHPG, one of the metabolites of

norepinephrine, are consistent with the hypothesis that turnover of norepinephrine is increased with short-term administration but that this does not persist with prolonged administration (Schildkraut, 1973). *Dopamine* levels and turnover do not seem to be affected by acute or chronic lithium administration (Bunney & Murphy, 1976).

Studies of the effects of lithium on *serotonin* metabolism have yielded conflicting results (Schildkraut, 1973). An increase in 5-hydroxyindoleactic acid in human cerebrospinal fluid was observed after treatment with lithium carbonate in two studies (Mendels, 1971; Wilk et al., 1972), but not in another (Bowers et al., 1969). It has been shown both to increase and decrease turnover, depending on the duration of treatment with lithium (Knapp & Mandell, 1973).

In some tissues, lithium has been shown to inhibit *cyclic-AMP* and it is felt that this may be the mechanism for its action on hormone systems (Friedman, 1973). Lithium has been shown to interact with cyclic-AMP mediated processes regulated to polypeptide hormones in the kidney, thyroid and CNS (Singer & Rotenberg, 1973).

It is thought that lithium may exert its effect by altering *membrane transport* mechanisms (Bunney & Murphy, 1976). Bunney and Murphy have postulated two possible mechanisms: a presynaptic mechanism leading to a functional decrease of dopamine and norepinephrine (Bunney et al., 1972) and a post-synaptic neuronal receptor hypothesis suggesting that lithium might stabilize the synaptic effects of norepinephrine and dopamine on receptors (Bunney & Murphy, 1975).

DOSE RESPONSE DATA

Because of the complex relationship between lithium and sodium excretion, dose/serum level interrelationships can be quite variable and require careful monitoring. It takes about 5 days before a steady state is reached. Prien, et al. (1971) found there was little correlation between blood level and clinical response once blood levels exceed 1.0 mEq/liter, though blood levels of less than 0.9 mEq/liter seem to be ineffective clinically. Though there have been no careful studies in children, pediatric studies have reported clinical effects to occur in about the same serum range as for adults (see Table 1 below).

Based on empirical clinical evidence, it is usually suggested that blood levels be maintained at a level of 0.9-1.4 mEq/liter for treatment of acute manic episodes and at a level of 0.7-1.1 mEq/liter for chronic preventive maintainence. Blood levels are usually obtained 12 hours after the last dose since earlier estimations may be spuriously high. If obtained after 18 hours they will be 0.1-0.2 mEq/liter lower (Schou, 1973).

TIME RESPONSE DATA

When used in the treatment of acute manic episodes, full therapeutic effect usually develops in 6 to 10 days. However, it may take weeks to months before full protection against depressive relapses is achieved (Schou, 1976). Pediatric studies have similarly reported 7-10 days delay before therapeutic effect is noted.

Clinical Effects

ELECTROENCEPHALOGRAM (EEG)

Platman and Fieve (1969) looked at EEG effects in 45 patients, all with a long history of affective illness. Studies were double-blind and investigated the effects of placebo, lithium, chlorpromazine and imipramine. They found more abnormal EEGs with lithium than with placebo, though more than half of the EEGs in the lithium treated group were normal. Abnormalities were not related to sex, age, serum lithium level, clinical state or outcome. The conclusion was that the EEG changes were not necessary for clinical benefit but rather represented a nonspecific toxic effect. Johnson (1969) found a much closer correlation with EEG changes and toxic clinical effect in a study of 10 patients. *In many patients, toxic clinical symptoms were found to correlate more closely with EEG changes than with serum levels.* Also, latent focal changes and epileptic potential are easily exaggerated during treatment (Itil & Akpinar, 1971).

EEG effects of lithium have not been studied systematically in pediatric populations. There has been a single report, however, of the development of paroxysmal EEG abnormalities in a child under treatment with lithium carbonate which seemed clearly related to drug treatment (Brumback et al., 1975).

Kupfer et al. (1970) reported no change in *total sleep time* in patients receiving lithium though they note decreased amount of REM sleep with reciprocal increases in Stages 3 and 4. However, these were depressed patients who had sleep alterations before receiving lithium so the significance of these findings is uncertain, particularly since Brebbia et al. (1969) found no change in sleep cycle with lithium in normal and remitted manic-depressive patients.

Studies of auditory and visual evoked cortical responses (EP) have suggested that patients with affective illness have relatively greater increases in evoked response amplitudes with increasing stimulus intensity, an abnormality which was normalized by lithium and associated with therapeutic improvement (Buchsbaum et al., 1971). However, lithium produced no significant change in the amplitude or latency of the AER in a study with 9 hyperactive children maintained on 0.8-1.2 mEq/l (Greenhill et al., 1973).

CARDIOVASCULAR

T wave depression suggestive of changes in cardiac excitability has been the most consistent effect of lithium on the EKG (Demers & Heninger, 1970). These effects are accentuated in poisoning and at high serum levels. At extremely high levels, prolongation of the QT interval can occur (Horowitz & Fisher, 1969). Pulse irregularities and hypotension have also been reported (Shopsin & Gerson, 1973).

GASTROINTESTINAL AND NEUROMUSCULAR

Patients receiving lithium frequently report anorexia, nausea, vomiting, diarrhea, constipation, dry mouth and metallic taste (Gershon & Shopsin, 1973).

The effects of lithium on neurotransmitter systems would lead one to expect various neuromuscular effects—indeed, tremor, weakness, ataxia, muscle fasiculations and twitching, clonic movements, choreoathetotic movements and hyperactive reflexes have all been noted, though to a variable degree (Shopsin & Gershon, 1973).

ENDOCRINE

Lithium has been shown to result in a deficiency of circulating *thyroid hormone* and can produce goiter and even clinical hypothyroidism (Shopsin & Gershon, 1973); thyropituitary response in such patients usually leads to enhanced levels of endogenous TSH. As indicated above, these changes are probably mediated through inhibition of the cyclic AMP system. There have also been case reports of hypoparathyroidism developing in patients on lithium and subsiding after the drug was discontinued (Christensson, 1976). Lithium also has effects on *carbohydrate metabolism* and treatment has been shown to lead to a decreased tolerance to glucose (Shopsin & Gershon, 1973). Serum *growth hormone* concentrations in hospitalized psychiatric patients have been reported to show significant elevations during lithium treatment. There appears to be evidence of an increase in plasma *cortisol* levels during subacute ingestion of lithium but there have not been definitive long-term studies (Shopsin & Gershon, 1973).

Polyuria, polydipsia and even *diabetes insipidus* syndromes are frequently encountered in patients receiving lithium. The cause is unclear and suggestions that inhibition of adenyl cyclase and vasopressin as the basis cannot explain adequately the full range of phenomena observed. The area is considered an important one for further investigation (Shopsin & Gershon, 1973).

BLOOD

Lithium can produce a leukocytosis though the mechanism is not clear (Shopsin & Gershon, 1973).

ACTIVITY

While lithium causes a marked reduction in activity in manic adults, no studies have monitored motor activity *per se* in children receiving lithium, though there have been a few clinical reports of reduction in restlessness.

COGNITIVE FUNCTION

Subjective feelings of muddleheadedness and mental confusion were reported by normal adults taking usual therapeutic doses of lithium carbonate and objective decrements in two cognitive tests (Digit Symbol and Halstead-Reitan Trail making) were noted (Judd et al., 1977a, b). Thus, it is extremely important that any future studies of lithium in children include objective measures of cognitive function (see Chapter 3).

ACADEMIC ACHIEVEMENT

This has not been looked at systematically in lithium studies in children. While some clinical reports mention improved functioning in school, this has not been demonstrated objectively. The decrement in cognitive function noted in normal adults (above) calls for careful study of this area in children.

BEHAVIOR

A variety of behavior has been reported improved by lithium in children in the handful of open and controlled clinical trials, including periodic excitement, aggressivity, restlessness, and emotional instability. However, most of the studies have not utilized the reliable or formal measures detailed in Chapter 2 and their conclusions must be considered highly tentative. Reports with adults indicate that some patients may become more *reflective* on lithium (Tupin & Smith, 1973) and think more before acting. Changes in children responding to lithium in this area have not been studied in detail, but measures of this reflective dimension (see Chapter 3) would be well worthwhile in impulsive, aggressive children.

MOOD AND SELF-IMAGE

Though lithium has not been studied using self-reports (see Chapter 2) with children, clinical observations in individual cases suggest that some children with periodic depression, anger and agitation may be helped by lithium. This is in accord, also, with a specific effect on mood swings in young, emotionally unstable female adults demonstrated with lithium (Rifkin et al., 1972).

Lithium may cause irritability in therapeutic doses in adults, but this does not appear to have been a particular difficulty with children and adolescents so far. However, this effect may be hard to distinguish from the target symptoms in a behavior disordered child. Sheard et al. (1976) noted that some of their adult patients experienced depressions when their violence was diminished and it is possible that this too occurs in children but has gone unnoticed.

Treatment Emergent (Side) Effects

SHORT-TERM

Lithium is a potentially toxic substance and concern about treatment emergent effects and the need for monitoring blood levels has limited its use in child psychiatry. A particular problem with lithium treatment is that mild to moderate side effects are common even with nontoxic and quite low serum lithium concentrations. *The most frequent are nausea, diarrhea, muscular weakness, tremor, blurred vision, drowsiness, polyuria and polydipsia.* There are not sufficient data really to compare treatment emergent effects in children with those found in adults. However, in the children treated by Campbell et al. (1972), toxicity occurred in relatively low blood levels of lithium, and Dostal and Zvolsky (1970) noted that polydipsia and polyuria were prominent in their adolescent patients during lithium treatment.

Lithium poisoning generally occurs when serum lithium rises to values above 2 mEq/liter. The onset is usually gradual and primarily affects the nervous system. Symptoms include sluggishness, slurred speech, and anorexia; vomiting and coma may develop.

As the treatment emergent symptoms seen with therapeutic blood levels of lithium are qualitatively similar to those of toxicity, they must be treated with considerable caution. Because there is no known antidote to lithium, treatment of toxicity has to be largely directed toward individual symptoms such as infection, dehydration and electrolyte imbalance.

LONG-TERM

As the conditions for which lithium is used in childhood and adolescence are chronic disturbances, long-term treatment is likely once initial short-term response has been demonstrated. For this reason, the physician must be aware of long-term complications of lithium treatment which result from metabolic and endocrine effects of lithium maintenance. These have been discussed in detail above. *Euthyroid goiter, hypothyroidism and diabetes insipidus-like syndromes* are the most common effects of chronic lithium treatment, but, fortunately, are reversible when lithium therapy is discontinued.

Drug Interactions

Lithium should not be given together with any compound that contains *iodides* as this will interact with lithium to produce goiter. Thus in the pediatric age group, particular care should be taken not to use lithium with cough medications and bronchodilators which commonly contain iodide. Treatment with *diuretics* which act on the proximal tubule leads to a fall of renal lithium clearance and to lithium accumulation unless the lithium dosage is reduced concomitantly. *Antipsychotics* by their chemoreceptor antiemetic action (see Chapter 8) may suppress the clinically valuable nausea which commonly heralds the onset of lithium toxicity. *Sodium* intake needs careful control to prevent unexpected variations in serum levels of lithium.

Clinical Indications

ESTABLISHED INDICATIONS

None.

POSSIBLE INDICATIONS

1) *Manic-Depressive Illness and Periodic Disorders.* This is disputed or, at best, extremely rare in childhood and rare in adolescence. However, a

criteria for childhood mania has been defined by Weinberg and Brumback (1976) and individual case reports have described children with cyclic attacks of excitement and depression who seem to respond to lithium treatment (Berg et al., 1974; Feinstein & Wolpert, 1973; Kelly et al., 1976; van Krevelen & van Voorst, 1959; Warneke, 1975).

Frommer (1968) reported on 19 cases who, in addition to seeming depressed, had periodic violent temper outbursts alternating with brief states of reasonableness or a condition of continuous, unconstructive mechanical activity. She gave lithium, in some cases combined with amitriptyline, and reported that most of the 19 responded remarkably well. However, Frommer did not monitor blood levels of lithium and gave small doses (100-250 mg/day) which probably did not reach therapeutic levels. This polypharmacy (see Chapter 7) does not help evaluate results.

2) *Aggressiveness.* As in adults, there has been interest in a possible antiaggressive effect of lithium in retarded, and/or behavior disordered children (Dostal & Zvolsky, 1970; Dyson & Barcai, 1970; Lena & O'Brien, 1975). These clinical case reports are of interest as aggressive disorders (see Chapter 5) are common among child psychiatric populations while manic-depressive illness is not. Dostal and Zvolsky (1970) found considerable improvement in 14 severely retarded aggressive adolescents in an open study using a ward behavior rating scale. A few controlled trials have been carried out since that time.

3) *Other Conditions.* Annell (1969a) reported excellent results in 11 of 12 patients aged 10 to 18 years, 3 of whom had been admitted to the hospital for treatment before age 10. A further series of 5 patients with onset of difficulties before age 10 who responded to lithium was also reported by the same investigator (Annell, 1969b). Though patients in the latter series were described as manic-depressive, they had a variety of symptoms including sleep disorders, night terrors, and frequent somatic complaints such as stomachaches and headaches. Diagnosis is thus contentious, proper measures of drug effect (see Chapter 2) were not obtained and blood levels not reported, although unlike Frommer's (1968), doses were probably in the therapeutic range (600-1200 mg/day).

These clinical reports suggest that there may be some child psychiatric disorders manifest by cyclic behavioral outbursts alternating with withdrawal, and that these may, in some cases, respond to lithium.

PROBABLE NON-INDICATIONS

1) *Hyperactivity.* Two studies of lithium treatment with hyperactive children (Greenhill et al., 1973; Whitehead & Clark, 1970) failed to show

a significant effect of lithium on hyperactivity. However, the favorable report by Dyson and Barcai (1970) in 2 hyperactive children whose parents were lithium responders suggests that such an admittedly uncommon subgroup of hyperactive children might well be responders, though an attempt by one of the authors (JR) who tried to replicate this finding in 4 hyperactive children, all of whom who had either a lithium responding parent or a positive family history of manic-depressive illness, failed to find any response to a 4-week trial of lithium carbonate treatment at adequate therapeutic doses.

2) *Psychosis*. Lithium was not found helpful in childhood psychosis or infantile autism (Campbell et al., 1972). However, this represents an isolated study, and a subgroup with a high degree of associated aggressive and/or self-mutilating behavior might be found to respond; such cases should be specifically selected for study.

SUMMARY

Table 1 summarizes the small number of controlled trials of lithium in children and adolescents for various indications.

As can be seen from Table 1, several different populations of children and, more particularly, adolescents may possibly benefit from lithium. While *symptoms* such as emotionality, mood swings, and outbursts of aggressive behavior seem most promising, *diagnostic* groups are far from clear. Furthermore, in some cases improvement appears to be nonspecific as, for example, in the Gram and Rafaelsen (1972) study; patients whose psychopathology was not cyclic responded to lithium in a general way compared to placebo. Hyperactivity and childhood psychoses do not appear responsive.

Contraindications

Children receiving diuretics, or children on low sodium diets and/or with renal, cardiovascular or sodium metabolism diseases should not be given lithium (see Drug Interactions) because of possible faulty excretion leading to toxicity.

Dosages and Precautions

Several writers have reported that children and adolescents may require almost adult doses (900-1500 mg/day) to reach adequate plasma levels (Berg et al., 1974; Greenhill et al., 1973; Warneke, 1975), and, in general, doses reported seem to approximate adult doses. With young children

TABLE 1

Controlled Studies of Lithium in Psychiatric Disorders of Childhood and Adolescence

Authors	N	Age	Diagnosis-Description	Dose (Serum Level)	Results & Comments
Whitehead & Clark, 1970	7	5-9	All hyperactive Two also psychotic	6-10 mg/lb day	Possibly single-blind. Unquantified results. No difference between placebo and lithium. Six children also received thioridazine (0.6-1.5 mg/lb).
Campbell, et al., 1972	10	3-6	Childhood Schizophrenia (6) Behavior Disorder (2) Chronic Brain Syndrome (1) Infantile Autism (1)	450-900 mg/day 0.25-1.9 mEq/1	Single-blind crossover, compared to chlorpromazine (9-45 mg/day). No significant difference for the group between lithium and chlorpromazine.
Gram & Rafaelsen, 1972	18	8-22	Pupils at special school for psychotic children	12-30 mEq/day 0.6-1.0 mEq/1	Double-blind crossover, lithium vs. placebo. Six months of each treatment. Lithium superior by global ratings of parents ($p < .05$), School ($p < .001$). Two patients improved in mood shifts. Others improved in a nonspecific way.
Rifkin, et al., 1972	21	Adolescent Females	"Emotionally Unstable Character Disorder"	0.6-1.5 mEq/1	Double-blind crossover, 6-week treatment. Lithium superior to placebo using a global measure of mood swings ($p < .002$).
Greenhill, et al., 1973	9	9-14	Hyperactive, nonresponders to other drugs	0.8-1.2 mEq/1	Double-blind, 3-month comparison with dextroamphetamine and placebo. No significant treatment differences. Two children showed marked but transient improvement on lithium.
Sheard, et al., 1976	66	16-24	Prisoners in maximum security institution, nonpsychotic, with chronic assaultive behavior	0.6-1.0 mEq/1	Double-blind crossover, 1-3 months lithium or placebo. Significantly fewer major infractions of institutional rules on lithium ($p < .01$).

(under 6), however, somewhat smaller doses were needed to reach therapeutic blood levels (Campbell et al., 1972). The usual starting dose is 300 mg/day in divided doses in older children and 150 mg in younger children, to be increased by 150 mg daily until blood levels reach 0.8-1.2 mEq/liter. Blood should be obtained in the morning before the first lithium tablet is taken, and 10-12 hours after the previous lithium dose.

As children may not reliably report side effects, and as toxicity of lithium can be life-threatening, children should be checked carefully each day during initial treatment weeks. While Greenhill et al. (1973) found only transient initial drowsiness in their hyperactive group during 3 months of outpatient treatment, others have been impressed by the continuing toxicity of lithium in young children (Campbell et al., 1972; Dostal & Zvolsky, 1970). Careful attention to sodium balance is also necessary during treatment but there is no substitute for alertness on the part of parents to early signs of toxicity and for regular estimates of serum level despite children's objection to them. It goes without saying, too, in view of the risks and of the necessity for frequent blood tests, that any prospective clinical and research gains must be substantial.

Unlike most other psychotropic drugs, lithium may be stopped abruptly without any apparent withdrawal effects.

Summary and Conclusions

There is increasing interest in lithium in pediatric psychopharmacology, stemming from two sources. First, high-risk research has led to new awareness of the possible relevance of family history of manic-depressive illness and of drug response to a more rational drug treatment of children. Secondly, residential treatment centers and correctional facilities are plagued with the question of how to control outbursts of violence and chronic aggressive behavior without obtunding the patient. Studies of lithium in children and adolescents are somewhat encouraging in both these considerations. In particular, lithium may prove preferable to phenothiazines (see Chapter 8) for behavioral control, especially in retarded patients. However, in contrast to the situation in adults, in children, to date, lithium effects seem to have been disappointingly symptomatic rather than specific. The studies on aggressive outbursts in adolescents and adults, for example, indicate that diagnostic entities like psychosis or retardation do not predict lithium response. In short, there is no reason at this point to equate lithium responsiveness with manic-depressive or some equivalent illness in childhood, though future work needs considerable refinement. Studies on the antiaggressive properties of lithium should distinguish between periodic outbursts and chronic aggressive behavior, as well as between aggressivity with a marked affective component and aggressivity without affectivity, since to this date, it remains only speculative whether or not cyclicity and/or affectivity, so important in adults, can predict clinical response to lithium in an aggressive child or adolescent. Nevertheless, from a theoretical point of view, interest would still lie in the possible ability of lithium to treat childhood symptoms occurring in offspring of manic-depressive lithium responsive parents. These need not be symptoms which are among Weinberg and Brumback's (1976) criteria for true childhood mania which seems rare. Studies of such children with a variety of presenting complaints should be undertaken to investigate this possibility.

In general lithium must be regarded as an interesting, though potentially toxic, experimental drug with several possible but no firm indications in pediatric psychopharmacology.

ANTIANXIETY (SEDATIVE) DRUGS*

(CNS DEPRESSANTS)

Introduction

In spite of the antiquity and ubiquity of sedative drugs, much of their pharmacology and psychopharmacology is shrouded in mystery, particularly where children are concerned. Much of what follows in this section is a distillate of various papers and texts, notably Abel (1974), Goodman and Gilman (1975), Greenblatt and Shader (1974), Efron et al. (1968), Kalinowsky and Hippius (1969). In some places, a degree of closure over areas of confusion and uncertainty (as, for example, in the discussion of the antimuscarinic drugs) has been exercised in the belief that this is necessary in a text of this type.

Anxiolysis and Sedation

Because of the universal properties of all drugs which are capable of relieving anxiety (*anxiolysis*), this seems simply a "side effect" of depression of CNS function (Irwin, 1968) which, in its mildest form, begins with sedation and at its extremity terminates in coma and death. In its turn, *depression* of CNS function is simply the negative axis of a continuum of arousal of which the other is *stimulation* leading to excitement, convulsions and, likewise, death. *Sleep* is a complex circadian neurophys-

---

* This and succeeding sections have been contributed by John S. Werry, M.D.

iological event of recurring approximately 90-minute cycles of decreasing, then increasing levels of arousal, a necessary prelude to which seems to be a reduced state of sensory stimulation. Under ordinary circumstances, this state of quietude is produced by individual and social rituals and by psychological means. However, it is also possible to produce sleep by depressing the level of arousal *pharmacologically*, though in so doing, the naturally occurring neurophysiological nature of sleep is nearly always distorted. For the purpose of this review it will be assumed *that sleep is a state of reduced arousal in which there is some approximation to the normally recurring cycles in the level of arousal, but which is characterized by arousability or production of a wakeful state through sufficient stimulation*.

Depression of CNS function can be achieved *pharmacologically* by a variety of substances and *neurophysiologically* in changes in various systems. The effect of any drug will, however, interact with the preexisting state of arousal in the nervous system, the prevalent mood, the social and psychological context and the individual's personality and particular physiology. Predicting the effect of sedative drugs, therefore, is an extremely complex business which obviously will not only vary from individual to individual, but from situation to situation.

THE STAGES OF ANESTHESIA

The spectrum of CNS depression by pharmacological means is seen, in its purest if somewhat accelerated form, in the induction of of anesthesia for surgical purposes. Mild sedation or drowsiness—which, except in unpleasant moods or situations, is ordinarily perceived as pleasant and the source of a great deal of human effort, ingenuity and expenditure—progressively gives way to sleep, then to loss of consciousness, the onset of which is signaled by irregular breathing, increases in muscle tone and importantly, a *delirious state* in which the patient may struggle, shout and become quite violent. If depression of the CNS is continued, unconsciousness deepens, muscle tone relaxes, breathing steadies, reflexes are successfully lost and true general anesthesia obtains. If further extended, deep coma and, ultimately, death from depression of vital functions controlling cardiovascular and respiratory systems supervenes.

The goal in pharmacotherapy varies according to the circumstances—in many instances, it will be simply to produce a mild degree of sedation which relieves anxiety but permits normal function to continue or which maximizes the chances of sleep supervening—in others, as in very disturbed, violent or panic-stricken patients, rapid unconsciousness may be

Antimanic, Antianxiety, Hallucinogenic Drugs

sought. The choice of route of administration and dose of drug will therefore depend on the particular therapeutic goal in mind.

General Pharmacology of Depressant Drugs

The effect of different sedative or depressant drugs varies according to their effects on neurotransmitter and biochemical mechanisms, the concentration of the drug in particular neurones or neurophysiological systems due to selective uptake, configuration of the blood supply, cell size and type, vulnerability, particular types of cell organization (for example, polysynaptic systems are particularly sensitive to central depressants), the functional state of the cell, etc. (see also Chapter 1). Add to this the enormous complexity of the brain, in particular the intricacy and mutual interdependency of its many functional systems, and it will be readily understandable that while *CNS depression has a common core, the action of any class of sedative drugs will also have elements of specificity of which 4 are of particular concern:*

1) The fineness of effect or the margin of safety—low with barbiturates and high with the benzodiazepines.

2) Associated actions such as production of extrapyramidal and autonomic effects characteristic of the antipsychotics (see Chapter 8) or respiratory depression with barbiturates and opiates or analgesia with opiates and to a lesser extent, alcohol.

3) Induction of enzymes leading to the development of tolerance and necessity of increased dosage and, in some cases, to physiological dependence.

4) Pharmacokinetic properties (see Chapter 1), notably volatility, which enables exhibition of the drug by inhalation resulting in rapid induction and dissipation of effect particularly desirable in anesthesiology; lipid solubility which, if very high as with thiopentone (Pentothal) or diazepam (Valium), leads under ordinary circumstances to rapid induction and dissipation of effect and hence suitability for intravenous administration; ability to penetrate the blood/brain barrier (see Chapter 1), etc.

Physiological Basis of Sedation

There are 4 main ways in which sedation may be produced physiologically:

1) Inhibition of the system responsible for the maintenance of wakefulness (the reticular activating system—RAS) which produces its effect by nonspecific energizing of the CNS.

2) Inhibition of vigilance. As used here, the term vigilance implies a *selective attention* as, for example, in anxiety or worry over some particular thing.

3) Inhibition of sensory stimuli through such mechanisms as muscle relaxation and reduction of incoming sensory stimuli.

4) General depression of all CNS activity.

It is obvious that 2 and 3 are equally amenable to non-pharmacological and pharmacological alteration.

Cellular Action of Sedatives

A number of mechanisms have been identified, but it is unclear how many of these are due to the action of the drug or secondary to sedation or simply coincidental. As noted above, it is remarkable how little is known about the fundamental cellular action of the sedatives even of ancient drugs, like alcohol and opium. As noted in Chapter 1, mechanisms posited for pyschotropic drugs in general and for the sedatives in particular are:

1) *Membrane stabilisation* which makes induction of a neuronal discharge more difficult. It seems likely that general depressants like barbiturates, anesthetics and perhaps alcohol (as well as, incidentally, the antiepileptics—see Chapter 9) act this way.

2) Interference with *neurotransmitters*. As discussed in Chapter 1, this may be by mimicking, competitive inhibition, interference with activation, inactivation or synthesis or diffusion. While there are some exceptions, drugs which interfere with neurotransmitters can nearly all produce neurological-type side effects of which interference with autonomic function is one of the more conspicuous.

3) General depression of cell metabolism, by interference with oxidative or other general energy systems. While it was once believed this was the basis of the action of such drugs as alcohol and barbiturates, it now seems likely that this is not important in normal clinical dosage.

Tranquilization v. Sedation

The term tranquilizer is now part of everyday parlance but no term is less sensible of clear meaning. It stems from the time of introduction of the first antipsychotics or neuroleptics (see Chapter 8) and, as noted there, originated in animal studies, later confirmed, at least partially, in humans, which suggested that the behavioral depression produced was strikingly different from that associated with traditional general sedatives such as the barbiturates or alcohol. There appeared to be a curious unconcern with the environment, ready rousability and lack of *disinhibition*. This latter phenomenon consists of the release of behaviors previously suppressed through punishment or other aversive consequences and would appear to be the basis of anxiolysis. The human paradigm of disinhibition is, of course, seen in all those things for which alcohol is favored—reduction of tension, social lubrication, self-confidence, a sense of well-being etc.—as well as in those for which it is vilified, such as an increase in truculence and belligerence, loss of judgment, insight and social sensitivity. Much has been made recently of the capacity of sedative drugs such as diazepam (Valium) to *release aggression*. In fact, there should be neither a sense of mystification or astonishment at such a phenomenon, if it is kept clearly in mind that the *sedatives release behavior ordinarily suppressed through aversive contingencies whether real or anticipated* (shame, guilt). Thus in the aggregate there must be a mixture of behaviors released, some desirable and others which would be better kept suppressed. The balance between these two will depend on the individual concerned, his basic mood state, and the aggressiveness or otherwise of the situation and or culture in which he finds himself.

The term tranquilization given to the behavior state produced by antipsychotic drugs soon attracted camp followers. In the 1950's a group of miscellaneous drugs such as meprobamate (Miltown, Equanil), the diphenylmethane derivatives (hydroxyzine and other antihistamines) and the benzodiazepines appeared, for which claims (later proven to be false) were made of a similar ability to produce sedation without disinhibition, dependence or depression of cognitive function characteristic of traditional sedatives. This resulted in the application of the term *major tranquilizers* to the drugs now called antipsychotics, while the new group of drugs, so obviously pharmacologically different, were termed *minor tranquilizers*.

While the distinction between the major tranquilizers and other sedatives is clear because the former have antipsychotic activity, neurological side effects and fail to produce disinhibition, most of the claimed differences between the so-called minor tranquilizers and other sedatives have been elided with more intensive study. (There is a possible exception in the antimuscarinic drugs—see below.) Greenblatt and Shader (1974, pp. 43-44) attempt a redefinition of minor tranquilizers as follows: *minor tranquilizers and sedatives are drugs which attenuate the behavioral consequences of frustration, fear and punishment (that is, produce disinhibition) but minor tranquilizers achieve this state in doses which are not neurotoxic*. In short, then, this is not a qualitative distinction as the term implies, but rather a *quantitative* toxic-to-effective dosage ratio. There is also an inherent danger to this definition, in that it may be misinterpreted to mean that the minor tranquilizers are not, in fact, ever neurotoxic. This is, of course, simply not the case. Another weakness in the definition is that it in no way clarifies the position of the antimuscarinic or antihistaminic drugs. These *do* produce neurological (mostly autonomic) effects in non-hypnotic doses which, while hardly as dramatic as, say, the alcohol-type *intoxication* characterizing general depressants, can nevertheless still be quite distressing. All these factors make irrefutable the conclusion, repeated intermittently for several years (e.g., Irwin, 1968), that the term minor tranquilizer should be abandoned as pharmacologically misleading.

Classification of Antianxiety (Sedative) Drugs

A simplified classification will be followed here and is adapted from that in Goodman and Gilman (1975):

1) *General Depressants.* These include alcohol, anesthetic agents, barbiturates, chloral hydrate, opiates, etc.

2) *Selective Depressants.* Benzodiazepines and propanediols, though the legitimacy of the latter in this group is contentious.

3) *Antimuscarinic Sedatives.*

General Depressants

Little will be said about this group, though historically, whether brandy or laudanum, they have been used for centuries to quiet fussy infants. The barbiturates have been discussed in detail in Chapter 9 to which readers are referred and they provide a typical model of the pharmacology and action of most general depressants.

A few summary points will suffice:

1) The general depressants vary greatly in pharmacokinetic properties and this influences such factors as the speed of onset (and dissipation) of their sedative action, being highest, because of the route of administration with gaseous, volatile or highly lipid soluble substances (such as thiopentone) when given intravenously. Induction of general anesthesia is only a special case of sedation rapidly induced, profound in depth and, ideally, equally rapidly dissipated.

2) Probably, though by no means certainly (McNair, 1973), antianxiety action implies depression of psychomotor function except in states of high arousal where this depression may appear as improved performance.

3) Given in anything above modest doses, progressively more distinctive and severe neurotoxicity (usually reversible) develops affecting a wide range of higher CNS and motor function exemplified in the familiar stages of alcoholic intoxication.

4) All can produce sleep but, in so doing, the normal neurophysiological pattern of sleep is distorted, notably the suppression of REM sleep and decrease in the amount of very deep (stage 4) sleep. The compensatory or rebound increases in these may cause distressing symptoms upon withdrawal.

5) All are potentially life-threatening in *overdosage* and upon sudden *withdrawal* after chronic high dose administration. Paradoxically, while the former is the greatest, the latter is least with the opiates. The speed at which these withdrawal symptoms develop varies with the duration of action of the drug.

6) All can produce dependence both psychological and physical which varies from drug to drug in the speed and intensity with which this develops. It is high with opiates and low with alcohol and other sedatives.

7) All can induce, to a varying degree, enzyme induction in the liver which results in tolerance and increases interactions with other drugs.

8) Side effects and additional pharmacological actions (e.g., analgesia) vary, and range from hepatotoxicity to those resulting from peculiarities of metabolism (e.g., the production of toxic formaldehyde with alcohol) and with contaminants such as other alcohols and organic substances in different sources of alcohol.

9) All act synergistically with other CNS depressants and many other drugs acting on the CNS, often with potentially life-threatening results.

INDICATIONS AND CONTRAINDICATIONS

These are discussed for all sedatives in a section which follows. It may be noted in passing that glue and petrol sniffing is simply the self-induction of a state of rapid sedation by the use of volatile solvents which resemble the general anesthetic agents and it differs qualitatively little from the fashionable ether or nitrous oxide parties held by Victorian notables. In spite of the dramatic nature of sniffing, largely a function of the rapidity with which sedation is induced, the toxicity of most volatile solvents (as with most drugs of abuse) has been exaggerated and is fortunately low—the greatest risk comes from accidents associated with intoxication. Fortunately too, though the mode of intake of the sedative substance (through the lungs) produces a rapid degree of sedation, it also leads to an equally rapid discontinuation of inhalation and return to consciousness and normality. Societies which place a high premium on the chemical production of sedation, whether by alcohol or drugs, can scarcely be surprised when their young members try to achieve a similar result by whatever means lie at hand.

Selective Depressants

Members of this group derive their name from 1) the rather uncertainly demonstrated selectivity of their depressant action in which *subcortical* structures are said to figure prominently though by no means to the exclusion of cortical depression, and 2) a greater dose response range or gradient (see Chapter 1). There are two main groups in this class: first, the *benzodiazepines*, which more clearly fulfill these two requirements than the second, the *propanediols*, which after the heady heights of the Eisenhower era when they took Washington by storm, have suffered an eclipse though by no means a total demise.

Fig. 1

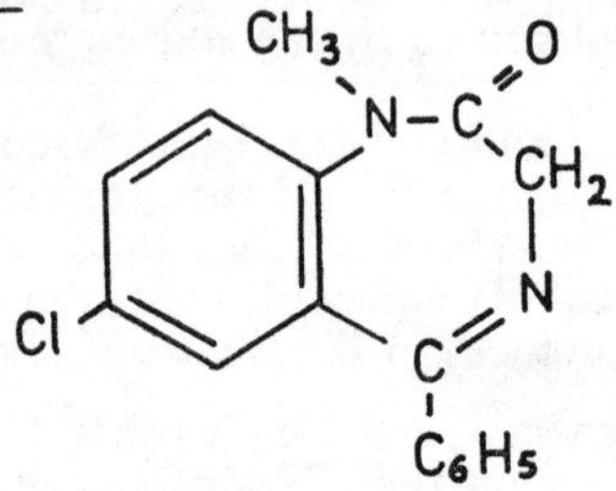

DIAZEPAM
(Valium)

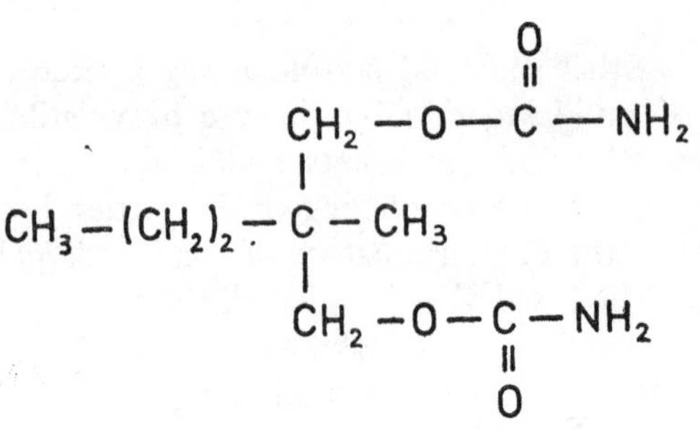

MEPROBAMATE
(Miltown, Equanil)

Chemical Structures

These are set out in Figure 1.

The benzodiazepines in common use are diazepam (Valium), chlordiazepoxide (Librium), oxazepam (Serepax, Serax)—the active metabolite of diazepam, nitrazepam (Mogadon) and flurazepam (Dalmane), the latter two of which are used primarily as hypnotics rather than anxiety agents. The popular propanediols are meprobamate (Equanil, Miltown) and tybamate (Solacen, Tybatran).

BENZODIAZEPINES

Because of their current insignificance, the propanediols will not be discussed in any detail.

Much of what follows is extracted from Greenblatt and Shader's (1974) comprehensive monograph on benzodiazepines and from Byck (1975).

PHARMACOLOGY

With the exception of oxazepam, the benzodiazepines are rapidly and completely absorbed. Oxazepam is poorly absorbed so that despite its being the active metabolite of diazepam, doses needed are some 20 times higher. However, benzodiazepines are poorly absorbed intramuscularly.

While a single acute dose of benzodiazepine such as a diazepam has a relatively short half-life, successive doses lead to half-lives of well in excess of 24 hours and in some cases as long as 72 hours. This can lead to accumulation and delayed toxicity. The only benzodiazepine in common use which may not have this property is oxazepam which may be related to its lack of metabolism into active principles. Benzodiazepines are, in general, highly lipid soluble and, as a result, they are rapidly distributed into the brain which is, of course, rich in lipid tissue. Intravenous administration produces high brain levels and consequent sedative effects in a few seconds but, as is characteristic of all highly lipid soluble drugs (see Chapter 1), this may be followed by a rapid fall of levels and dissipation of effect within a few minutes as rather more even tissue distribution occurs.

Metabolism varies from drug to drug and influences cumulative properties. Diazepam and chlordiazepoxide have intermediate metabolites which are pharmacologically active and so does nitrazepam to a lesser extent, while oxazepam and flurazepam have none. There is some evidence, also, that some of the cumulative property is due to binding in the gut wall (independent of route administration) and subsequent slow release. As

Greenblatt and Shader (1974) point out, the differences between various benzodiazepines are largely *pharmacokinetic* rather than *therapeutic* and relate principally to duration of effect, with flurazepam and oxazepam being the shortest and hence the most suitable for short-lived sedation such as hypnosis though, curiously, oxazepam seems seldom used for such while the long-acting nitrazepam is.

Most are ultimately conjugated with glucuronic acid in the liver and excreted by the kidney, though there is also some hydroxylation too. Dose response relationships, it can be seen, will depend on the frequency and route of administration and on the drug concerned, but *cumulation* is the rule except as noted. However, generally speaking, the greatest strength of the benzodiazepines lies in their relativly *flat* dose response curve (Chapter 1) so that there is a much higher margin between clinical effect and neurotoxicity than with most other drugs.

As far as children are concerned, there is little pharmacokinetic data, as usual, but such as there are suggest that any differences are likely to be along predictable, quantitative directions due to faster metabolism and, in younger children, to higher fat/water ratios, all of which are likely to make children somewhat more resistant, except in the neonatal period (see Chapter 1).

Serum levels can, with some difficulty, be estimated quite accurately by GLC methods (Greenblatt and Shader, 1974).

The pharmacology of the propanediols in man and animals is very similar to that of the barbiturates (Byck, 1975) which has been discussed in detail in Chapter 9.

SITES AND MODE OF ACTION

While the benzodiazepines rapidly penetrate the blood/brain barrier and are widely distributed throughout the brain, little is known of the cellular action responsible for their pharmacological properties though they do have a number of effects upon cell metabolism and on biogenic amines. While they resemble general depressants in their antiepileptic effect and effect on cortical function as judged from EEG changes and depression of higher CNS functions, in other respects their claim to a selective action is substantial, notably 1) a depression of the limbic system concerned with emotions, sometimes picturesquely, though not always accurately, described as *chemical amygdylectomy*, and 2) a capacity to produce centrally some degree of muscle relaxation at considerably below the general anesthetic levels required of most general depressants such as the barbiturates.

Despite some neurophysiological effects suggestive of a selective depressant action, the exact site and mechanism of action of the propanediols is unknown but clinically typical, general sedative reactions predominate.

CLINICAL EFFECTS

Central nervous system effects of the benzodiazepines consist of *sedation* including *disinhibition* (see above). Although intoxication of the alcohol type and unconsciousness result from increasing dosage, the benzodiazepines are unique in that death from even colossal overdosage is almost unknown except *where other depressant drugs have also been taken*. As noted, EEG changes resemble those of other sedative drugs, as do the effects upon the neurophysiology of sleep (reduction in REM or dreaming time and in the amount of deep (stage 3 and 4) sleep). However, it is disputed whether the rebound increase in REM sleep, characteristic of other hypnotics and responsible for excessive dreaming upon withdrawal and, often, some of the resistance to patient's stopping, occurs with the benzodiazepines too. The frequency of hangovers, though, seems similar to that with hypnotics. Also disputed is whether or not tolerance to the hypnotic effect so typical of the other hypnotics develops with benzodiazepines, though such data as there are suggest that they may maintain their effect (Kales & Kales, 1974).

Depression and slowing of psychomotor function also occur as with other sedatives. In adults, clear evidence of psychomotor depression, with notably increased reaction time, is regularly noted in the laboratory after 40-50 mg of chlordiazepoxide, 2-4 mg of lorazepam (Ativan), 5-10 mg of diazepam and nitrazepam. However, effect of antianxiety drugs on performance is not independent of the level of arousal or anxiety (Levitt, 1968, see Chapter 3), and an improvement of performance may actually result in highly stressed individuals. Though enzyme induction similar to that caused by many sedatives such as barbiturates has been observed in animals, it has not been demonstrated in humans, making the possibility of drug interactions somewhat less.

Muscle relaxation, objectively demonstrable by EMG recordings and subjectively reported, also occurs in clinical dosage to a variable degree and seems to be largely central in origin though, like with the propanediols, some of this is produced at the level of spinal reflexes. It is doubtful this latter has much clinical significance.

Effects on *activity* are unclear though trials in hyperactivity in children have not been impressive and as might be expected from the disinhibiting ability of these drugs, an increase in activity has been reported. Effects on *systems other than those mediated* through the nervous system are remarkably absent with this group of drugs.

The propanediols resemble the benzodiazepines in their clinical effects except that they lack any usable anticonvulsant or muscle relaxant action, and, *most importantly, are much more neurotoxic,* being fatal in adults in doses as low as 12 G (30 tablets).

TREATMENT EMERGENT (SIDE) EFFECTS

The commonest unwanted or treatment emergent side effects are those which stem directly from the *sedative* effect, namely drowsiness, disinhibition, incoordination. Psychological and physical *dependence* can develop but certainly there is no greater risk of this than with sedatives such as barbiturates, propanediols and alcohol. Because of tissue binding and slow metabolism into active substances, withdrawal symptoms may take longer (a week or more) to develop, and for the same reason are unlikely to be as serious as with barbiturates or propanediols.

The most serious treatment emergent effects are *withdrawal seizures,* but, again, these are characteristic of all sedatives.

Greenblatt and Shader (1974) warn that, though the benzodiazepines appear relatively innocuous as far as serious side effects like agranulocytosis are concerned, much further monitoring is required before this apparent innocence can be affirmed.

The propanediols are similar though they are more neurotoxic, withdrawal symptoms are more rapid and severe, there is a rather high (3.4%) frequency of allergic skin reactions and, perhaps because of their longer history, serious blood dyscrasias have been reported, though no more frequently than with most psychotropic drugs.

DRUG INTERACTIONS

The only important drug interactions of benzodiazepines are with other sedatives or drugs affecting the central nervous system, including, paradoxically, the stimulants. Thus, in cases of life-threatening overdose or high clinical dosage of other drugs acting on the CNS, the benzodiazepines, while innocuous on their own, can act synergistically to produce serious coma or death.

Meprobamate, like barbiturates and unlike benzodiazepines, induces liver enzymes which increases the probability of drug interaction (and tolerance) though tybamate with a half-life of 3 hours is said to lack this property.

Antimuscarinic (Antihistaminic) Sedatives

This is a group of closely related substances, the sedative action of which is most probably due, in part, though not entirely, to the blockage of the central (muscarinic) action of acetylcholine, one of the neurotransmitter substances. The choice of the term antimuscarinic as a single classificatory grouping is novel to this review, but seems to do most justice to what is the probable basis of much of their sedative action.

Most of the members of this group are antihistamines of the H1 blocking type and include diphenhydramine (Benadryl), promethazine (Phenergan), hydroxyzine (Atarax, Vistaril) but also include the prototype antimuscarinics atropine and scopolamine (Hyoscine), the latter found in a number of non-prescription type sedatives readily available throughout the world. The antihistamines are probably amongst the most widely used sedatives for the control of sleep disorders in children (see below).

PHARMACOLOGY

1) *Pharmacokinetics.* These substances are readily absorbed, the onset of their sedative action is rapid and the duration of action varies according to the particular substance and frequency of dosage with most having a relatively short serum half-life (about 6 hours) and duration of sedative action, though good information in the latter respect is remarkably sparse. Distribution is widespread, but some tissues (for example, lung in the case of diphenhydramine) seem selectively to concentrate the drugs.

2) *Sites and Modes of Action.* These substances have a number of actions only one of which is sedation. As noted, their grouping here is based on an antimuscarinic action which resembles the central action of atropine and hyoscine. While their cellular action is unclear, it is presumably by reduction in some way of the efficacy or supply of acetylcholine.

3) *Clinical Effects.* CNS effects are characterized by antimuscarinic actions similar to those seen with atropine and hyoscine, namely a) *sedation* which is usually weak and to which tolerance develops fairly rapidly; b) *delirium, excitation*—the production of this effect is common with higher doses of hyoscine and atropine. It seems to be less frequently reported with the antihistamine group; c) *antiemetic action* of the chemoreceptor type but also in some cases of the motion-induced type; d) various peripheral and *autonomic blocking effects* such as dry mouth, blurring of vision, etc.; e) *anti-Parkinson effects;* f) possibly a weak

ataractic or true tranquilizing effect (it is not possible in the state of the literature to resolve this issue and it is simply something which has been posited as a possibility by this reviewer).

Effects on the gastrointestinal tract include nausea, vomiting and diarrhoea and are probably nervous system effects related to anticholinergic activity, notably vagal blocking.

Most of the drugs also possess an antihistamine action against H1 type receptors and a local anesthetic action.

In reviewing this list of clinical effects and comparing it with those of the antipsychotic drugs (Chapter 8) it will be seen that, apart from a true antipsychotic action and the production of extrapyramidal symptoms, there is a remarkable similarity in the spectrum of effects. The literature on these drugs when used as sedatives is so inadequate that it is not possible to state whether or not disinhibition occurs or, in short, whether the sedative action resembles that of the central nervous system depressants or is rather more closely tied to that of the antipsychotic drugs, or is unique.

It is the opinion of this reviewer that it is much more likely that the sedative action resembles that of the antipsychotics than that of the general or selective CNS depressants. As a result, the general impression in the literature that the anti-anxiolytic action of these drugs is at best weak, rapidly dissipated and not proven is consistent with the type and quality of sedation generally considered as an undesirable side effect with the antipsychotic drugs of the sedative type (e.g., chlorpromazine and thioridazine).

CLINICAL INDICATIONS AND CONTRAINDICATIONS

See below.

Clinical Indications of Antianxiety Drugs

Because of the similarity of such indications for all drugs, these will be discussed as a whole rather than drug by drug.

PROBABLE INDICATIONS—SLEEP INDICATIONS

a) *Insomnia and Night Waking.* These are common in children, especially in younger children. While a search must be made for physical and psychological causes, it seems that 10% of infants never really settle into a routine of sleeping and that some degree of waking subsequently recurs for a few weeks in a large percentage of children (perhaps over half) at age 5-9 months, even though they have established the usual regular sleep pattern within a few weeks of birth (Carey, 1974; Guilleminault & Anders, 1976). Later, children wake to nightmares. It is obvious that where sleep disturbances are an *acute phenomenon* of some magnitude and unrelated to pain or removable psychological factors, an effective hypnotic given for a few nights should be effective in inducing sleep, as it is in adults. Almost any of the sedatives mentioned could, in theory, fulfill this role but the paucity of properly controlled studies makes this statement less than certain. A wide range of hypnotics is used by family doctors and pediatricians who usually encounter this problem, ranging from chloral hydrate to barbiturates and the benzodiazepines but the most popular would seem to be the antihistamines diphenhydramine (Benadryl), hydroxyzine (Atarax, Vistaril) and the sedative phenothiazines (CPZ and thioridazine). One controlled study (Russo et al., 1976) showed that diphenhydramine 1 mg/kg was superior to placebo in decreasing sleep onset latencies and number of awakenings in 50 children aged 2-12 over the period of a week but did not prolong actual length of total sleeping time, probably because the action of the drug is only 4-6 hours. Side effects were minimal. How effective this drug would be over a longer period of time is not possible to state though as a general principle, *the treatment of insomnia should be short,* and it would be predicted that antimuscarinic sedatives would be no more immune from the development of tolerance than other sedatives.

There are no good data relating to other agents but it would be predicted that while general and selective depressants would be effective, too, disinhibition and, in excessive dose, delirium, could prove a problem. It is a sad commentary, considering the frequency of the problem and the undoubted frequency with which sedatives are used in children, that there are almost no usable data. More studies are urgently needed. In the meantime, the first choice should be diphenhydramine or possibly hydroxyzine which seems similar pharmacologically and clinically, with the short acting benzodiazepines (flurazepam and oxazepam) worthy of study, particularly in view of their effectiveness and freedom from side effects. The role of the sedative-type antipsychotics, chlorpromazine and thioridazine, is unclear but this reviewer predicts that they will be no more useful than the antimuscarinics and considerably more neurotoxic and unpleasant (see Chapter 8).

Where insomnia, nightmares and waking appear to be due to *separation anxiety* (see Chapter 5), imipramine should be tried first (see Chapters 5 and 7).

b) *Night Terrors and Somnambulism.* It is important that these be distinguished from insomnia, simple waking or nightmares, since they are neurophysiologically different, occurring as Stage 4 sleep is terminating and lighter stages beginning, in a typical 90-minute cycle (Guilleminault & Anders, 1976; Kales & Kales, 1974). The child with night terrors or somnambulism is characteristically difficult to rouse and, if roused, is amnesic for the episode. In general, these episodes are *not* truly psychiatric in origin (Guilleminault & Anders, 1976) but seem related to immaturity of the CNS and, except in exceptional cases, disappear with age. Further, they do not inconvenience the child, though sleep walking may be dangerous in a hazardous environment. The answer then, will be pharmacological only in exceptional cases and a benzodiazepine such as flurazepam would appear to be the drug of choice since it has proven able to shorten the duration of Stage 4 sleep in adults, probably (though not certainly) without the disadvantages of development of tolerance and overdose hazards of other sedatives.

SUMMARY

1) Much of irritability and sleeplessness in children is due to physical or psychological distress which will not be relieved pharmacologically and, in certain instances, underlying physical conditions may be dangerously masked by the use of sedatives.

2) Unlike adults wishing to sleep, the indications for sedation in children are usually the needs of parental control over a resistant child. As a result of this and also of the underlying causes of the sleeplessness such as anxiety or simple wakefulness, doses required in many cases will be high. This carries with it the high probability of producing disinhibition, followed, if pressed, by the induction of the second or delirious stage of anesthesia. This fundamental pharmacological fact is, no doubt, responsible for the reputation that the general depressants such as the barbiturates have for causing behavioral deterioration and excitement rather than sedation in children. Antihistaminics may not exhibit these problems but if their action really does resemble that of other antimuscarinic substances, delirium could be a problem in high doses.

3) If given over any extended period, tolerance develops with loss of initial effect, increased dosage and risk of production of dependency with all sedatives except possibly, though improbably, the benzodiazepines. Further, when given on a chronic basis, most, if not all, sedatives produce distortions of the normal neurophysiology of sleep which ultimately may even result in a drug dependent insomnia (Gilleminault & Anders, 1976; Kales & Kales, 1974).

4) Undesirable effects such as impairment of cognitive and motor function, often extending well beyond the actual period of sleep, are to be expected with most sedatives, even in hypnotic doses.

5) Withdrawal symptoms, especially in children prone to seizures, can be serious, as is the result of accidental poisoning (except with benzodiazepines).

6) The use of medication may prevent the development of alternative better methods by parents and interfere with parent-child coping mechanisms.

In general, then, the handling of most sleep disorders will lie in the relief of pain, physical or psychological, the acceptance of the normality, inevitability and transitory nature of much of it, and the recognition that some of it is a matter of family training. Only occasionally, therefore, will pharmacological treatment be indicated and, except in true separation anxiety, only on a short-term basis. Generally, sleep disorders offer a challenge for good diagnosis, good parenting and sensible advice, not for resorting to drugs which not only are often unsuccessful but have a variety of undesirable effects.

POSSIBLE INDICATIONS

1) *Anxiety*. This is a symptom not a diagnostic entity. If associated with psychosis, antipsychotics are indicated, not antianxiety drugs; if with school phobia or other separation anxiety disorders (see Chapter 5), imipramine is the drug of first choice though if this fails, a benzodiazepine may be tried for the acute situational anxiety. Other anxiety states have been poorly studied. There is, as yet, no proof that the antimuscarinic drugs are effective antianxiety agents though, as noted, they may be useful as hypnotics. Reviews by Gittelman-Klein (1978b), Freeman (1970), and Campbell (1975) attest to the lack of adequately controlled literature in this area. Further, two of the very few adequate studies (Cytryn et al., 1960; Eisenberg et al., 1961) suggest that a sedative in this case was no better than placebo or psychotherapy in producing relief of anxiety disorders in children. Therefore, it must be stated that there is as yet no proven role for antianxiety drugs in the various disorders of childhood in which anxiety figures prominently, though extrapolation of their clearly demonstrated superiority over placebo in adults suggests that the benzodiazepines are worthy of further study in children (Gittelman-Klein, 1978b), particularly in non-psychotic withdrawn states where disinhibition may facilitate the learning of socially advantageous behaviors. Such pharmacological treatment, though, should be seen as only

a *catalyst* within a behavior modification or other psychotherapeutic program.

2) *Other Childhood Conditions.* In a fashion characteristic of pediatric psychopharmacology, most studies of antianxiety agents have been used in a hotchpotch of diagnostic conditions, in uncontrolled circumstances, without good measures of drug effect and often in obfuscating combinatin with other drugs. There is no firm evidence that the antianxiety drugs have any usefulness in psychoses (pervasive developmental disorders and schizophrenia), in behavior disorders (conduct and attention deficit disorders), or stereotyped movement disorders such as tics (Campbell, 1975; Freeman, 1970; Gittelman-Klein, 1978b; Greenblatt & Shader, 1974). Rumor has it that they actually make children with attention deficit disorders (hyperactivity) worse and there is some evidence for this (Conners et al., 1965; Ounsted, 1955).

Diphenhydramine is also reputed to have a role in behavior disorders of a more severe kind, particularly in younger children (Campbell, 1975) but most of this evidence is uncontrolled, based on small samples and emanates from a single center (Bellevue Hospital) (Freeman, 1970). It would, however, seem worthy of further study since its sedative effects are probably free from disinhibition.

Conclusions

The role of the sedative or antianxiety drugs is one of the poorest researched areas in pediatric pyschopharmacology. These drugs may be occasionally useful in sleep disorders, acutely disturbed children, and in non-psychotic anxiety. The antimuscarinic type sedatives seem to be the most popular but their role is no more properly established than that of the virtually unexplored, attractively safe benzodiazepines. Both seem worthy of further investigation but only under properly controlled circumstances in properly defined and homogeneous diagnostic groups. In general, however, anxiety in children is situational rather than sustained and exquisitely sensitive to psychological maneuvers (Eisenberg et al., 1961; Gittelman-Klein, 1978b).

HALLUCINOGENS

(PSYCHOTOMIMETICS, PSYCHEDELICS)

Introduction

This group of drugs, variously named, is characterized less by any hallucinogenic capacity, which is ordinarily weak and common to many drugs acting on the CNS, than by an ability "reliably to induce . . . states of altered perception, thought and feeling that are not (or cannot be) experienced otherwise except in dreams or at times of religious exaltation" (Jaffe, 1975). This capacity stands in contrast to that of other drugs which produce these states only irregularly, idiosyncratically, in toxic doses or incidentally to their major therapeutic action.

While the hallucinogens have figured socially and religiously in other cultures for centuries (Ray, 1972), their introduction into austere, puritanical achievement-oriented Western societies in the last half-century has many of the features not of a pharmacological event but of a religious Reformation. Theses of Devil Incarnate advanced by the Established Order have been matched in intemperateness and absurdity only by Elixir of Life notions of the Psychedelic Zealots. The social controls and resources of the Orthodox have, to date, given them a premium on persecution, but there is reason to believe, as for example, from the behavior of the Puritans in Massachusetts, that if the Heretics were to gain power, the town water supply would be hallucinogenated, liquor and tobacco stores outlawed and replaced by State Head shops. For such is the nature of Man!

It is of interest to note that tobacco, chocolate and coffee evoked similar polarization in their day (Ray, 1972).

Types and Structures

The number of potential hallucinogens is high and newcomers are always appearing on the street. But, as is so often the case with drugs, the first ones to be introduced often prove to be the safest and most effective. For the past two decades or more, the favorites have been *cannaboids* from marihuana and the easily synthesised *lysergic acid diethylamide* (LSD) discovered by accident in a Swiss pharmaceutical laboratory. Mescaline from the mushroom peyote, DMT, psilocybin, bufotenin, morning glory and so on for various reasons (availability, toxicity, etc.), has lagged considerably far behind. All the above substances belong to one of three groups 1) *cannaboids*, 2) *indolealkylamines* related to the biogenic amine serotonin (the majority), or 3) substituted *phenethylamines* related to the catecholamines dopamine and the epinephrines. The pharmacological distinctiveness of cannaboids from other hallucinogens is disputed (Byck, 1975; Jaffe, 1975) though there can be no doubt about social differences in use and acceptability.

Many street hallucinogens are not, in fact, true hallucinogens, but antimuscarinics (see this chapter) resembling atropine, stimulants or central depressants. It is not uncommon for the belladonna alkaloids atropine, hyoscine or stramonium, readily available over the counter in proprietary hypnotic and antiemetic preparations, to be passed off as LSD or spliced into reefers for dealer profit. Some of the erroneous information about the dangers of the hallucinogens may stem from this source.

Patterns of Use

There is good reason to believe that the use of LSD, in the U.S. at least, has declined greatly in the last few years (Jaffe, 1975; Ray, 1972). This decline has been more than matched by an ever-increasing use of cannabis which in several U.S. states and Canada enjoys a legal-but-not-quite status rather similar to that of alcohol during Prohibition or to underage drinking. The hallucinogens are far outstripped as public health and social problems, of course, by tobacco and alcohol and one could well argue that the million or more dollars spent by the U.S. government to eradicate the wild marihuana growing along the Illinois Central Railroad tracks would have been much better spent on preventive programs for tobacco and alcohol.

Pharmacology

The hallucinogens vary greatly in 1) *potency*—LSD is by far the strongest, the dose being only micrograms, while smoked, home-grown marihuana is quite weak which is the basis of some of its apparent distinctiveness from other hallucinogens; 2) *route of administration*—sniffing and smoking produce faster intoxication, faster recovery and hence the possibility of finer tuning of his state by the user than with orally ingested drugs; 3) *duration of action*—the half-life of LSD is 2-3 hours though its effects may persist for 8-12 hours. Despite its conversion to active metabolites and high lipid solubility which should, in theory, lead to cumulation seen, for example, with the benzodiazepines (see this chapter), cannabis appears to remain a short-acting drug, the effect of which is 2-3 hours. Mescaline is the longest acting common hallucinogen (Jaffe, 1975).

Because of the resemblance of the state they produce to schizophrenia, the stronger hallucinogens such as LSD have been sometimes called *psychotomimetics* and have received a great deal of experimental study in search for a biochemical cause of this disorder. In spite of this, their site and mode of action are still unclear. The most popular theory is that they have a serotonin-like action (Byck, 1975; Snyder et al., 1974) though, since the action of serotonin in the CNS is unclear, this is not particularly enlightening at the moment. Other theories suggest dopamine (Snyder et al., 1974) or octopamine actions. These latter theories derive in part from the ability of antipsychotic drugs to block the action of these biogenic amines (see Chapter 8).

Clinical Effects

CENTRAL NERVOUS SYSTEM

As already noted, the striking clinical effect is *altered consciousness, perception, thinking and feeling*. While there is certainly some similarity between this state and schizophrenia, especially acute schizophrenia, there are also significant differences, notably the preponderance of visual over auditory hallucinations and the (relative) preservation of awareness and insight with the hallucinogens (Snyder et al., 1974). Though, as Snyder et al. (1974) point out, these differences might well be elided if hallucinogens were to be given regularly over a period comparable to that of schizophrenia, natural experiments provided by the chronic use of marihuana in India and the West Indies (see Ray, 1972, various Canadian, English and U.S. governmental reports) and the failure unequivocally to demonstrate long-term ill-effects of LSD use (Jaffe, 1975) make this seem unlikely. The state produced by the hallucinogens differs from that of a *toxic delirium* producible by a wide variety of psychotropic and other substances active on the CNS, in that while visual and tactile hallucinations and illusions are features of both, the degree of disorientation and confusion is much greater in toxic delirium as are incidental side effects due to the toxicity of the drug.

The exact intensity, content and reaction in this state of altered consciousness depend on the drug, the dose, the route of administration, the personality and the mood of the user and the social situation in which the drug is taken. Of these, the social and personal factors seem overriding in normal social doses (Ray, 1972). Disinhibition, so characteristic of the central and selective depressant sedatives (see this chapter) and responsible for many of the social problems of alcohol, does not seem to occur with hallucinogens though the power of the social situation to influence the resultant behavior can be seen in the contrast between the nodding, introverted Western pothead and the Assassins of the Orient (Ray, 1972).

OTHER SYSTEMS

All hallucinogens have centrally and peripherally mediated autonomic effects, largely sympathomimetic (alpha-adrenergic) (see Chapter 6) but these seldom are of serious clinical significance. Individual drugs may have additional peculiar effects such as suffusion of the conjunctivae with cannabis, vomiting with mescaline and antidiuresis with LSD (Byck, 1975), all equally benign.

Treatment Emergent (Side) Effects

This term is somewhat inappropriate here since treatment is scarcely an appropriate term—unwanted effects would be better. Two of the more remarkable features of the hallucinogens are their *physical safety* repeatedly revealed in official publications throughout the English speaking world and the vehemence with which this has been denied and disputed, usually by public figures whose careers have been distinguished largely by conservatism and a persistent belief that the Nation is on the point of political or moral collapse from forces without or within. There may be good reasons for not taking hallucinogens but *physical risks* including chromosomal abnormalities (apart from accidents) are not among them (Byck, 1975; Jaffe, 1975). On the other hand, pseudohallucinogens such as antimuscarinics (see this chapter) and combinations of hallucinogens with other psychotropic substances can be dangerous, though there are no fatalities in which the hallucinogens have been shown unequivocally to have played a major role (Ray, 1972; Yolles, 1970).

Physical side effects are usually mild, short-lived and related to sympathomimetic action—tremor, weakness, dizziness, nausea, etc.

PSYCHOLOGICAL

While physical effects are minor, there can be no doubt about the ability of these drugs to produce unpleasant and, rarely, dangerous (because of accidents) psychological states. As noted, these are dependent less on the drug than on the person, his mood and stability, and the situation. Compared with the dangerous drugs, opiates and alcohol, these are, however, relatively infrequent and minor. One of the difficulties of assessing psychological side effects is the propensity of the psychologically frail and uneasy to see solutions to their current ills in drugs (e.g., Rosenberg, 1969; Smart & Jones, 1970). *While psychological ill-effects—mostly panic states (the bad trip) during the action of the drug which, as already noted, are relatively short for most of these drugs—are indisputable, any long-term ill-effects such as schizophreniform psychoses and impairment of abstract thinking ability are still a matter of controversy and quite unproven* (Jaffe, 1975; Ray, 1972).

The best established long-term ill-effect is the *flashback* (Stanton &

Bardoni, 1972) which, however, is not necessarily unpleasant or confined to the hallucinogens. During this, emotionally charged experiences first occurring during a drug state recur spontaneously at irregular intervals.

There is nothing mysterious in this phenomenon—emotionally strong experiences of any kind can stamp themselves indelibly on the memory in a sort of one trial conditioning. Phobias, panic states and religious and poetic ecstatic experiences are examples which may be instigated without pharmacological means.

The treatment of the psychological distress caused by hallucinogens is aimed primarily at the relief of anxiety, usually by talking down and reassurances. Since the user may have taken other substances or the purity of the hallucinogen may be in doubt, only in extreme states and then only cautious use of a safe anxiolytic like diazepam may be indicated (Jaffe, 1975). Antipsychotics should be used with caution except in true psychotic states since street drugs may contain significant amounts of antimuscarinics and the bad trip may be, in fact, a toxic delirium. Some antipsychotics have strong antimuscarinic actions of their own and may thus exaggerate the delirious state (Shader, 1975, also Chapter 8).

The question of dependence arises. While physical dependence does not seem to occur (Jaffe, 1975)—in fact, LSD is said to lose its effect ultimately—psychological dependence can and does occur with the hallucinogens though they are probably no more likely to produce this than most other drugs such as alcohol, aspirin or benzodiazepines and considerably less so than the most potent in this respect, namely opiates and stimulants. With the variety of psychotropic substances available, the common mixed use of drugs and the highly abnormal personalities of persons who become dependent on drugs, it is debatable if any one substance (outside those which produce rapid physical dependence) will have much influence on the *total number* of persons dependent on drugs other than opiates.

Indications and Contraindications

In contrast to adult psychiatry, where the strong hallucinogens such as LSD have been used in almost every known disorder though without conspicuous success, LSD and its congener, methysergide, have been tried in pediatric psychopharmacology only in the Pervasive Developmental Disorders (psychoses). Most, but not all, these studies have emanated from one center known for its rather heroic approach to the treatment of these disorders (see Campbell, 1975).

These studies have mostly been informal and the results inconclusive or a mixture of gains (in alertness and responsiveness) and losses (anxiety and disorganization). In general, *autistic* children seem to have responded slightly better than older *schizophrenic* children; but any usefulness in the former condition needs further establishing and it is significant that no studies appear to have been done for 10 years. Cannabis does not appear to have been tried in pediatric psychopharmacology.

Summary

Hallucinogens are of interest in pediatric psychopharmacology only as a research tool and because of the possibilities of their accidental ingestion by small children (e.g., Samuelsson, 1974) and of self-administration by older children. Medically they are relatively benign, though like all intoxicants, their use is to be actively discouraged because of the possibilities of accidents, panic states, flashbacks and as yet undiscovered long-term effects. Such a pious statement, however, denies something elemental in human nature—the need to enrich or enjoy experiences by making those distinctively human qualities attributable to the highest CNS functions distorted or less efficient. If adults sanction this ethos for themselves, they must not be surprised if their children adopt it too, using whatever new means may lie at hand. Experimentation by the young may have its perils but it is also the mechanism by which societies adapt and change. Any problem presented by the hallucinogens pales into insignificance beside that of tobacco and alcohol. The relationship between a drug, its availability, attempts to prohibit it and its pattern of use and abuse is extremely complex and only the naive and politicians see this problem simplistically (Jaffe, 1975; Ray, 1972).

MISCELLANEOUS SUBSTANCES

Levodopa (L-Dopa). This is a precursor of dopamine (Goodman & Gilman, 1975) which is itself a neurotransmitter and also a precursor of another, norepinephrine. In adults it is used in the treatment of Parkinson's disease and in children has been tried in the Pervasive Developmental Disorders notably autism, with conflicting results (Campbell, 1975; Ritvo et al., 1971). As might be predicted from the close relationship of levodopa to the stimulants, the changes reported are rather similar, most conspicuously an increase in energy and alertness. It may appear surprising that levodopa has been used little or not at all in hyperactivity where the stimulants are so useful (see Chapter 6), but dopaminergic side effects such as nausea, orthostatic hypotension and abnormal involuntary movements akin to tardive dyskinesia (see Chapter 8) can occur. Concern about these and possible long-term consequences of the stimulation of growth hormone which levodopa also produces (Goodman & Gilman, 1975) are no doubt responsible, though all these effects are dose-dependent. Parkinson's disease, which is the source of most of the information on side effects, requires rather higher doses than might be necessary in hyperactivity.

Thyroid. This seems to be a hardy chestnut having once been popular in the management of mental retardation (Freeman, 1970). Lately, the most powerful of the naturally occurring thyroid hormones, triodothyronine or T3 has attracted some interest in the treatment of autism and schizophrenia in children from the Bellevue group. They reported it to produce behavioral and cognitive stimulation, paradoxically most marked in those children who had slightly elevated thyroid function (Campbell, 1975). However, the changes were not dramatic and hardly surprising in view of the general increase in body metabolic rate produced by thyroid, usually considered undesirable or unsafe except in hypothyroidism.

Vitamins. These are a miscellaneous group of dietary essentials (that is, not able to be synthesised within the body from other food substances). Their metabolic roles vary and their grouping together is simply one of history and a common origin in foodstuffs. Physicians cannot but be bemused by the mystical qualities with which vitamins are imbued by the lay public who seem to comprehend neither their abundance in modern diets and their toxic potential when given in excess. Vitamins have a respectable history in psychiatry since it was discovered that pellagra, which at one time filled the psychiatric hospitals in the Southern U.S., was due in part to vitamin deficiency. Since that signal success, however, efforts to re-establish a therapeutic role for them in psychiatric disorders have failed despite the efforts of Linus Pauling, Nobel Laureate in Chemistry, who has espoused a Canadian idea of megavitamin therapy for schizophrenia. In this view, there is a relative shortage of vitamins, notably of niacin, one of the B group, because of certain metabolic inefficiencies which necessitate large amounts of the vitamin to produce normal metabolic rates. While systematic American and Canadian studies (see Klein & Gittelman-Klein, 1976) have been consistently negative, this seems to have done little to discourage enthusiasts, including Pauling. Two trials, one of which was well controlled, have failed to show any role for megavitamin therapy in childhood schizophrenia (see Campbell, 1975). Rimland (1975), whose data come from informal clinical studies on individual children, not his own work, where other drugs have often been used as well, claims that the results in autism, if modest, are sufficiently encouraging to warrant proper investigation. Autism is one of the most distressing and intractable conditions in child psychiatry and it has an understandable propensity of attracting enthusiastic claims for treatment which usually do not withstand close scrutiny.

Glutamic Acid. Like thyroid, this essential amino acid (protein building substance) was once popular as a learning facilitator in mental retardation (Freeman, 1970) but fell into disuse despite an exhaustive review by Vogel et al. (1963) strongly supporting its effectiveness. There is some evidence that its simple derivative, 1-glutamate, may act as a neurotransmitter and, further, is found in high concentrations in the forebrain (Goodman & Gilman, 1975), so that there is a possible pharmacological rationale for any psychotropic action. More careful work is needed, not only to affirm its efficacy but also its safety and its distinctiveness from a number of substances such as stimulants and thyroid which seem to be able to stimulate cognitive processes, though to a limited and evanescent degree (see Chapter 3).

Chelating Substances. These have the capacity to bind heavy metals and assist in their excretion. Recent work has suggested that some cases of hyperactivity in children may be due to subclinical lead poisoning (see Werry, in press b) and one controlled study reported improvement in some children with these substances (David et al., 1976). This interesting work requires replication but would be predicted to be useful, at best, in only a minority of hyperactive children and not necessarily to obviate the need for other treatments, since some of the damage due to lead would be irreversible.

Other Substances. Freeman (1970) lists several other chemical substances used at various times in exceptional children and it would seem that there is and will be no end to possible psychotropic substances. Most, however, will prove to be ships passing in the night and substantive advances are likely to come only from a better understanding of brain function and any derangements of it in psychopathological disorders of childhood. One thing is clear, though: The burden of proof must pass from critic to proposer of a treatment. The recent Feingold dietary management of hyperactivity (see Chapters 4 and 6) is a case in point. At the time of writing, this treatment has attained near-epidemic proportions in the U.S. and Australia but has only meagre scientific support (Conners et al., 1976), most carefully controlled studies being negative (see Werry, 1976). While the Feingold hypothesis that 1) salicylates and certain other food additives can, in genetically predisposed individuals, interfere with the synthesis of prostaglandins, vital metabolic substances for most cells, and 2) that such interference, if it occurs, can result in hyperactivity, is tenable, it seems to have assumed the status of dogma despite the fact that it remains only an hypothesis, not a proven fact. The time has come when to promulgate a treatment to an anxious and credulous public before it has been properly tested following FDA periatric guidelines (see Chapter 4) should be regarded as a possible breach of medical ethics.

REFERENCES

AARSKOG, D., FEVANG, F., KLOVE, H., STOA, K., & THORSEN, T. The effect of the stimulant drugs, dextroamphetamine and methylphenidate on secretion of growth hormone in hyperactive children. *Journal of Pediatrics*, 1977, 90:136-139.
ABEL, E. *Drugs and Behavior: A Primer in Neuropsychopharmocology*. New York: Wiley, 1974.
ADNITT, P. Hypoglycemic action of monoamineoxidase inhibitors. *Diabetes*, 1968, 17:628-633.
AHMAD, S., LAIDLAW, J., HOUGHTON, G., & RICHENS, A. Involuntary movements caused by phenytoin intoxication in epileptic patients. *Journal of Neurology, Neurosurgery and Psychiatry*, 1975, 38:225-231.
ALDERTON, H. Imipramine in childhood nocturnal enuresis: Relationship of time of administration to effect. *Canadian Psychiatric Association Journal*, 1967, 12:197-203.
ALDERTON, H. & HODDINOTT, B. A controlled study of the use of thioridizine in the treatment of hyperactive and aggressive children in a children's psychiatric hospital. *Canadian Psychiatric Association Journal*, 1969, 9:239-247.
ALEXANDER, F.: The dynamics of psychotherapy in the light of learning theory. *American Journal of Psychiatry*, 1963, 120:440-448.
ALEXANDERSON, B., and SJOQVIST, F. Individual differences in the pharmacokinetics of monomethylated tricyclic antidepressants; role of genetic and environmental factors, and clinical importance. *Annals of the New York Academy of Sciences*, 1971, 179:739-751.
AL-KAISI, A. & McGUIRE, R. The effect of sulthiame on disturbed behaviour in mentally subnormal patients. *British Journal of Psychiatry*, 1974, 124:45-49.
ALPERN, D. M. Questions of ethics. *Newsweek*, June 14, 1976, 21-22; 25-26; 27-28.
ALVARES, A. P., KAPELNER, S., SHIGERU, S. & ATTALLAH, K. Drug metabolism in normal children, lead poisoned children and normal adults. *Clinical Pharmacology and Therapeutics*, 1975, 17:179-183.
AMAN, M. Cognitive and social differences between normal and specific learning disability children. Submitted for publication, 1977.
AMAN, M. & SPRAGUE, R. The state-dependent effects of methylphenidate and dextroamphetamine. *Journal of Nervous and Mental Disease*, 1974, 158:268-279.
AMAN, M. & WERRY, J. The effects of methylphenidate and haloperidol on the heart rate and blood pressure of hyperactive children with special reference to time of action. *Psychopharmacologia*, 1975a, 43:163-168.
AMAN, M. & WERRY, J. Methylphenidate in children: Effects upon cardiorespiratory function on exertion. *International Journal of Mental Health*, 1975b, 4:119-131.
AMDISEN, A. Variation of serum lithium concentration during the day in relation to treatment control, absorptive side-effects, and the use of slow-release tablets. *Acta Psychiatrica Scandinavica*, 1969, 207:55-58.

American Academy of Pediatrics, (Council on Child Health): Medication for hyperkinetic children. *Pediatrics*, 1975, 55:560-561.

American College of Neuropsychopharmacology. Drug therapy neurological syndromes associated with antipsychotic drug use. *New England Journal of Medicine*, 1973, 289:20-23.

An International Glossary of Anticonvulsants. (3rd ed). London: International Bureau for Epilepsy, 1977.

ANDERMANN, F. & ROBB, J. Absence status. *Epilepsia*, 1972, 13:177-187.

ANDERSON, R., HALCOMB, C., & DOYLE, R. The measurement of attentional deficits. *Exceptional Children*, 1973, 39:534-540.

ANNELL, A. Lithium treatment of children and adolescents. *Acta Psychiatrica Scandinavica*, 1969a, 207:19-30.

ANNELL, A. Manic-depressive illness in children and effect of treatment. *Acta Paedopsychiatrica*, 1969b, 36:292-301.

ANNESLEY, P. Nardil response in a chronic obsessive-compulsive. *British Journal of Psychiatry*, 1969, 115:748.

APPELMAN, M. A. The legal issues involved in the use of stimulants on hyperactive school children. Doctoral dissertation, University of Minnesota, 1974.

ARANDA, J., SITAR, D., PARSONS, W., LOUGHNAN, P., & NEIMS, A.: Pharmacokinetic aspects of theophylline in premature newborns. *New England Journal of Medicine*, 1976, 295:413-416.

ARNOLD, L., HUESTIS, R., SMELTZER, D., SCHEIB, J., WEMMER, D., & COLNER, G. Levoamphetamine v. dextroamphetamine in minimal brain dysfunction. *Archives of General Psychiatry*, 1976, 33:292-301.

ARNOLD, L., KIRILCUK, V., CORSON, S., & CORSON, E.: Levoamphetamine and dextroamphetamine: Differential effect on aggression and hyperkinesis in children and dogs. *American Journal of Psychiatry*, 1973, 130:165-170.

ARNOLD, E. & MAGNIN, D. Fluphenazine in the treatment of disturbed mentally retarded children. *Medical Journal of Australia*, 1967, 1:758-760.

ARNOLD, L., WENDER, P., MCCLOSKEY, K., & SNYDER, S. Levoamphetamine and dextroamphetamine: Comparative efficacy in the hyperkinetic syndrome: Assessment by target symptoms. *Archives of General Psychiatry*, 1972, 27:816-822.

ARONOFF, M. S., EVANS, R., & DURRELL, J. Effect of lithium salts on electrolyte metabolism. *Journal of Psychiatric Research*, 1971, 8:139-159.

ASBERG, M. Treatment of depression with tricyclic drugs—pharmacokinetic and pharmacodynamic aspects. *Pharmakopsychiatrie*, 1976, 9:18-26.

AYD, F. A survey of drug-induced extrapyramidal reactions. *Journal of the American Medical Association*, 1961, 175:1054-1060.

AYD, F. Haloperidol: Fifteen years of clinical experience. *Diseases of the Nervous System*, 1972, 33:459-469.

AYD, F. *Rational Psychopharmacology and the Right to Treatment*. Baltimore: Waverley Press, 1975.

BADHAM, J., BARDON, L., REEVES, P., & YOUNG, A. A trial of thioridazine in mental deficiency. *British Journal of Psychiatry*, 1963, 109:408-410.

BAER, L. Lithium absorption, distribution, renal handling, and effect on body electrolytes. In: S. Gershon and B. Shopsin (Eds.), *Lithium ion: Its Role in Psychiatric Treatment and Research*. New York: Plenum Press, 1973, 33-49.

BAER, L., PLATMAN, S., KASSIR, S., & FIEVE, R. Mechanisms of renal lithium handling and their relationship to mineralocorticoids: A dissociation between sodium and lithium ions. *Journal of Psychiatric Research*, 1971, 8:91-105.

BAIR, H. & HEROLD, W. Efficacy of chlorpromazine in hyperactive mentally retarded children. *Archives of Neurology and Psychiatry*, 1955, 74:363-364.

BAKER, M. & WINOKUR, G. Cerebrospinal fluid lithium in manic disease. *British Journal of Psychiatry*, 1966, 112:163-165.

BALDWIN, R. & KENNY, T. Thioridazine in the management of organic behavior disturbances in children. *Current Therapeutic Research*, 1966, 8:373-377.
BALDWIN, R. & PETERS, J. Hematologic complications from tranquilizers in children. *Southern Medical Journal*, 1968, 61:1072-1075.
BALLARD, J., BOILEAU, R., SLEATOR, E., MASSEY, B., & SPRAGUE, R. Cardiovascular responses of hyperactive children to methylphenidate. *Journal of the American Medical Association*, 1976, 236:2870-2874.
BARBER, B. The ethics of experimentation with human subjects. *Scientific American*, 1976, 234:(2), 25-31.
BARCAI, A. Predicting the response of children with learning disabilities and behavior problems to dextroamphetamine sulfate. The clinical interview and the finger twitch test. *Pediatrics*, 1971, 47:79-80.
BARKER, R. The effects of psychotropic drugs on psychological testing. *Psychological Bulletin*, 1968, 69: 377-387.
BARKER, P. & FRASER, I. A controlled trial of haloperidol in children. *British Journal of Psychiatry*, 1968, 114:855-857.
BARKLEY, R. Predicting the response of hyperkinetic children to stimulant drugs: A review. *Journal of Abnormal Child Psychology*, 1976, 4:327-348.
BARKLEY, R. A review of stimulant drug research with hyperactive children. *Journal of Child Psychology and Psychiatry*, 1977, 18:137-165.
BARKLEY, R. & CUNNINGHAM, C. Do stimulant drugs improve the academic performance of hyperkinetic children? A review of outcome research. *Clinical Pediatrics*, in press.
BARKLEY, R. & JACKSON, T. Hyperkinesis, autonomic nervous system activity and stimulant drug effects. *Journal of Child Psychology and Psychiatry*, in press.
BARKLEY, R. & ULLMAN, D. A comparison of objective measures of activity and distractibility in hyperkinetic and nonhyperkinetic children. *Journal of Abnormal Child Psychology*, 1975, 3:231-244.
BASSTRUP, P. & SCHOU, M. Lithium as a prophylactic agent: Its effect against recurrent depressions and manic-depressive psychosis. *Archives of General Psychiatry*, 1967, 16:162-172.
BATTIG, W. Procedural problems in paired-associate learning research. *Psychonomic Monograph Supplement*, 1965, 1.
BEAUDRY, P. & GIBSON, D. Effect of trifluoperazine on the behavior disorders of children with malignant emotional disturbances. *American Journal of Mental Deficiency*, 1960, 64:823-826.
BECK, L., LANGFORD, W., MACKAY, M., & SUM, G. Childhood chemotherapy and later drug abuse and growth curve: A follow up study of 30 adolescents. *American Journal of Psychiatry*, 1975, 132:436-438.
BEDELL, J. & ROITZSCH, J. The effects of stress on state and trait anxiety in emotionally disturbed, normal and delinquent children. *Journal of Abnormal Child Psychology*, 1976, 4:173-178.
BELL, J. H. The family that fought back. *McCall's*, May 1977, 26, 30, 32, 34, 36, 40.
BELL, R., WELLER, G., & WALDROP, M. Newborn and preschooler: Organisation of behavior and relations between periods. *Monographs of the Society for Research in Child Development*, 1971, 36: Serial No. 142.
BELLMAN, M. Treatment of phenothiazine drug intoxication with benztropine. *Archives of Diseases in Childhood*, 1974, 49:664-665.
BENDER, L. Instructions for the use of Visual Motor Gestalt Test. The American Orthopsychiatric Association, Inc., 1946.
BENDER, L. & COTTINGTON, F. The use of amphetamine sulfate (benzedrine) in child psychiatry. *American Journal of Psychiatry*, 1942, 99:116-121.
Benskin v. Taft City School District C.A. No. 136795 (Sup. Ct., Kern Co., Cal. filed Sept. 1975).

BERG, I., HULLIN, R., ALLSOPP, M., O'BRIEN, P., & MACDONALD, R. Bipolar manic-depressive psychosis in early adolescence. *British Journal of Psychiatry*, 1974, 125:416-417.

BERGMAN, A. & WERNER, R. Failure of children to receive penicillin by mouth. *New England Journal of Medicine*, 1963, 268:1334-1338.

BETTSCHART, et al., unpublished findings, 1969. Quoted by Remschmidt (1976).

BIALER, I., DOLL, L., & WINSBERG, B. A modified Lincoln-Oseretsky Motor Development Scale: Provisional standardization. *Perceptual and Motor Skills*, 1974, 38: 599-614.

BICHONSKI, R. The changes of physico-chemical properties of blood of mentally retarded children after pharmacotherapy. *Journal of Pharmacy and Pharmacology*, 1973, 25:231-235.

BICKEL, M. Poisoning by tricyclic antidepressant drugs. *International Journal of Clinical Pharmacology*, 1975, 11:145-176.

BICKEL, M. & WEDER, H. Buccal absorption and other properties of pharmacokinetic importance of imipramine and its metabolites. *Journal of Pharmacy and Pharmacology*, 1969, 21:160-168.

BIRCH, H. & BELMONT, L. Auditory-visual integration in normal and retarded readers. *American Journal of Orthopsychiatry*, 1964, 34:852-861.

BIRCH, H. & BELMONT, L. Auditory-visual integration in brain-damaged and normal children. *Developmental Medicine and Child Neurology*, 1965, 7:135-144.

BLACKLIDGE, V. & EKBLAD, R. The effectiveness of methylphenidate hydrochloride (Ritalin) on learning and behavior in public school educable mentally retarded children. *Pediatrics*, 1971, 47:923-926.

BLACKWELL, B. & CURRAH, J. The psychopharmacology of nocturnal enuresis. In: I. Kolvin, R. McKeith, and S. Meadow (Eds.), *Bladder Control and Enuresis*. Clinics and Developmental Medicine Nos. 48/49. London: Heinemann, 1973, pp. 231-257.

BLANK, M. & BRIDGER, W. Deficiencies in verbal labeling in retarded readers. *American Journal of Orthopsychiatry*, 1966, 36:840-847.

BLANK, M., WEIDER, S., & BRIDGER, W. Verbal deficiencies in abstract thinking in early reading retardation. *American Journal of Orthopsychiatry*, 1968, 38:823-832.

BOELHOUWER, C., HENRY, C., & GLUECK, B. Positive spiking: A double blind control study on its significance in behavior disorders, both diagnostically and therapeutically. *American Journal of Psychiatry*, 1968, 125:473-481.

BOGOCH, S. & DREYFUS, J. *The Broad Range of Use of Diphenylhydantoin*. New York: Dreyfus Medical Foundation, 1970.

BOGOCH, S. & DREYFUS, J. *DPH, 1975*. New York: Dreyfus Medical Foundation, 1975.

BOILEAU, R., BALLARD, J., SPRAGUE, R., SLEATOR, E., & MASSEY, B. Effects of methylphenidate on cardio-respiratory responses in hyperactive children. *Research Quarterley*, 1976, 47:590-596.

BOOKER, H. Idiosyncratic reactions to antiepileptic drugs. *Epilepsia*, 1975, 16:171-181.

BOSCO, J. J. & ROBIN, S. S. (Eds.). *The Hyperactive Child and Stimulant Drugs*. Chicago: University of Chicago Press, 1977.

BOWERS, JR., M., HENINGER, G., & GERBODE, F. Cerebrospinal fluid 5-hydroxyindoleacetic acid and homovanillic acid in psychiatric patients. *International Journal of Neuropharmacology*, 1969, 8:255-262.

BOXER, C., HERZBERG, J., & SCOTT, D. Has sodium valproate hypnotic effects? *Epilepsia*, 1976, 17:367-370.

BRADLEY, C. The behavior of children receiving benzedrine. *American Journal of Orthopsychiatry*, 1937, 94:577-585.

BRAITHWAITE, R., GOULDING, R., THEANO, G., BAILEY, J., & COPPEN, A. Plasma concentration of amitriptyline and clinical response. *Lancet*, 1972, 1:1297-1300.

BREBBIA, D., ALTSHULER, Z., & KLINE, N. Lithium and the electroencephalogram during sleep. *Diseases of the Nervous System*, 1969, 30:541-546.
BRECKENRIDGE, A. & ORME, M. Clinical implications of enzyme induction. *Annals of the New York Academy of Sciences*, 1971, 179:421-431.
BRIANT, R., BLACKWELL, E., WILLIAMS, F., DAVIES, D., & DOLLERY, C. The metabolism of sympathomimetic bronchodilator drugs by the perfused dog lung. *Xenobiotica*, 1973, 3:787-799.
British Medical Journal. Hyperactive children. *British Medical Journal*, 1973, 1:305-306. Editorial.
British Medical Journal. Tranquilizers causing aggression. *British Medical Journal*, 1975, 1:113-114.
BROMAN, S., NICHOLS, P., & KENNEDY, W. *Preschool I.Q.: Prenatal and Early Developmental Correlates.* Hillsdale, New Jersey: Lawrence Erlbaum, 1975.
BROWN, J. L. & BING, S. R. Drugging children: Child abuse by professionals. In: G. P. Koocher (Ed.), *Children's Rights and the Mental Health Professionals.* New York: Wiley, 1976.
BROWN, D., WINSBERG, B., BIALER, I., & PRESS, M. Imipramine therapy and seizures. *American Journal of Psychiatry*, 1973, 130:210-212.
BROWN, G. L., EBERT, M. H., HUNT, R. D., BUNNEY, W. E. Amphetamine blood levels, behavior and activity in minimal brain dysfunction. Presented. at APA, Toronto, 1977.
BROWN, T. C. Overdosage—the rise and fall of tricyclic antidepressants. *Australian Paediatric Journal*, 1975, 11:190-194.
BROWN, T., DRIEFUSS, F., DYKEN, P., GOODE, D., PENRY, J., PORTER, R., WHITE, B., & WHITE, P. Ethosuximide (Zarontin) in the treatment of absence (petit mal) seizures. *Neurology* 1975, 25:515-525.
BRUCK, C. Battle lines in the Ritalin war. *Human Behavior*, August 1976, 23-33.
BRUMBACK, R., WEINBERG, W., & HERJANIC, B. Epileptiform activity in the electroencephalogram induced by lithium carbonate. *Pediatrics*, 1975, 56:831-834.
BRUUN, R., SHAPIRO, A., SHAPIRO, E., SWEET, R., WAYNE, H., & SOLOMON, G. A follow-up of 78 patients with Gilles de la Tourette's Syndrome. *American Journal of Psychiatry*, 1976, 133:944-947.
BUCHANAN, R., TURNER, J., MOYER, C., & HEFFELFINGER, J. Single daily dose of diphenylhydantoin in children. *Journal of Pediatrics*, 1973, 83:479-483.
BUCHSBAUM, M., GOODWIN, F., MURPHY, D., & BORGE, G. AER in affective disorders. *American Journal of Psychiatry*, 1971, 128:19-25.
BUCHSBAUM, M., & WENDER, P. Average evoked responses in normal and minimally brain dysfunctioned children treated with amphetamine: A preliminary report. *Archives of General Psychiatry*, 1973, 29:764-770.
Bulletin of the Johns Hopkins Hospital. Diphenylhydantoin toxicity leading to psychiatric hospitalization. *Bulletin of the Johns Hopkins Hospital*, 1964, 115:417-418.
BUNNEY, W., JR., GOODWIN, F., & MURPHY, D. The switch process in manic-depressive illness. III. Theoretical implications. *Archives of General Psychiatry*, 1972, 27:312-317.
BUNNEY, W., JR., & MURPHY, D. Strategies for the systematic study of neurotransmitter receptor functions in man. In: E. Usdin and W. Bunney, Jr. (Eds.), *Pre- and Post-Synaptic Receptors.* New York: Marcel Dekker, 1975, 283-311.
BUNNEY, W., JR. & MURPHY, D. Neurobiological considerations on the mode of action of lithium carbonate in the treatment of affective disorders. *Pharmakopsychiatrie Neuro-psychopharmakologie*, 1976, 9:142-147.
BURDOCK, E. & HARDESTY, A. Children's Behavior Inventory Clinical Profile. *Psychopharmacology Bulletin*—Special Issue on Pharmacotherapy with Children, 1973, 71-84.

BURK, W. & MENOLASCINO, F. Haloperidol in emotionally disturbed, mentally retarded individuals. *American Journal of Psychiatry*, 1968, 124: 1589-1591.

BURNESS, F. Fluphenazine ("Anatensol") in the treatment of disturbed mentally retarded children. *Medical Journal of Australia*, 1968, 1:241.

BURNS, J. & SHORE, P. Biochemical effects of drugs. *Annual Review of Pharmacology*, 1961, 1:79-104.

BUROS, O. *The Seventh Mental Measurements Yearbook.* Highland Park, N.J.: Gryphon Press, 1972.

BURROWS, G., DAVIES, B., & SCOGGINS, B. Plasma concentration of nortryptiline in depressive illness. *Lancet*, 1972, 2:619-623.

BUTTER, H. & LAPIERRE, Y. The effect of methylphenidate on sensory perception and integration in hyperactive children. *International Pharmacopsychiatry*, 1974, 9:235-244.

BUTTER, H. & LAPIERRE, Y. The effect of methylphenidate on sensory perception in varying degrees of hyperkinetic behaviour. *Diseases of the Nervous System*, 1975, 36:286-288.

BYCK, R. Drugs in the treatment of psychiatric disorders. In: L. Goodman and A. Gilman (Eds.), *The Pharmacological Basis of Therapeutics*, (5th ed.). New York: Macmillan, 1975, pp. 152-200.

CADE, J. Lithium slats in the treatment of psychotic excitement. *Medical Journal of Australia*, 1949, 2:349-352.

CALNE, D., CHASE, T., & BARBEAU, A. (Eds.). *Advances in Neurology*, Vol. 9: *Dopaminergic Mechanisms*. New York: Raven Press, 1975.

CAMP, B. & SMERLING, L. Review of preschool behavior rating scales. In *Guidelines for Evaluation of Psychoactive Agents in Infants and Children*. Rockville, Maryland: U.S. Food and Drug Administration. DHEWS—in press.

CAMP, J., BIALER, I., PRESS, M., & WINSBERG, B. The physical and neurological examination for soft signs (PANESS): Pediatric norms and comparisons between normal and deviant boys. *Psychopharmacology Bulletin*, 1977, 13(2):39-41.

CAMPBELL, M. Biological interventions in psychoses of childhood. *Journal of Autism and Childhood Schizophrenia*, 1973, 3:347-373.

CAMPBELL, M. Pharmacotherapy in early infantile autism. *Biological Psychiatry*, 1975, 10:399-423.

CAMPBELL, M., FISH, B., KOREIN, J., SHAPIRO, T., COLLINS, P., & KOH, C. Lithium and chlorpromazine: A controlled crossover study of hyperactive severely disturbed young children. *Journal of Autism and Childhood Schizophrenia*, 1972, 2:234-263 (a).

CAMPBELL, M., FISH, B., SHAPIRO, T., & FLOYD, A., JR. Thiothixene in young disturbed children: A pilot study. *Archives of General Psychiatry*, 1970, 23, 70-72.

CAMPBELL, M., FISH, B., SHAPIRO, T., & FLOYD, A., JR. A study of molindone in disturbed preschool children. *Current Therapeutic Research*, 1971, 13:28-33 (b).

CAMPBELL, M., FISH, B., SHAPIRO, T., & FLOYD, A., JR. Acute responses of schizophrenic children to a sedative and "stimulating" neuroleptic: A pharmacologic yardstick. *Current Therapeutic Research*, 1972, 14:759-766 (b).

CAMPBELL, M. & SMALL, A. M. Drug treatment of mental disorders. In: L. L. Simpson (Ed.), *The Use of Psychotherapeutic Drugs in the Treatment of Mental Illness*. New York: Raven Press, 1976, pp. 209-236.

CAMPBELL, S., DOUGLAS, V., & MORGENSTERN, G. Cognitive styles in hyperactive children and the effect of methylphenidate. *Journal of Child Psychology and Psychiatry*, 1971, 12:55-67(a).

CANTWELL, D. *The Hyperactive Child—Diagnosis, Management, Current Research.* New York: Spectrum, 1975.

CANTWELL, D. The hyperkinetic syndrome. In: M. Rutter and L. Hersov (Eds.), *Child Psychiatry—Modern Approaches*. Oxford: Blackwell, 1976, pp. 524-555.

References

CANTWELL, D. P. CNS activating drugs in the treatment of hyperactive children. In: J. Brady and H. Brodie (Eds.), *Controversy in Psychiatry*. Philadelphia: W. B. Saunders Company, in press.

CAREY, W. Night waking and temperament in infancy. *Journal of Pediatrics*, 1974, 84:756-758.

CARLSSON, A., FUXE, K., HAMBERGER, B., & LINDQVIST, M. Biochemical and histochemical studies on the effects of imipramine-like drugs on central and peripheral catecholamine neurons. *Acta Physiologica Scandanavia*, 1966, 67:481-497.

CARON, H. & ROTH, H. Patients' cooperation with a medical regime. *Journal of the American Medical Association*, 1968, 203:922-929.

CARROLL, H. The remedial teaching of reading: An evaluation. *Remedial Education*, 1972, 7:10-15.

CASE, W., RICKLES, K., & BAZILIAN, S. Diphenylhydantoin in neurotic anxiety. *American Journal of Psychiatry*, 1969, 126:254-255.

CASTENEDA, A., MCCANDLESS, B., & PALERMO, D. The children's form of the manifest anxiety scale. *Child Development*, 1956, 27:317-326.

CAVERS, D. F. The legal control of the clinical investigation of drugs: Some political, economic, and social questions. In: S. R. Graubard (Ed.), *Ethical Aspects of Experimentation with Human Subjects*. Daedalus, 1969, 98:427-448.

CEREGHINO, J., BROCK, J., VAN METER, J., PENRY, J., SMITH, L., & WHITE, B. Carbamazepine for epilepsy. A controlled prospective evaluation. *Neurology*, 1974, 24:401-410.

CHALAS, G. & BRAUER, W. Tourette's disease: Relief of symptoms with R 1625. *American Journal of Psychiatry*, 1962, 20:283-284.

CHALMERS, T. Symposium on adverse reactions to psychotropic drugs. *Psychopharmacology Bulletin*, 1965, 3:3-19.

CHANG, R., WOOD, A., DIXON, W., CONNEY, A., ANDERSON, K., EISEMAN, M., & ALVARES, A. Antipyrine: Radioimmunoassay in plasma and saliva following administration of a high dose and a low dose. *Clinical Pharmacology and Therapeutics*, 1976, 20:219-226.

CHAO, D., SEXTON, J., & DAVIES, S. Convulsive equivalent syndrome of childhood. *Journal of Paediatrics*, 1964, 64:499-508.

CHAPEL, J., BROWN, N., & JENKINS, R. Tourette's disease: Symptomatic relief with haloperidol. *American Journal of Psychiatry*, 1964, 121:608-610.

CHARNEY, E., BYNUM, R., ELDREDGE, D., FRANK, D., MACWHINNEY, J., MCNAB, M., SCHEINER, A., SUMPTER, E., & IKER, H. How well do patients take oral penicillin? A collaborative study in private practice. *Paediatrics*, 1967, 40:188-195.

CHASE, T. Antipsychotic drugs, dopaminergic mechanisms and extrapyramidal function in man. In: G. Sedvall, B. Uvnäs, and Y. Zotterman (Eds.), *Antipsychotic Drugs: Pharmacodynamics and Pharmacokinetics*. New York: Pergamon Press, 1976.

CHAUNDRY, M. & POND, D. Mental deterioration in epileptic children. *Journal of Neurology, Neurosurgery and Psychiatry*, 1961, 24:213-219.

CHRISTENSEN, D. Effects of combining methylphenidate and a classroom token system in modifying hyperactive behavior. *American Journal of Mental Deficiency*, 1975, 80:266-276.

CHRISTENSEN, D. & SPRAGUE, R. Reduction of hyperactive behavior by conditioning procedures alone and combined with methylphenidate (Ritalin). *Behaviour Research and Therapy*, 1973, 11:331-334.

CHRISTENSSON, T. Lithium, hypercalcemia and hyperparathyroidism. *Lancet*, 1976, 2:144.

CLAY, M. *The Early Detection of Reading Difficulties a Diagnostic Survey*. Auckland, N.Z.: Heinemann Educational Books, 1975.

CLEMENT-CORMIER, Y., KABABIAN, J., PETZOLD, G., & GREENGARD, P. Dopamine-sensitive andenylate cyclase in mammalian brain: A possible site of action of antipsychotic drugs. *Proceedings of the National Academy of Sciences,* 1974, 71:1113-1117.

COATSWORTH, J. *Studies on the Clinical Efficiency of Marketed Antiepileptic Drugs.* NINDS Monograph No. 12. Washington: U.S. Government Printing Office, 1971.

COHEN, M. N. & SPRAGUE, R. L. Survey of drug usage in two midwestern institutions for the retarded. Paper presented at the Gatlinburg Conference on Research in Mental Retardation, Gatlinburg, Tennessee, March 1977 .

COHEN, N., DOUGLAS, V. & MORGENSTERN, G. The effect of methylphenidate on attentive behavior and autonomic activity in hyperactive children. *Psychopharmacologia* 1971, 22:282-294.

COLE, A. & FRIED, F. Favorable experiences with imipramine in the treatment of neurogenic bladder. *Journal of Urology,* 1972, 107:44-45.

COLE, J. Peeking through the double blind. In: D. Efron, J. Cole, J. Levine, and J. Wintenborn (Eds.), *Psychopharmacology: A Review of Progress,* 1957/67. Washington: U.S. Public Health Service Publication, 1968, pp. 979-984.

CONNERS, C. A teacher rating scale for use in drug studies with children. *American Journal of Psychiatry,* 1969, 126:152-156.

CONNERS, C. Symptom patterns in hyperkinetic, neurotic and normal children. *Child Development,* 1970, 41:667-682.

CONNERS, C. K. Recent drug studies with hyperkinetic children. *Journal of Learning Disabilities,* 1971, 4:476-483.

CONNERS, C. Rating scales for use in drug studies with children. *Psychopharmacology Bulletin. Special Issue*—Pharmacotherapy of children, 1973a, 24-84.

CONNERS, C. K. What parents need to know about stimulant drugs and special education. *Journal of Learning Disabilities,* 1973b, 6:349-351.

CONNERS, C. Minimal brain dysfunction and psychopathology in children. In: A. Davids (Ed.), *Child Personality and Psychopathology: Current Topics,* Vol. 2. New York: Wiley, 1975a, pp. 137-168.

CONNERS, C. A placebo-crossover study of caffeine treatment of hyperkinetic children. *International Journal of Mental Health,* 1975b, 4:132-143.

CONNERS, C. Rating scales for use in drug studies with children. In: *Assessment Manual.* Rockville, Md: Early Clinical Drug Evaluation Unit, National Institute of Mental Health, 1976a.

CONNERS, C. Classification and treatment of childhood depression and depressive equivalents. In: D. Gallant and G. Simpson (Eds.), *Depression: Behavioral, Biochemical, Diagnostic and Treatment Concepts.* New York: Spectrum, 1976b, pp. 181-196.

CONNERS, C. Global rating scales for childhood psychopharmacology. In *Guidelines for Psychoactive Agents in Infants and Children.* Rockville, Md.: Food and Drug Administration DHEW—in press.

CONNERS, C. & EISENBERG, L. The effects of methylphenidate on symptomatology and learning in disturbed children. *American Journal of Psychiatry,* 1963, 120:458-464.

CONNERS, C., EISENBERG, L., & BARCAI, A. Effect of dextroamphetamine in children. *Archives of General Psychiatry,* 1967, 17:478-485.

CONNERS, C., EISENBERG, L., & SHARPE, L. Effects of methylphenidate (Ritalin) on paired-associate learning and Porteus maze performance in emotionally disturbed children. *Journal of Consulting Psychology,* 1964, 28:14-22.

CONNERS, C., EISENBERG, L., & SHARPE, L. A controlled study of the differential application of outpatient psychiatric treatment for children. *Japanese Journal of Child Psychiatry,* 1965, 6:125-132.

CONNERS, C., GOYETTE, C., SOTHWICK, D., LEES, J., & ANDRULONIS, P. Food additives

REFERENCES

and hyperkinesis: A controlled double-blind experiment. *Pediatrics*, 1976, 58: 154-166.
CONNERS, C., KRAMER, R., ROTHSCHILD, G., SCHWARTZ, L., & STONE, A. Treatment of young delinquent boys with diphenylhydantoin sodium and methylphenidate—a controlled comparison. *Archives of General Psychiatry*, 1971, 24:156-160.
CONNERS, C. & ROTHSCHILD, G. Drugs and learning in children. In: J. Hellmuth (Ed.), *Learning Disorders*. Vol. III, Special Child Publications, 1968, 191-223.
CONNERS, C., ROTHSCHILD, G., EISENBERG, L., STONE, L., & ROBINSON, E. Dextroamphetamine in children with learning disorders. *Archives of General Psychiatry*, 1969, 21:182-190.
CONNERS, C. K., TAYLOR, E., MEO, G., KURTZ, M. A., & FOURNIER, M. Magnesium pemoline and dextroamphetamine: A controlled study in children with minimal brain dysfunction. *Psychopharmacologia*, 1972, 26:321-336.
CONNERS, C. & WERRY, J. Pharmocotherapy of psychopathology in children. In: H. Quay and J. Werry (Eds.), *Psychopathological Disorders of Childhood* (2nd Ed.). New York: Wiley—in press.
CONRAD, W., DWORKIN, E., SHAI, A., & TOBIESSEN, J. Effects of amphetamine therapy and prescriptive tutoring on the behavior and achievement of lower class hyperactive children. *Journal of Learning Disabilities*, 1971, 4:509-517.
CORDES, C. Chronic drug intoxication causing pseudo-retardation in a young child. *Journal of the American Academy of Child Psychiatry*, 1973, 12:215-222.
CORRODI, H., FUXE, K., & SCHOU, M. The effect of prolonged lithium administration on cerebral monoamine neurons in the rat. *Life Sciences*, 1969, 8:643-651.
COSTA, E., GESSA, G. L., & SANDLER, M. (Eds.). *Serotonin—New Vistas Biochemistry and Behavioral and Clinical Studies*. New York: Raven Press, 1974.
COURTNEY, P. Review of the wide range achievement test. In: O. Buros, (Ed.), *The Third Mental Measurements Yearbook*. New Brunswick, N.J.: Rutgers University Press, 1949, pp. 46-47.
CRAFT, M. Tranquilizers in mental deficiency: Chlorpromazine. *Journal of Mental Deficiency Research*, 1957, 1:91-95.
CREE, J., MEYER, J., & HAILEY, D. Diazepam in labour. Its metabolism and effect on the clinical condition and thermogenesis of the newborn. *British Medical Journal*, 1973, 4:251-255.
CROMWELL, R., BAUMEISTER, A., & HAWKINS, W. Research in activity level. In: N. Ellis (Ed.), *Handbook of Mental Deficiency*. New York: McGraw-Hill, 1963.
CROSBY, K. Attention and distractibility in mentally retarded and intellectually average children. *American Journal of Mental Deficiency*, 1972, 77:46-53.
CUATRECASAS, P.: Criterion for and pitfalls in the identification of receptors. In: E. Usdin and W. Bunney, Jr. (Eds.), *Pre- and Postsynaptic Receptors*. New York: Marcel Dekker, Inc., 1975.
CUNNINGHAM, M., PILLAI, V., & BLACHFORD ROGERS, W. Haloperidol in the treatment of children with severe behaviour disorders. *British Journal of Psychiatry*, 1968, 114:845-854.
CURRY, S. Determination of nanogram quantities of CPZ and some of its metabolites in plasma using gas-liquid chromatography. *Analytical Chemistry*, 1968, 40:1251-1255.
CURRY, S. Plasma protein binding of chlorpromazine. *Journal of Pharmacy and Pharmacology*, 1970, 2:193-197.
CURRY, S. Action and metabolism of chlorpromazine. In: D. Davies and B. Pritchard (Eds.), *Biological Effects of Drugs in Relation to Their Plasma Concentrations*. Baltimore: University Park Press, 1973.
CURRY, S. *Drug Disposition and Pharmacokinetics*. Oxford: Blackwell Scientific Publishing, 1974.
CUTTS, K. K. & JASPER, H. H. Effects of benzedrine sulfate and phenobarbital on

behavior problem children with abnormal electroencephalograms. *Archives of Neurology and Psychiatry*, 1939, 41:1138-1145.

CYTRYN, L., GILBERT, A., & EISENBERG, M. The effectiveness of tranquilizing drugs plus supportive psychotherapy in treating behavior disorders of children: A double-blind study of eighty outpatients. *American Journal of Orthopsychiatry*, 1960, 30:113-129.

DABBOUS, I. & BERGMAN, A. Neurologic damage associated with phenothiazines. *American Journal of Diseases of Children*, 1966, 111:291-296.

DALBY, M. Antiepileptic and psychotropic effects of carbamazepine (Tegretol) in the treatment of psychomotor epilepsy. *Epilepsia*, 1971, 12:325-334.

DALLY, P. *Anorexia Nervosa*. London: William Heineman, 1969.

DALY, D. Ictal manifestations of complex partial seizures. In: J. Penry and D. Daly (Eds.), *Complex Partial Seizures and Their Treatment*. Advances in Neurology No. 10. New York: Raven Press, 1975.

DARLING, H. The treatment of ambulatory adolescent schizophrenia with acetophenazine. *American Journal of Psychiatry*, 1963, 120, 68-69.

DAS, J. Patterns of cognitive ability in nonretarded and retarded children. *American Journal of Mental Deficiency*, 1972, 77:6-12.

DAVID, O., HOFFMAN, S., SVERD, J., CLARK, J., VOELLER, K. Lead and hyperactivity. Behavioral response to chelation: A pilot study. *American Journal of Psychiatry*, 1976, 133:1155-1158.

DAVIDS, A. An objective instrument for assessing hyperkinesis in children. *Journal of Learning Disabilities*, 1971, 4:499-501.

DAVIDSON, P. O. & COSTELLO, C. G. $N=1$: *Experimental Studies of Single Cases*. New York: van Nostrand, 1969.

DAVIES, B., BURROWS, G., & SCOGGINS, B. Plasma nortriptyline and clinical response. *Australia and New Zealand Journal of Psychiatry*, 1975, 9:249-253.

DAVIS, K., SPRAGUE, R., & WERRY, J. Stereotyped behavior and activity level in severe retardates: The effect of drugs. *American Journal of Mental Deficiency*, 1969, 73:721-727.

DAVIS, M. S. Variation in patients' compliance with doctors' orders. Analysis of consequence between survey responses and the results of empirical investigations. *Journal of Medical Education*, 1966, 41:1037-1048.

DAYTON, P. G., READ, J. M., & ORG, V. Physiological disposition of methylphenidate C^{14} in man. *Federation Proceedings*, 1970, 29:345.

DE LA CRUZ, F., FOX, B., & ROBERTS, R. (Eds.). Minimal brain dysfunction. *Annals of the New York Academy of Sciences*, 1973, 205:1-396.

DELAHUNT, W. D. Biomedical research: A view from the state legislature. *Hastings Center Report*, April 1976, 25-26.

DEMERS, R. & HENINGER, G. Electrocardiographic changes during lithium treatment. *Diseases of the Nervous System*, 1970, 31:674-679.

DENHOFF, E. Natural life history of children with minimal brain dysfunction. *Annals of the New York Academy of Science*, 1973, 205:188-205.

DENHOFF, E. & KING, J. Fluphenazine dihydrochloride elixir as an adjunct in management of cerebral dysfunction syndromes. *Clinical Medicine*, 1965, 72:837-843.

Diagnostic and Statistical Manual of Mental Disorders. II. Washington, D.C., American Psychiatric Association, 1968.

DIMASCIO, A., SOLTYS, J., & SHADER, R. Psychotropic drug side effects in children. In: R. Shader and A. DiMascio (Eds.), *Psychotropic Drug Side Effects*. Baltimore: Williams and Wilkins, 1970.

DIOKNO, A. C., HYNDMAN, C. W., HARDY, D. A., LAPIDES, J. Comparison of action of imipramine and propantheline on detrusor contraction. *Journal of Urology*, 1972, 107:42-43.

DIVOKY, D. Toward a nation of sedated children. *Learning*, 1973, March, 6-13. *Experi-*

ments and Research with Humans: Values in Conflict (National Academy of Sciences Book Number 0-309-02347-5). *Washington*, D.C.: U.S. Government Printing Office, 1975.

DODRILL, C. Diphenylhydantoin serum levels, toxicity and neuropsychological performance in patients with epilepsy. *Epilepsia*, 1975a, 16:593-600.

DODRILL, C. Effects of sulthiame upon intellectual, neuropsychological, and social functioning abilities among adult epileptics: Comparison with diphenylhydantoin. *Epilepsia*, 1975b, 16:617-625.

DOSTAL, T. & ZVOLSKY, P. Antiaggressive effect of lithium salts in severely mentally retarded adolescents. *International Pharmacopsychiatry*, 1970, 5:203-207.

DOUGLAS, V. Stop, look and listen: The problem of sustained attention and impulse control in hyperactive and normal children. *Canadian Journal of Behavioural Science*, 1972, 4:259-282.

DOUGLAS, V. Differences between normal and hyperkinetic children. In: C. Conners (Ed.), *Clinical Use of Stimulant Drugs in Children*. Excerpta Medica, Amsterdam, American Elsevier Publishing Co., 1974, pp. 12-23.

DYKMAN, R., ACKERMAN, P., CLEMENTS, S., & PETERS, J. Specific learning disabilities: An attentional deficit syndrome. In: H. Mykelbust (Ed.), *Progress in Learning Disabilities*, Vol. II. New York: Grune & Stratton, 1971.

DYSON, L. & BARCAI, A. Treatment of children of lithium-responding parents. *Current Therapeutic Research*, 1970, 12:286-290.

EBERT, M. H., VAN KAMMEN, D. P., & MURPHY, D. L. Plasma levels of amphetamine and behavioral response. In: L. A. Gottschalk and S. Merlis, (Eds.), *Pharmacokinetics of Psychoactive Drugs*. New York: Spectrum Publications, 1976.

ECDEU. *Assessment Manual*. Rockville, Md.: National Institute of Mental Health, 1976.

EEG-OLOFSSON, O. The development of the electroencephalogram in normal children from the age of 1 through 15 years. 14 and 6 Hz positive spike phenomenon. *Neuropädiatrie*, 1971, 2:405-427.

EFRON, D., COLE, J., LEVINE, J., & WITTENBORN, R. (Eds.). *Psychopharmacology: A Review of Progress 1957-1967*. Washington, D.C.: U.S. Government Printing Office, 1968.

EHRENPREIS, S. & KOPIN, I. (Eds.). *Reviews of Neuroscience*, Vol. 1. New York: Raven Press, 1974.

EHRLICH, R. A neurological complication in children on phenothiazine tranquilizers. *Canadian Medical Association Journal*, 1959, 81:241-243.

EISENBERG, L., GILBERT, A., CYTRYN, L., & MOLLING, P. The effectiveness of psychotherapy alone and in conjunction with perphenazine or placebo in the treatment of neurotic and hyperkinetic children. *American Journal of Psychiatry*, 1961, 117:1088-1093.

EISENBERG, L., LACHMAN, R., MOLLING, P., LOCKNER, A., MIZELLE, J., & CONNERS, C. A psychopharmacologic experiment in a training school for delinquent boys. *American Journal of Orthopsychiatry*, 1963, 33:431-447.

ELLINGSON, R. The incidence of EEG abnormality among patients with mental disorders of apparently nonorganic origin: A critical review. *American Journal of Psychiatry*, 1954, 111:263-275.

ELLIS, M., WITT, P., REYNOLDS, R., & SPRAGUE, R. Methylphenidate and the activity of hyperactive children in the informal setting. *Child Development*, 1974, 45:217-220.

ELLIS, N. & PRYER, R. Quantification of gross bodily activity in children with severe neuropathology. *American Journal of Mental Deficiency*, 1959, 63:1034-1037.

ENGELHARDT, D. CNS consequences of psychotropic drug withdrawal in autistic children: A follow-up report: Paper presented at ECDEU meeting, Miami, Florida, May 23-24, 1974.

ENGELHARDT, D., POLIZOS, P., & MARGOLIS, T. The drug treatment of childhood psychosis. In: W. Smith (Ed.), *Drugs, Development and Cerebral Function.* Springfield, Ill., Charles C Thomas, 1972.

ENGELHARDT, D., POLIZOS, P., WAIZER, J., & HOFFMAN, S. A double-blind comparison of fluphenazine and haloperidol. *Journal of Autism and Childhood Schizophrenia,* 1973, 3:128-137.

EPSTEIN, L., LASAGNA, L., CONNERS, C., & RODRIGUEZ, A. Correlation of dextroamphetamine excretion and drug response in hyperkinetic children. *Journal of Nervous and Mental Disease,* 1968, 146:136-146.

ESEN, F. & DURLING, D. Thorazine in the treatment of mentally retarded children. *Archives of Pediatrics,* 1956, 73:168-173.

EVELOFF, H. Psychopharmacologic agents in child psychiatry. *Archives of General Psychiatry,* 1966, 14:472-481.

FABISCH, W. Chlorpromazine and epilepsy. *Lancet,* 1955, 1:1277.

FALCONER, M. & DAVIDSON, S. Coarse features in epilepsy as a consequence of anticonvulsant therapy. *Lancet,* 1973, 2:1112-1114.

FANN, W. Dyskinesias with tricyclic antidepressants. *British Journal of Psychiatry,* 1976, 128:490-493.

FANN, W., LAKE, C., GUBER, C., & MCKENZIE, G. Cholinergic suppression of tardive dyskinesia. *Psychopharmacologia,* 1974, 37:101-107.

FARAJ, B. A., ISRAILI, Z. H., PEREL, J. M., JENKINS, M. L., HOLTZMAN, S. G., COCINILL, S. A., & DAYTON, P. G. Metabolism and disposition of methylphenidate ^{14}C: Studies in man and animals. *Journal of Pharmacological and Experimental Therapeutics,* 1974, 191:535-547.

FARETRA, G., DOOHER, L., & DOWLING, J. Comparison of haloperidol and fluphenazine in disturbed children. *American Journal of Psychiatry,* 1970, 126:1670-1673.

FDA. Guidelines for evaluation of psychoactive agents in infants and children. Rockville, Md.: Food and Drug Administration (DHEW)—in press.

FDA rapped for delay on drugs. *Science,* 1975, 189:864.

FEINSTEIN, S. & WOLPERT, E. Juvenile manic-depressive illness. *Journal of the American Academy of Child Psychiatry,* 1973, 12:123-136.

FINCH, A., KENDALL, P., & MONTGOMERY, L. Multidimensionality of anxiety in children: Factor structure of the Children's Manifest Anxiety Scale. *Journal of Abnormal Child Psychology,* 1974, 4:331-336.

FINE, R. Clinical experience with trifluoperazine in the severely retarded. *Journal of Neuropsychiatry,* 1964, 5:370-372.

FINGL, E.: Absorption, distribution, and elimination: Practical pharmacokinetics. In: D. Woodbury, J. Penry, and R. Schmidt (Eds.), *Antiepileptic Drugs.* New York: Raven Press, 1972.

FINK, M. Quantitative electroencephalography and human pharmacology. *Electroencephalography and Clinical Neurophysiology,* 1959, 11:398.

FINKEL, M. J. Instruction booklet and form for the IND. *Psychopharmacology Bulletin,* 1973, 9:(3), 73-82.

FINNERTY, R., SOLTYS, J., & COLE, J. The use of D-amphetamine with hyperkinetic children. *Psychopharmacologia,* 1971, 21:302-308.

FISH, B. Drug therapy in child psychiatry: Pharmacological aspects. *Comprehensive Psychiatry,* 1960, 1:212-227.

FISH, B. The "one child, one drug" myth of stimulants in hyperkinesis. *Archives of General Psychiatry,* 1971, 25:193-203.

FISH, B., CAMPBELL, M., SHAPIRO, T., & FLOYD, A., JR. Comparison of trifluperidol, trifluoperazine and chlorpromazine in preschool schizophrenic children: The value of less sedative antipsychotic agents. *Current Therapeutic Research,* 1969, 11:589-595 (a).

FISH, B., CAMPBELL, M., SHAPIRO, T., & WEINSTEIN, J. Preliminary findings on thiothixene compared to other drugs in psychotic children under five years. In: H. Lehmann and T. Ban (Eds.), *The Thioxanthenes: Modern Problems of Pharmacopsychiatry.* Basel: Karger, 1969(b).

FISH, B. & SHAPIRO, T. A typology of children's psychiatric disorders: I. Its application to a controlled evaluation of treatment. *Journal of the American Academy of Child Psychiatry,* 1965, 4:32-52.

FISH, B., SHAPIRO, T., & CAMPBELL, M. Long-term prognosis and the response of schizophrenic children to drug therapy: A controlled study of trifluoperazine. *American Journal of Psychiatry,* 1966, 123:32-39.

FLAHERTY, J. Effect of chlorpromazine medication on children with severe emotional disturbance. *Delaware Medical Journal,* 1955, 27:180-184.

FLEISCHHAUER, J. & VAN RIEZEN, H. Studies on clinical and pharmacological spectra of the tetracyclic compound mianserin. *Arzneimittel-Forschung* (Aulendorf), 1974, 24:1129-1131.

FORSMAN, A. & ÖHMAN, R. Some aspects of the distribution and metabolism of haloperidol in man. In: G. Sedvall, B. Uvnäs, and Y. Zotterman (Eds.), *Antipsychotic Drugs: Pharmacodynamics and Pharmacokinetics.* New York: Pergamon Press, 1976(a).

FORSMAN, A. & ÖHMAN, R. Pharmacokinetic studies on haloperidol in man. *Current Therapeutic Research,* 1976b, 20:319-336.

FOULKS, J., MUDGE, G., GILMAN, A. Renal excretion of cation in the dog during infusion of isotonic solutions of lithium chloride. *American Journal of Physiology,* 1952, 168:642.

FRANKENBURG, W. & CAMP, B. *Pediatric Screening Tests.* Springfield, Ill.: Charles C Thomas, 1975.

FRAS, I. & KARLAVAGE, J. The use of methylphenidate and imipramine in Gilles de la Tourette's disease in children. *American Journal of Psychiatry,* 1977, 134:195-197.

FREED, H., ABRAMS, J., & PEIFER, C., JR. Reading disability: A new therapeutic approach and its implications. *Journal of Clinical and Experimental Psychopathology and Quarterly Review of Psychiatry and Neurology,* 1959, 3:251-259.

FREED, H. & PEIFER, C. Treatment of hyperkinetic emotionally disturbed children with prolonged administration of chlorpromazine. *American Journal of Psychiatry,* 1956, 113:22-26.

FREEDMAN, A. Drug therapy in behavior disorders. *Pediatric Clinics of North America,* 1958, 5:573-594.

FREEDMAN, A., EFFRON, A., & BENDER, L. Pharmacotherapy in children with psychiatric illness. *Journal of Nervous and Metnal Disease,* 1955, 122:479-486.

FREEDMAN, D. Report of the conference on the use of stimulant drugs in the treatment of behaviorally disturbed young school children. *Psychopharmacology Bulletin,* 1971, 7:23-29.

FREEMAN, R. Special education and the electroencephalogram: Marriage of convenience. *Journal of Special Education,* 1967, 2:61-73.

FREEMAN, R. Psychopharmacology and the retarded child. In: F. Menolascino (Ed.), *Psychiatric Approaches to Mental Retardation.* New York: Basic Books, 1970.

FREEMAN, R. D. Minimal brain dysfunction hyperactivity, and learning disorders: Epidemic or episode? In: J. J. Bosco and S. S. Robin (Eds.), *The Hyperactive Child and Stimulant Drugs.* Chicago: University of Chicago Press, 1977.

FREIBERGS, V., DOUGLAS, V., & WEISS, G. The effect of chlorpromazine on concept learning in hyperactive children under two conditions of reinforcement. *Psychopharmacologia,* 1968, 13:299-310.

FRIEDMAN, E. Lithium's effect on cyclic AMP, membrane transport and cholinergic mechanisms. In: S. Gershon and B. Shopsin (Eds.), *Lithium ion: Its Role in Psychiatric Treatment and Research.* New York: Plenum Press, 1973, pp. 33-49.

FRIEDMAN, R., DALE, E., & WAGNER, J. A long-term comparison of two treatment regimens for minimal brain dysfunction. *Clinical Pediatrics*, 1973, 12:666-671.

FRIEDHOFF, A. (Ed.). *Catecholamines and Behavior 1: Basic Neurobiology*. New York: Plenum Press, 1975(a).

FRIEDHOFF, A. (Ed.). *Catecholamines and Behavior 2: Neuropsychopharmacology*. New York: Plenum Press, 1975(b).

FRIIS-HANSEN, B. Body water compartments in children: Changes during growth and related changes in body composition. *Pediatrics*, 1961, 28:169-181.

FROMMER, E. Treatment of childhood depression with antidepressant drugs. *British Medical Journal*, 1967, 1:729-732.

FROMMER, E. Depressive illness in childhood. In: A Coppen and A. Walk (Eds.), *Recent Developments in Affective Disorders*. Kent: Headly Brothers, 1968, pp. 117-136.

FULDA, T. R. *Prescription Drug Data Summary*, 1974 (HEW Publication No. [SSA] 76-11928). Washington, D.C.: U.S. Government Printing Office, 1976.

GADOW, K. D. Pills and preschool: Medication usage with young children in special education. Paper presented at the Illinois Council for Exceptional Children, Chicago, October 1975.

GADOW, K. D. Psychotropic and anticonvulsant drug usage in early childhood special education programs I. Phase One: A preliminary report: Prevalence, attitude, training, and problems. Paper presented at the annual meeting of the Council for Exceptional Children, Chicago, April 1976. (ERIC Document Reproduction Service No. ED 125 198).

GADOW, K. D. Survey of medication usage with children in trainable mentally handicapped programs and teacher role in drug treatment. Doctoral dissertation. University of Illinois, 1977.

GALLAGHER, C. E. *Federal Involvement in the Use of Behavior Modification Drugs on Grammar School Children of the Right to Privacy Inquiry* (Hearing before a Subcommittee of the Committee on Government Operations No. 52-268). Washington, D.C.: U.S. Government Printing Office, 1970.

GAMSTORP, I. Treatment with carbamazepine: Children. In: J. Penry and D. Daly (Eds.), *Complex Partial Seizures and Their Treatment*. New York: Raven Press, 1975.

GAP. *Psychopathological Disorders in Childhood: Theoretical Considerations and a Proposed Classification*. New York: Group for the Advancement of Psychiatry, 1966.

GARATTINI, S., MARCUCCI, F., MORSELLI, P., & MUSSINI, E. The significance of measuring blood levels of benzodiazepines. In: B. Davies and B. Pritchard (Eds.), *Biological Effects of Drugs in Relation to Their Plasma Concentration*. London: Macmillan, 1973.

GARFIELD, S., HELPER, M., WILCOTT, R., & MUFFLY, R. Effects of chlorpromazine on behavior in emotionally disturbed children. *Journal of Nervous and Mental Disease*, 1962, 135:147-154.

GARFINKEL, B., WEBSTER, C., & SLOMAN, L. Methylphenidate and caffeine in the treatment of children with minimal brain dysfunction. *American Journal of Psychiatry*, 1975, 132:723-728.

GARRETTSON, L. & DAYTON, P. Disappearance of phenobarbital and diphenylhydantoin from serum of children. *Clinical Pharmacology and Therapeutics*, 1970, 11:674-678.

Gary W. v. State of Louisiana, No. 72 2412 (E.D. Louisiana, 1976).

GASTAUT, H. Clinical and electroencephalographical classification of epileptic seizures. *Epilepsia*, 1970, 11:102-113.

GEIGER, L. & LESSER, L. Ocular side effects of chlorpromazine in a child. *Journal of the American Medical Association*, 1967, 202:916.

GERSHON, S. & SHOPSIN, B. *Lithium, its Role in Psychiatric Research and Treatment.* New York: Plenum, 1973.
GILL, M. & UEDA, C. Novel method for the determination of pediatric dosages. *American Journal of Hospital Pharmacy,* 1976, 33:389-392.
GITTELMAN-KLEIN, R. Pilot clinical trial of imipramine in hyperkinetic children. In: C. K. Conners (Ed.), *Clinical Use of Stimulant Drugs in Children.* Amsterdam: Excerpta Medica, 1974, pp. 192-201.
GITTELMAN-KLEIN, R. Stimulant drug treatment of hyperkinesis. In: D. Klein and R. Gittelman-Klein (Eds.), *Progress in Psychiatric Drug Treatment* (Vol. I). New York: Brunner/Mazel, 1975.
GITTELMAN-KLEIN, R. Personal communication, March 15, 1977.
GITTELMAN-KLEIN, R.: Validity of projective tests for psychodiagnosis in children. In: R. Spitzer & D. Klein (Eds.), *Critical Issues in Psychiatric Diagnosis.* New York: Raven Press, 1978, pp. 141-166 (a).
GITTELMAN-KLEIN, R. Psychopharmacological treatment of anxiety disorders, mood disorders, and tic disorders of childhood. In: M. Lipton, A. DiMascio & K. Killam (Eds.), *A Review of Psychopharmacology: A Second Decade of Progress.* New York: Raven Press, 1978, pp. 1471-1480 (b).
GITTELMAN-KLEIN, R. & KLEIN, D. Controlled imipramine treatment of school phobia. *Archives of General Psychiatry,* 1971, 25:204-207.
GITTELMAN-KLEIN, R. & KLEIN, D. School phobia: Diagnostic considerations in the light of imipramine effects. *Journal of Nervous and Mental Disease,* 1973, 156: 199-215.
GITTELMAN-KLEIN, R. & KLEIN, D. Are behavioral and psychometric changes related in methylphenidate-treated, hyperactive children? *International Journal of Mental Health,* 1975, 4:182-198.
GITTELMAN-KLEIN, R. & KLEIN, D. Methylphenidate effects in learning disabilities: Psychometric changes. *Archives of General Psychiatry,* 1976, 33:655-664.
GITTELMAN-KLEIN, R. KLEIN, D., ABIKOFF, H., KATZ, S., GLOISTEN, A., & KATES, W. Relative efficacy of methylphenidate and behavior modification in hyperkinetic children: An interim report. *Journal of Abnormal Child Psychology,* 1976a, 4:361-380.
GITTELMAN-KLEIN, R., KLEIN, D., KATZ, S., SARAF, K., & POLLACK, E. Comparative effects of methylphenidate and thioridazine in hyperkinetic children. I. Clinical results. *Archives of General Psychiatry,* 1976b, 33:1217-1231.
GLASER, G. Diphenylhydantoin toxicity. In: D. Woodbury, J. Penry and R. Schmidt (Eds.), *Antiepileptic Drugs.* New York: Raven Press, 1972.
GLASS, G. V., WILSON, V. L., & GOTTMAN, J. M. *Design and Analysis of Time-Series Experiments.* Boulder: Colorado Associated University Press, 1974.
GLASSMAN, A., HORWIC, M., & PEREL, J. Plasma binding of imipramine and clinical outcome. *American Journal of Psychiatry,* 1973, 130:1367-1369.
GLASSMAN, A. & PEREL, J. Plasma levels and tricyclic antidepressants. *Clinical Pharmacology Therapy,* 1974, 16:198-200.
GLAVIN, J., QUAY, H., & WERRY, J. Behavioral and academic gains of conduct problem children in different classroom settings. *Exceptional Children,* 1971, 37:441-446.
GODDARD, J. L. The medical business. *Scientific American,* 1973, 229(3):161-166.
GODDARD, J. L. & ALLAN, F. N. Regulations of the U.S. Food and Drug Administration. In: W. G. Clark and J. del Guidice (Eds.), *Principles of Psychopharmacology.* New York: Academic Press, 1970.
GOLDBERG, S., HALMI, K., ECKERT, E., CASTER, R., & DAVIS, J. Cyproheptadine in anorexia nervosa. Paper presented at the annual meeting of the American Psychiatric Association, Toronto, Canada, May 1-7, 1977.
GOLDFARB, W. Factors in the development of schizophrenic children: An approach

to subclassification. In: J. Romano (Ed.), *The Origins of Schizophrenia*. Amsterdam: Excerpta Medica, 1960, pp. 70-91.

GOLDMAN, D. Prolonged treatment of psychotic states. *Diseases of the Nervous System*, 1968, 29:51-57 (Suppl. to #3).

GOLDSTEIN, A., ARONOW, L., & KALMAN, S. *Principles of Drug Action: The Basis of Pharmacology*. New York: John Wiley & Sons, 1974.

GOODMAN, L. & GILMAN, A. (Eds.). *The Pharmacological Basis of Therapeutics*. (5th Ed.). New York: Macmillan, 1975.

GORDON, M. *Psychopharmacological Agents* (Vol. II). New York: Academic Press, 1967.

GOTTMAN, J. M., MCFALL, R. M., & BARNETT, J. T. Design and analysis of research using time series. *Psychological Bulletin*, 1969, 72:229-306.

GOTTSCHALK, C., BIENER, R., NOBLE, E., BIRCH, H., WILBERT, D., & HIESER, J. Thioridazine plasma levels and clinical response. *Comprehensive Psychiatry*, 1975, 16:323-337.

GRAHAM, P. Depression in pre-pubertal children. *Developmental Medicine and Child Neurology*, 1974, 16:340-349.

GRAHAM, P. & RUTTER, M. The reliability and validity of the psychiatric assessment of the child. II. Interview with the parent. *British Journal of Psychiatry*, 1968, 114:581-592.

GRAM, L. & RAFAELSEN, J. Lithium treatment of psychotic children and adolescents. *Acta Psychiatrica Scandinavica*, 1972, 48:253-260.

GREEN, J., TROUPIN, A., HALPERN, L., FRIEL, P., & KANAREK, P. Sulthiame: Evaluation as an anticonvulsant. *Epilepsia*, 1974, 15:329-349.

GREENBERG, A. & COLEMAN, M.: Depressed 5-hydroxyindole levels associated with hyperactive and aggressive behavior. *Archives of General Psychiatry*, 1976, 33: 331-336.

GREENBERG, L., DEEM, N., & MCMAHON, S. Effects of dextroamphetamine, chlorpromazine and hydroxyzine on behavior and performance in hyperactive children. *American Journal of Psychiatry*, 1972, 129:532-539.

GREENBERG, L. & YELLIN, A. Blood pressure and pulse changes in hyperactive children treated with imipramine and methylphenidate. *American Journal of Psychiatry*, 1975, 132:1325-1326.

GREENBERG, L., YELLIN, A., SPRING, C., & METCALF, M. Clinical effects of imipramine and methylphenidate in hyperactive children. *International Journal of Mental Health*, 1975, 4:144-156.

GREENBLATT, D., ALLEN, M., KOCK-WESER, J., & SHADER, R. Accidental poisoning with psychotropic drugs in children. *American Journal of Diseases of Children*, 1976, 130:507-511.

GREENBLATT, D. & SHADER, R. *Benzodiazepines in Clinical Practice*. New York: Raven Press, 1974.

GREENBLATT, D. & SHADER, R. Drugs interactions in psychopharmacology. In: R. Shader (Ed.), *Manual of Psychiatric Therapeutics*. Boston: Little Brown, pp. 269-279, 1975.

GREENBLATT, S. & SHADER, R. Acute poisoning with psychotropic drugs. In: I. Shader and A. DiMascio (Eds.), *Psychotropic Drug Side Effects*. Baltimore: Williams & Wilkins Co., 1970.

GREENGRASS, P., WALDMEIR, P., IMHOF, P., & MAITREJ, L. Comparison of the effects of maprotiline, and clomipramine on serotonin uptake and tryptophan binding in plasma. *Biological Psychiatry*, 1976, 11:91-100.

GREENHILL, L. L., PUIG-ANTICH, J., SASSIN, J. & SACHAR, E. J.: Hormone and growth responses in hyperkinetic children on stimulant medication. *Psychopharmacology Bulletin*, 1977, 13(2):33-36.

GREENHILL, L., RIEDER, R., WENDER, P., BUCHSBAUM, M., & ZAHN, T. Lithium car-

bonate in the treatment of hyperactive children. *Archives of General Psychiatry*, 1973, 28:636-640.
GRINSPOON, L. & SINGER, S. B. Amphetamines in the treatment of hyperkinetic children. *Harvard Educational Review*, 1973, 43:515-555.
GROH, C., ROSENMAYR, F., & BIRBAUMER, N. Psychotrope Wirkung von Carbamazepin bei nicht-epileptischen Kindern. *Medizinische Monatsschrift*, 1971, 25:329-333. Quoted by Remschmidt (1976).
GROSS, M. Caffeine in the treatment of children with minimal brain dysfunction or hyperkinetic syndrome. *Psychosomatics*, 1975, 16:26-27.
GROSS, M. Growth of hyperkinetic children taking methylphenidate, dextroamphetamine, or imipramine, desipramine. *Pediatrics*, 1976, 58:423-431.
GROSSMAN, H. J., WARREN, S., BEGAB, M., EYMAN, R., NIHAIRA, K., & O'CONNOR, G. *Manual on Terminology and Classification in Mental Retardation*. Baltimore, Md.: American Association for Mental Deficiency, 1973.
GROVES, P., WILSON, C., YOUNG, S., & REBEC, G. Self inhibition by dopaminergic neurons. *Science*, 1975, 190:522-529.
GUEY, J., CHARLES, C., COQUERY, C., ROGER, J., & SOULAYROL, R. Study of psychological effects of ethosuximide (Zarontin) on 25 children suffering from petit mal epilepsy. *Epilepsia*, 1967, 8:129-141.
Guidelines for the conduct of clinical trials. *Psychopharmacology Bulletin*, 1974, 10(4): 70-91.
GUILLEMINAULT, C. & ANDERS, T. Sleep disorders in children. In: I. Schulman (Ed.), *Advances in Pediatrics* (Vol. 22). Chicago: Yearbook Medical Publishers, 1976, p. 151-174.
HAGGERTY, R. & ROGHMANN, K. Non-compliance and self-medication. Two neglected aspects of pediatric pharmacology. *Pediatric Clinics of North America*, 1972, 19:101-115.
HALGREN, B. Enuresis—a clinical and genetic study. *Acta Psychiatrica et Neurologica Scandinavica*, 1957, 32: Supplement No. 114.
HALLIDAY, R., ROSENTHAL, J., NAYLOR, H., & CALLAWAY, E. Average evoked potential predictors of clinical improvement in hyperactive children treated with methylphenidate: An initial study and replication. *Psychophysiology*, 1976, 13: 429-440.
HAMILTON, M. *Lectures on the Methodology of Clinical Research* (2nd ed). Edinburgh: Churchill Livingstone, 1974.
HANSSON, E. & CASSANO, G. Distribution and metabolism of antidepressant drugs. *Proceedings of the 1st International Symposium*, Milan, 1966, p. 10, International Congress Series, No. 122 (Excerpta Medical Foundation, Amsterdam, 1967).
HART, J., HILL, H., BYE, C., WILKINSON, R., & PECK, A. The effects of low doses of amylobarbitone sodium and diazepam on human performance. *British Journal of Clinical Pharmacology*, 1976, 3:289-298.
HAWARD, L. Effects of sodium diphenylhydantoin and pemoline upon concentration: A comparative study. In: W. Smith (Ed.), *Drugs and Cerebral Function*. Springfield, Illinois: Charles C Thomas, 1970.
HAWARD, L. Effects of DPH (Sodium diphenylhydantoinate) upon concentration in pilots. *Revue Medicale Aéronautique Spatiale*, 1973, 12:372-374.
HAYES, T. A. Role of the FDA. In: J. G. Langan (Chair.), *Workshop on Psychotropic Drugs and the Mentally Retarded*. Symposium presented at the meeting of the American Association on Mental Deficiency, Portland, Ore., 1975.
HAYES, T. A., PANITCH, M. L., & BARKER, E. Imipramine dosage in children. A comment on "Imipramine and Electrocardiographic Abnormalities in Hyperactive Children." *American Journal of Psychiatry*, 1975, 132:546-547.
HAYWOOD, H. C. The ethics of doing research . . . and of not doing it. *American Journal of Mental Deficiency*, 1977, 81:311-318.

HELPER, M., WILCOTT, R., & GARFIELD, S. Effects of chlorpromazine on learning and related processes in emotionally disturbed children. *Journal of Consulting Psychology*, 1963, 27:1-9.

HENDLEY, E. & SNYDER, S. Relationship between the action of monoamine oxidase inhibitors on the noradrenaline uptake system and their antidepressant activity. *Nature*, 1968, 220:1330-1331.

HERJANIC, B., HERJANIC, M., BROWN, F., & WHEATT, T. Are children reliable reporters? *Journal of Abnormal Child Psychology*, 1975, 3:41-48.

HERSEN, M. & BARLOW, D. H. *Single-case Experimental Designs. Strategies for Studying Behavior Change.* New York: Pergamon, 1976.

HERSHEY, N. & MILLER, R. D. *Human Experimentation and the Law.* Germantown, Md.: Aspen Systems Corp., 1976.

HETHERINGTON, E. & MARTIN, B. Family interaction factors. In: H. Quay and J. Werry (Eds.), *Psychopathological Disorders of Childhood* (2nd ed). New York: Wiley—in press.

HIMWICH, H., COSTA, E., RINALDI, F., & RUDY, L. Trifluopromazine and trifluoperazine in the treatment of disturbed mentally defective patients. *American Journal of Mental Deficiency*, 1960, 64:711-712.

HOAKEN, P. & KANE, F. Unusual brain syndrome with diphenylhydantoin and pentobarbital. *American Journal of Psychiatry*, 1963, 120:282-283.

HOFFMAN, S., ENGELHARDT, D., MARGOLIS, R., POLIZOS, P., WAIZER, J., & ROSENFELD, R. Response to methylphenidate in low socioeconomic hyperactive children. *Archives of General Psychiatry*, 1974, 30:354-359.

HOLLIS, J. Chlorpromazine: Direct measurement of differential behavioral effect. *Science*, 1968, 159:1487-1489.

HOLLIS, J. & ST. OMER, V. Direct measurement of psychopharmacologic response: Effects of chlorpromazine on motor behavior of retarded children. *American Journal of Mental Deficiency*, 1972, 76:397-407.

HOLLISTER, L. Clinical use of psychotherapeutic drugs II: Antidepressant and antianxiety drugs and special problems in the use of psychotherapeutic drugs. *Drugs*, 1972, 4:361-410.

HOLLISTER, L. Adverse reactions to psychotherapeutic drugs. In: L. Simpson (Ed.), *Drug Treatment of Mental Disorders.* New York: Raven Press, 1976.

HORENSTEIN, S. Reserpine and chlorpromazine in hyperactive mental defectives. *American Journal of Mental Deficiency*, 1957, 61:525-529.

HORNYKIEWICZ, O. Parkinson induced by dopaminergic antagonists. In: D. Calne, T. Chase, and A. Barbeau (Eds.), *Advances in Neurology, Vol. 9: Dopaminergic Mechanisms.* New York: Raven Press, 1975.

HOROWITZ, L. & FISHER, G. Acute lithium toxicity. *New England Journal of Medicine*, 1969, 281:1369.

HUESSY, H. & COHEN, A. Hyperkinetic behaviors and learning disabilities followed over 7 years. *Pediatrics*, 1976, 57:4-10.

HUESSY, H. & WRIGHT, A. The use of imipramine in children's behavior disorders. *Acta Paedopsychiatrica*, 1970, 37:194-199.

HUESTIS, R., ARNOLD, E., & SMELTZER, D. Caffeine versus methylphenidate and d-amphetamine in minimal brain dysfunction: A double blind comparison. *American Journal of Psychiatry*, 1975, 132:868-871.

HUNT, B., FRANK, T., & KRUSH, T. Chlorpromazine in the treatment of severe emotional disorders of children. *American Journal of Diseases of Children*, 1956, 91:268-277.

HUNTER, H. & STEPHENSON, G. Chlorpromazine and trifluoperazine in the treatment of behaviour abnormalities in the severely subnormal child. *British Journal of Psychiatry*, 1963, 109:411-417.

HUTT, S., JACKSON, P., BELSHAM, A., & HIGGINS, G. Perceptual-motor behavior in rela-

tion to blood phenobarbitone levels. A preliminary report. *Developmental Medicine and Child Neurology*, 1968, 10:626-632.
HUTT, C., JACKSON, P., & LEVEL, M. Behavioural parameters and drug effects. A study of a hyperkinetic epileptic child. *Epilepsia*, 1966, 7:250-259.
IDESTROM, C-M., SCHALLING, D., CARLQVIST, U., & SJOQVIST, F. Acute effects of diphenylhydantoin in relation to plasma levels. *Psychological Medicine*, 1972, 2:111-120.
INGRAM, T. & RATCLIFFE, S. Clinical trials of Ospolot in epilepsy. *Developmental Medicine and Child Neurology*, 1963, 5:313-315.
IREY, N. S. Adverse drug reactions and death. A review of 827 cases. *Journal of the American Medical Association*, 1976, 236:575-578.
IRWIN, S. Anti-neurotics: Practical pharmacology of the sedative-hypnotics and minor tranquilizers. In: D. Efron, J. Cole, J. Levine, and J. Wittenborn (Eds.), *Psychopharmacology: A Review of Progress 1957-1967*. Washington, D.C.: U.S. Government Printing Office, 1968, pp. 185-205.
ITIL, T. & AKPINAR, S. Lithium effect on human electroencephalogram. *Clinical Electroencephalography*, 1971, 2:89-102.
ITIL, T., HERRMANN, W., & AKPINAR, S. Prediction of psychotropic properties of lisuride Hydrogen maleate by quantitative pharmacoelectroencephalogram. *International Journal of Clinical Pharmacology*, 1975, 12:221-233.
IVERSON, L. How do antipsychotic drugs work? *Neurosciences Research Program Bulletin*, 1975, 13: supplement 29-51.
JAFFE, J. Drug addiction and drug abuse. In: L. Goodman and A. Gilman (Eds.), *The Pharmacological Basis of Therapeutics*. New York: Macmillan, 1975, pp. 284-324.
JANSSEN, P. Structure-activity relations (SAR) and drug design as illustrated with neuroleptic agents. In: G. Sedvall, B. Uvnäs, and Y. Zotterman (Eds.), *Antipsychotic Drugs: Pharmacodynamics and Pharmacokinetics*. New York: Pergamon Press, 1976.
JEAVONS, P. The effects of chlordiazepoxide on the electroencephalogram. *Epilepsia*, 1962, 3:110-116.
JEAVONS, P. Carbamazepine and the EEG. In: C. Wink (Ed.), *Tegretol in Epilepsy*. Manchester: Nicholls, 1973.
JEAVONS, P. The practical management of epilepsy. *Hospital Update*, 1975, 1:11-18.
JEAVONS, P. Behavioural effects of antiepileptic drugs (letter). *Developmental Medicine and Child Neurology*, 1976, 18:394-400.
JEAVONS, P., CLARK, J., & MAHESHWARI, M. Treatment of generalised epilepsies of childhood and adolescence with sodium valproate (Epilim). *Developmental Medicine and Child Neurology*, 1977, 19:9-25.
JEAVONS, P. & HARDING, G. *Photosensitive Epilepsy*. Clinics in Developmental Medicine No. 56. London: Spastics International Medical Publications and Heinemann, 1975.
JENKINS, R., NUR EDDIN, E., & SHAPIRO, I. Children's behavior syndromes and parental responses. *Genetic Psychology Monographs*, 1966, 74:261-329.
JOHNSON, C. Hyperactivity and the machine: The actometer. *Child Development*, 1971, 42:2105-2110.
JOHNSON, G. Lithium and the EEG: An analysis of behavioral, biochemical and electroencephalographic changes. *Electroencephalography and Clinical Neurophysiology*, 1969, 27:656-657.
JOHNSON, S. & BOLSTAD, O. Methodological issues in naturalistic observation: Some problems and solutions for field research. In: L. Hamerlynck, L. Handy, and E. Mash (Eds.), *Behavior Change: Methodology Concepts in Practice*, 4th Banff International Conference on Behavior Modification, Champaign. Illinois: Research Press, 1973, pp. 7-67.

JOHNSSON, G. & REGARDH, G. Clinical pharmacokinetics of β-adrenoceptor blocking drugs. *Clinical Pharmacokinetics*, 1976, 1:233-263.
JOHNSTON, A. & MARTIN, C. The clinical use of reserpine and chlorpromazine in the care of the mentally deficient. *American Journal of Mental Deficiency*, 1957, 62:292-294.
JOHNSTONE, E & MARSH, W. Acetylator status and response to phenelzine in depressed patients. *Lancet*, 1973, 1:567-570.
JONES, R., REID, J., & PATTERSON, G. Naturalistic observation in clinical assessment. In: P. McReynolds (Ed.), *Advances in Psychological Assessment* (Vol. 3). San Francisco: Jossey-Bass, 1976, pp. 42-95.
JUDD, L., HUBBARD, B., JANOWSKY, D., HUEY, L., & ATTEWELL, P. Lithium carbonate in normal subjects. *Archives of General Psychiatry*, 1977a, 34:346-354.
JUDD, L., HUBBARD, B., JANOWSKY, D., HUEY, L., & TAKAHASHI, K. The effect of lithium carbonate on the cognitive functions of normal subjects. *Archives of General Psychiatry*, 1977b, 34:355-357.
JULIANO, D. Conceptual tempo, activity and concept learning in hyperactive and normal children. *Dissertation Abstracts International*, 1974, 34A:4875.
KAGAN, J. Reflection-impulsivity and reading ability in primary grade children. *Child Development*, 1965, 36:609-628.
KALES, A. & KALES, J. Sleep disorders: Recent findings in the diagnosis and treatment of disturbed sleep. *New England Journal of Medicine*, 1974, 290:487-499.
KALINOWSKY, L. & HIPPIUS, H. *Pharmacological, Convulsive and Other Somatic Treatments in Psychiatry*. New York: Grune & Stratton, 1969.
KAMANO, D. Selective review of effects of discontinuation of drug treatment: Some implications and problems. *Psychological Reports*, 1966, 19:743-749.
KAMM, I. & MANDEL, A. Thioridazine in the treatment of behavior disorders in epileptics. *Diseases of the Nervous System*, 1967, 28:46-48.
KANNER, L. Autistic disturbances of affective contact. *The Nervous Child*, 1943, 2:217-250.
KANTO, J., ERKKOLA, R., & SELLMAN, R. Perinatal metabolism of diazepam. *British Medical Journal*, 1974, 1:641-642.
KAPLITZ, S. The use of perphenazine syrup in the severely disturbed mentally retarded child. *Illinois Medical Journal*, 1966, 130:785-787.
KASPAR, J., MILLICHAP, J., BACKUS, R., CHILD, D., & SHULMAN, J. A study of the relationship between neurological evidence of brain damage in children and activity and distractibility. *Journal of Consulting and Clinical Psychology*, 1971, 36:329.
KATZ, J. *Experimentation with Human Beings*. New York: Russell Sage Foundation, 1972.
KATZ, S., SARAF, K., GITTELMAN-KLEIN, R., & KLEIN, D. Clinical pharmacological management of hyperkinetic children. *International Journal of Mental Health*, 1975, 4:157-181.
KAZDIN, A. E. Statistical analysis for single-case experimental designs. In: M. Hersen and D. H. Barlow (Eds.), *Single-case Experimental Designs: Strategies for Studying Behavior Change*. New York: Pergamon, 1976.
KELLAWAY, G. and MCCRAE, E. Drug compliance in hospital practice. To be published (1977).
KELLY, D., GUIRGUIS, W., FROMMER, E., MITCHELL-HEGGS, N. & SARGANT, W. Treatment of phobic states with antidepressants. *British Journal of Psychiatry*, 1970, 116:387-398.
KELLY, J., KOCH, M., & BUEGEL, D. Lithium carbonate in juvenile manic-depressive illness. *Diseases of the Nervous System*, 1976, 37:90-92.
KENNY, T., CLEMMENS, R., HUDSON, B., LENTZ, G., CICCI, R., & NAIR, P. Characteristics of children referred because of hyperactivity. *Journal of Pediatrics*, 1971, 79:618-622.

KENNEDY, W. A. & SLOOP, E. W. Methedrine as an adjunct to conditioning of nocturnal enuresis in normal and institutionalized retarded subjects. *Psychological Reports,* 1968, 22:997.

KIRSCHNER, G. and KNOPF, I. Differences in the vigilance performance of second grade children as related to sex and achievement. *Child Development,* 1974, 45:490-495.

KIVALO, E. SEPPALAINEN, A-M., & LYDECKEN, K. The treatment of the agitated and most severe cases of cerebral injury and cerebral palsy with carbamazepine (Tegretol). *Nordisk Psykiatrisk Tidsskrift,* 1968, 22:44-52. Quoted by Remschmidt (1976).

KLAVERBOER, A. A neurobehavioral study in preschool children. *Clinics in Developmental Medicine,* No. 54. London: Heinemann, 1975.

KLAWANS, H., JR. The pharmacology of tardive dyskinesias. *American Journal of Psychiatry,* 1973, 130:82-86.

KLEIN, D. F. Delineation of two drug-responsive anxiety syndromes. *Psychopharmacologia,* 1964, 5:397-408.

KLEIN, D. F. The importance of diagnosis: An analysis and program. In: T. Rothman (Ed.), *Changing Patterns in Psychiatric Care.* New York: Crown Publishers, 1970.

KLEIN, D. F. Drug therapy as a means of syndromal identification and nosological revision. In: J. Cole, A. Freedman, and A. Friedhoff (Eds.), *Psychopathology and Psychopharmacology.* Baltimore: The Johns Hopkins Press, 1973, pp. 143-160.

KLEIN, D. F. & DAVIS J. *Diagnosis and Drug Treatment of Psychiatric Disorders.* Baltimore, Md.: Williams & Wilkins, 1969.

KLEIN, D. & GITTELMAN-KLEIN, R. Problems in the diagnosis of minimal brain dysfunction and the hyperkinetic syndrome. In: R. Gittelman-Klein (Ed.), *Recent Advances in Child Psychopharmacology.* New York: Human Sciences Press, 1975.

KLEIN, D. & GITTELMAN-KLEIN, R. *Progress in Psychiatric Drug Treatment* (Vol. 2). New York: Brunner/Mazel, 1976.

KLUGH, H. & JANSSEN, R. Discrimination learning by retardates and normals: Method of presentation and verbalization. *American Journal of Mental Deficiency,* 1966, 70:903-906.

KLUTCH, A. & HANNA, M. The urinary metabolites of imipramine in behavior disordered children. Submitted for publication, 1976.

KNAPP, S. & MANDELL, A. Short-and-long term lithium administration: Effects on the brain's serotonergic biosynthetic systems. *Science,* 1973, 180:645-647.

KNEEBONE, G. The use of sulthiame (Ospolot) in the epileptic child with the hyperkinetic syndrome. *Medical Journal of Australia,* 1968, 2:1096-1097.

KNIGHTS, R. Psychometric assessment of stimulant-induced behavior change. In: C. Conners (Ed.), *Clinical Use of Stimulant Drugs in Children.* Amsterdam: Excerpta Medica 1974, pp. 221-229.

KNIGHTS, R. & HINTON, G. The effects of methylphenidate (Ritalin) on the motor skills and behavior of children with learning problems. *Journal of Nervous and Mental Disease,* 1969, 148:643-653.

KNOBEL, M., WOLMAN, M., & MASON, E. Hyperkinesis and organicity in children. *Archives of General Psychiatry,* 1959, 1:310-321.

KNOPP, W., ARNOLD, L., ANDRAS, R., & SMELTZER, D. Predicting amphetamine response in hyperkinetic children by electric pupillography. *Pharmakopsychiatrie Neuro-Psychopharmakologie,* 1973, 6:158-166.

KOCH-WESER, J. & SELLERS, E. Drug interactions with coumarin anticoagulants. *New England Journal of Medicine,* 1971, 285:547-558.

KOCH-WESER J. & SELLERS, E. Binding of drugs to serum albumin. *New England Journal of Medicine,* 1976, 294:311-316.

KOLAKOWSKA, T., WILES, D., GELDER, M., & MCNEILLY, A. Clinical significance of plasma chlorpromazine levels. *Psychopharmacologia*, 1976, 49:101-107.
KOLBYE, A. C. First report of the preliminary findings and recommendations of the Interagency collaborative group on hyperkinesis. Washington, D.C.: U.S. Department of Health, Education, and Welfare, 1976.
KOLVIN, I. Psychosis in childhood: A comparative study. In: M. Rutter (Ed.), *Infantile Autism: Concepts, Characteristics and Treatment*. London: Churchill Livingstone, 1970.
KOOCHER, G. P. (Ed.). *Children's Rights and the Mental Health Professions*. New York: Wiley, 1976.
KOPPITZ, E. *The Bender Gestalt Test for Young Children*. New York: Grune & Stratton, 1964, pp. 5-11.
KOREIN, J., FISH, B., SHAPIRO, T., GEVNER, E., & LEVIDOW, L. EEG and behavioral effects of drug therapy in children. *Archives of General Psychiatry*, 1971, 24: 552-563.
KORSCH, B., GOZZI, E., & FRANCIS, V. Gaps in doctor-patient interaction and patient satisfaction. *Pediatrics*, 1968, 42:855-869.
KRAGER, J. M. & SAFER, D. J. Type and prevalence of medication used in the treatment of hyperactive children. *New England Journal of Medicine*, 1974, 291: 1118-1120.
KRAGH-SORENSON, P., ASBERG, M., & EGGERT-HANSEN, C.: Plasma-nortriptyline levels in endogenous depression. *Lancet*, 1973, 1:113-115.
KRAGH-SORENSON, P., HANSSON, E., BAASTRUP, P., & HVIDBERG, E. Relationship between antidepressant effect and plasma level of nortriptyline clinical studies. *Pharmakopsychiatrie*, 1976a, 9:27-32.
KRAGH-SORENSON, P., HANSSON, E., BAASTRUP, P., & HVIDBERG, E. Self-inhibiting action of nortriptyline's antidepressive effect at high plasma levels. *Psychopharmacologia*, 1976b, 45:305-312.
KRAKOWSKI, A. Amitriptyline in treatment of hyperkinetic children, a double-blind study. *Psychosomatics*, 1965, 6:355-360.
KUHN, V. & KUHN, R. Drug therapy for depression in children. In: A. Annell (Ed.), *Depressive States in Childhood and Adolescence*. New York: Halsted Press, 1972.
KUHN-GEBHARDT, V. Results obtained with a new antidepressant in children in depressive illness. In: A. Annell (Ed.), *Depressive States in Childhood and Adolescence*. New York: Halsted Press, 1972.
KUPFER, D. & BOWERS, M. REM sleep and central monoamine oxidase inhibition. *Psychopharmacologia*, 1972, 27:183-190.
KUPFER, D., WYATT, R., GREENSPAN, K., SCOTT, J., & SNYDER, F. Lithium carbonate and sleep in affective illness. *Archives of General Psychiatry*, 1970, 23:35-40.
KUPIETZ, S .S. & BALKA, E. B. Alterations in the vigilance performance of children receiving amitriptyline and methylphenidate pharmacotherapy. *Psychopharmacologia*, 1976, 50:29-33.
KUPIETZ, S. & RICHARDSON, E. Children's vigilance performance and inattentiveness in the classroom. *Journal of Abnormal Child Psychology*—in press.
KUTT, H. Mechanism of action of antiepileptic drugs. In: P. Vinken and G. Bruyn (Eds.), *Handbook of Clinical Neurology: 15, The Epilepsies*. Amsterdam and New York: North Holland Publishing Company and American Elsevier Publishing Co., Inc., 1974.
KUTT, H. & LOUIS, S. Untoward effects of anticonvulsants. *New England Journal of Medicine*, 1972, 286:1316-1317.
KUTT, H. & MCDOWELL, F. Management of epilepsy with diphenylhydantoin sodium. *Journal of the American Medical Association*, 1968, 203:969-972.
KUTT, H. & PENRY, J. Usefulness of blood levels of antiepileptic drugs. *Archives of Neurology*, 1974, 31:283-288.

References

LABAY, P. & BOYARSKY, S. The action of imipramine on the bladder musculature. *Journal of Urology*, 1973, 109:385-386.

LAMBERT, N. M., WINDMILLER, M., SANDOVAL, J., & MOORE, B. Hyperactive children and the efficacy of psychoactive drugs as a treatment intervention. *American Journal of Orthopsychiatry*, 1976, 46:335-352.

LANGHORNE, J., LONEY, J., PATERNITE, C., & BECHTOLD, H. Childhood hyperkinesis: A return to the source. *Journal of Abnormal Psychology*, 1976, 85:201-209.

LARSEN, S., ROGERS, D., & SOWELL, V. The use of selected perceptual tests in differentiating between normal and learning disabled children. *Journal of Learning Disabilities*, 1976, 9:85-90.

LASAGNA, L. The pharmaceutical revolution: Its impact on science and society. *Science*, 1969, 166:1227-1233.

LAUFER, M., DENHOFF, E., & SOLOMONS, G. Hyperkinetic impulse disorder in children's behavior problems. *Psychosomatic Medicine*, 1957, 19:38-49.

LAVECK, G. & BUCKLEY, P. The use of psychopharmacological agents in retarded children with behavior disorders. *Journal of Chronic Diseases*, 1961, 13:174-183.

LAVECK, G., DE LA, CRUZ, F., & SIMUNDSON, E. Fluphenazine in the treatment of mentally retarded children with behavior disorders. *Diseases of the Nervous System*, 1960, 21:82-85.

LAWLIS, M. A note on trifluoperazine in the management of hyperactive mentally retarded children. In: *Trifluoperazine; Clinical and Pharmacological Aspects*. Philadelphia: Lea & Febiger, 1958.

LEFKOWITZ, M. Effects of diphenylhydantoin on disruptive behaviour: Study of male delinquents. *Archives of General Psychiatry*, 1969, 20:643-651.

LEHR, D. J. & TATEL, D. Legal restrictions on the use of phenothiazines in institutions for the mentally retarded. In: J. G. Langan (Chair.), *Workshop on Psychotropic Drugs and the Mentally Retarded*. Symposium presented at the meetings of the American Association on Mental Deficiency, Portland, Ore., 1975.

LEISTYNA, J. & MACAULEY, J. Therapy of streptococcal infection. *American Journal of Diseases of Children*, 1966, 111:22-26.

LENA, B. & O'BRIEN, E. Success with lithium in a disturbed child. *Lancet*, 1975, 2:1307-1308.

LERER, R. & LERER, M. The effects of methylphenidate on the soft neurological signs of hyperactive children. *Pediatrics*, 1976, 57:521-525.

LESSER, E. Thalidomide and the pharmacologists. *New Scientist*, 1974, 62:472-473.

LEVANN, L. Trifluoperazine dihydrochloride: An effective tranquilizing agent for behavioural abnormalities in defective children. *Canadian Medical Association Journal*, 1959, 80:123-124.

LEVANN, L. Thioridazine (Mellaril) a psychosedative virtually free of side effects. *Alberta Medical Bulletin*, 1961, 26:144-147.

LEVANN, L. Haloperidol in the treatment of behavioural disorders in children and adolescents. *Canadian Psychiatric Association Journal*, 1969, 14:217-220.

LEVANN, L. Clinical comparison of haloperidol with chlorpromazine in mentally retarded children. *American Journal of Mental Deficiency*, 1971, 6:719-723.

LEVITT, E. *The Psychology of Anxiety*. Indianapolis: Bobbs-Merrill, 1968.

LEVY, G. Relationship between pharmacological effects and plasma or tissue concentration of drugs in man. In: B. Davies and B. Pritchard (Eds.), *Biological Effects of Drugs in Relation to their Plasma Concentrations*. Baltimore: University Park Press, 1973.

LEWIS, J. & YOUNG, R. Deanol and methylphenidate in minimal brain dysfunction. *Clinical Pharmacology and Therapeutics*, 1975, 17:534-540.

LEY, P. Patient compliance—a psychologist's viewpoint. *Prescribers Journal*, 1977, 17:15-20.

LIDDELL, D., WILLIAMS, F., & BRIANT, R. Phenazone (antipyrine) metabolism and distribution in young and elderly adults. *Clinical and Experimental Pharmacology and Physiology,* 1975, 2:481-487.

LINDSLEY, D. & HENRY, C. The effect of drugs on behavior and the electroencephalograms of children with behavior disorder. *Psychosomatic Medicine,* 1941, 4: 140-149.

LING, W., OFTEDAL, G., & WEINBERG, W. Depressive illness in childhood presenting as severe headache. *American Journal of Diseases of Children,* 1970, 120:122-124.

LINNOILA, M., VIUKARI, M., & HIETALA, O. Effect of sodium valproate on tardive dyskinesia. *British Journal of Psychiatry,* 1976, 129:114-119.

LIPMAN, R. Learning: Verbal, perceptual-motor, and classical conditioning. In: N. R. Ellis (Ed.), *Handbook of Mental Deficiency.* New York: McGraw-Hill, 1963, pp. 391-423.

LIPMAN, R. S. The use of psychopharmacological agents in residential facilities for the retarded. In: F. J. Menolascino (Ed.), *Psychiatric Approaches to Mental Retardation.* New York: Basic Books, 1970.

LIPMAN, R. S. NIMH-PRB support of research in minimal brain dysfunction in children. In: C. K. Conners (Ed.), *Clinical Use of Stimulant Drugs in Children.* The Hague: Excerpta Medica, 1974.

LIPMAN, R., COLE, J., PARK, L., & RICKELS, K. Sensitivity of symptom and non symptom-focused criteria of outpatient drug efficacy. *American Journal of Psychiatry,* 1965, 122:24-27.

LIU, M. Clinical experience with sulthiame (Ospolot). *British Journal of Psychiatry,* 1966, 112:621-628.

LIVINGSTON, S. Behavioural effects of antiepileptic drugs (Letter). *Developmental Medicine and Child Neurology,* 1976, 18:258-259.

LOGAN, W. & FREEMAN, J. Pseudodegenerative disease due to diphenylhydantoin intoxication. *Archives of Neurology,* 1969, 21:631-637.

LONEY, J. An indirect measure of self esteem and impulse control in elementary school children. *Psychology in the Schools,* 1972, 9:182-185.

LONEY, J., COMLY, H., & SIMON, B. Parental management, self-concept and drug response in minimal brain dysfunction. *Journal of Learning Disabilities,* 1975, 8:187-190.

LONEY, J., LANGHORNE, J., PATERNITE, C., WHALEY-KLAHN, M., BROEKER, C., & HACKER, M. The Iowa HABIT: Hyperkinetic/Aggressive Boys in Treatment. In S. Sells (Ed.), *Life History Research in Psychopathology*—in press.

LONEY, J., WHALEY-KAHN, M., & WEISSENBURGER, F. Responses of hyperactive boys to a behaviorally focused school attitude questionnaire. *Child Psychiatry and Human Development,* 1976, 6:123-133.

LOOKER, A. & CONNER, C. Diphenylhydantoin in children with severe temper tantrums. *Archives of General Psychiatry,* 1970, 23:80-89.

LOVELAND, N., SMITH, B., & FORSTER, F. Mental and emotional changes in epileptic patients on continuous anticonvulsant medication. *Neurology,* 1957, 7:856-865.

LOVELL, K., BYRNE, C., & RICHARDSON, B. A further study of the educational progress of children who had received remedial education. *British Journal of Educational Psychology,* 1963, 33:3-9.

LOWTHER, G. Clinical experience with trifluoperazine in low-grade mental defectives. *Canadian Medical Association Journal,* 1960, 82:1158-1160.

LUCAS, A. Gilles de la Tourette's disease in children: Treatment with phenothiazine drugs. *American Journal of Psychiatry,* 1964, 121:606-608.

LUCAS, A. Gilles de la Tourette's disease in children: Treatment with haloperidol. *American Journal of Psychiatry,* 1967, 124:243-245.

MACCOLL, K. Chlorpromazine hydrochloride (Largactil) in the treatment of the disturbed mental defective. *American Journal of Mental Deficiency,* 1956, 61:378-389.

MACKAY, M., BECK, L., & TAYLOR, R. Methylphenidate for adolescents with minimal

brain dysfunction. *New York State Journal of Medicine,* 1973, 73:550-554.
MacKeith, R. High activity and hyperactivity. *Developmental Medicine and Child Neurology,* 1976, 16:543-544.
MacLean, R. Imipramine hydrochloride (Tofranil) and enuresis. *American Journal of Psychiatry,* 1960, 117:551.
Mahony, D., Laferte, R., & Mahoney, J. Observations on sphincter-augmenting effect of imipramine in children with urinary incontinence. *Journal of Urology,* 1973, 1:317-323.
Maizels, M. Cation transfer in human red cells. In: A. Kleinzeller and A. Kotyk (Eds.), *Membrane Transport and Metabolism.* London: Academic Press, 1961.
Majluf, E. Drug therapy in infant psychiatry. *Journal of the American Medical Association,* 1957, 165:1472-1475.
Maletzky, B. d-Amphetamine and delinquency: Hyperkinesis persisting? *Diseases of the Nervous System,* 1974, 35:543-547.
Malitz, S. & Kazler, M. Are antidepressants better than placebo? *American Journal of Psychiatry,* 1971, 127:1605-1611.
Marholin, D. & Phillips, D. Methodological issues in psychopharmacological research: Chlorpromazine—A case in point. *American Journal of Orthopsychiatry,* 1976, 46:477-495.
Marjerrison, G., Jedlicki, S., Keogh, R., Hrychuk, W., & Poulakakis, G. Carbamazepine: Behavioral, anticonvulsant and EEG effects in chronically-hospitalised epileptics. *Diseases of the Nervous System,* 1968, 29:133-136.
Marks, I. & Gelder, M. Different ages of onset in varieties of phobias. *American Journal of Psychiatry,* 1966, 123:218-221.
Mattar, M., Markello, J., & Yaffe, S. Inadequacies in pharmacologic management of ambulatory children. *Journal of Pediatrics,* 1975, 87:137-141.
Maynard, R. Omaha pupils given 'behavior' drugs. *Washington Post,* June 29, 1970.
MBD, drug research and the schools. *The Hastings Center Report,* June 1976, 1-23.
McAndrew, J., Case, Q., & Treffert, D. Effects of prolonged phenothiazine intake on psychotic and other hospitalized children. *Journal of Autism and Childhood Schizophrenia,* 1972, 2:75-91.
McCabe, E. & McCabe, L. Dissociation of learning on stimulant-drug therapy. *The New England Journal of Medicine,* 1972, 287:825.
McDowell, J. The molecular structure of phenothiazine derivatives. In: I. Forrest, C. Carr, and E. Usdin (Eds.), *Phenothiazines and Structurally Related Drugs.* New York: Raven Press, 1974.
McLaughlin, B. A double-blind study involving 30 emotionally disturbed children (outpatients). *Psychosomatics,* 1964, 5:40-43.
McLellan, D. & Swash, M. Choreo-athetosis and encephalopathy induced by phenytoin. *British Medical Journal,* 1974, 2:204-205.
McNair, D. Anti-anxiety drugs and human performance. *Archives of General Psychiatry,* 1973, 29:611-617.
McNutt, B., Boileau, R., & Cohen, M. The effects of long term stimulant medication on the growth and body composition of hyperactive children. *Psychopharmacology Bulletin,* 1977, 13:36-38.
Meek, J., Fuxe, D., & Anden, N. Effects of antidepressant drugs of the imipramine type on central 5-hydroxytryptamine nerve transmission. *European Journal of Pharmacology,* 1970, 9:325-332.
Mellerup, E., Plenge, P., Ziegler, R., & Rafaelsen, O. Lithium effects on calcium metabolism in rats. *International Pharmacopsychiatry,* 1970, 5:258-264.
Melmon, K. Preventable drug reactions—causes and cures. *New England Journal of Medicine,* 1971, 284:1361-1368.
Mendels, J. Relationship between depression and mania. *Lancet,* 1971, 1:342.

MENDELSON, W., GILLIN, C., & WYATT, R. *Human Sleep and its Disorders.* New York: Plenum Press, 1977.
MENDELSON, W., JOHNSON, N., & STEWART, M. Hyperactive children as teenagers: A follow-up study. *The Journal of Nervous and Mental Disease,* 1971, 153:273-279.
MIKSZTAL, M. Chlorpromazine (Thorazine) and reserpine in residential treatment of neuropsychiatric disorders in children. *Journal of Nervous and Mental Disease,* 1956, 123:477-479.
MILLER, L. Method factors associated with assessment of child behavior: Fact or artifact. *Journal of Abnormal Child Psychology,* 1976, 4:209-220.
MILLER, R. Clinically important drug interactions. *Journal of the Maine Medical Association,* 1975, 66:18-25.
MILLICHAP, J. *The Hyperactive Child with Minimal Brain Dysfunction—Questions and Answers.* Chicago: Year Book Medical Publishers, 1975.
MILLICHAP, J., AYMAT, F., STURGIS, L., LARSEN, K., & EGAN, R. Hyperkinetic behavior and learning disorders. *American Journal of Diseases of Children,* 1968, 116:235-244.
MILLICHAP, J. & BOLDREY, E. Studies in hyperkinetic behavior. II. Laboratory and clinical evaluations of drug treatments. *Neurology,* 1967, 17:467-471.
MILLICHAP, J. & JOHNSON, F. Methylphenidate in hyperkinetic behavior: Relation of response to degree of activity and brain damage. In: C. Conners (Ed.), *Clinical Use of Stimulant Drugs in Children.* Amsterdam: Excerpta Medica, 1974, pp. 130-139.
MINTZ, M. FDA and Panalba: A conflict of commercial, therapeutic goals? *Science,* 1969, 165:875-881.
MIRKIN, B. Drug distribution in pregnancy. In: L. Boreus (Ed.), *Fetal Pharmacology.* New York: Raven Press, 1973, pp. 1-27.
MIRSKY, A. & KORNETSKY, C. On the dissimilar effects of drugs on the digit symbol substitution and continuous performance tests. A review and preliminary integration of behavioural and physiological evidence. *Psychopharmacologia,* 1964, 5:161-177.
MISUREC, J., NAHUNEK, K., & RODOVA, A. EEG changes in treatment with maprotiline. *Activitas Nervosa Superior (Praha),* 1973, 15:110.
MODELL, W., SCHILD, H. O., & WILSON, A. *Applied Pharmacology.* Philadelphia: W. B. Saunders Company, 1976.
MOFFATT, W., SIDDIQUI, A., & MACKAY, D. The use of sulthiame with disturbed mentally subnormal patients. *British Journal of Psychiatry,* 1970, 117:673-678.
MOHLER, D., WALLIN, D., & DREYFUS, E. Studies in the home treatment of streptococcal diseases. *New England Journal of Medicine,* 1955, 252:1116-1118.
MOLLING, P., LOCKNER, A., SAULS, R., & EISENBERG, L. Committed delinquent boys. *Archives of General Psychiatry,* 1962, 7:70-79.
MONTAGU, J. The hyperkinetic child: Behaviour, electrodermal and EEG investigation. *Developmental Medicine and Child Neurology,* 1975, 17:299-305.
MONTAGU, J. & SWARBRICK, L. Effect of amphetamines in hyperkinetic children: Stimulant or sedative? A pilot study. *Developmental Medicine and Child Neurology,* 1975, 17:293-298.
MONTGOMERY, L. & FINCH, A. Validity of two measures of anxiety in children. *Journal of Abnormal Child Psychology,* 1974, 2:293-298.
Moos, R. Conceptualizations of human environments. *American Psychologist,* 1973, 28:652-665.
Moos, R. *The Family Environment Scales.* Consulting Psychologists' Press, 1974.
MORENA, D. & LITROWNIK, A. Self-concept in educable mentally retarded and emotionally handicapped children: Relationship between behavioral and self-report indices and an attempt at modification. *Journal of Abnormal Child Psychology,* 1974, 2:281-292.

MURPHY, D., BRAND, E., GOLDMAN, J., BAKER, M., WRIGHT, L., VAN KAMMEN, D., & GORDON, E. Platelet and plasma amine oxidase inhibition and urinary amine excretion changes during phenelzine treatment. *Journal of Nervous and Mental Disease*, in press.

MURRAY, E. & JACOBSON, L. The nature of learning in traditional and behavioral psychotherapy. In: A. E. Bergin and S. L. Garfield (Eds.), *Handbook of Psychotherapy and Behavior Change: An Empirical Analysis*. New York: John Wiley, 1971, pp. 709-747.

MURRAY, M. Behavioral management in pediatrics. Applications of operant learning theory to problem behaviors of children. *Clinical Pediatrics*, 1976, 15:465-477.

NEEDLEMAN, H. L. & WABER, D. Amitryptiline therapy in patients with anorexia nervosa. *Lancet*, 1976, 2:580.

NEISWORTH, J., KURTZ, P., JONES, R., & MADLE, R. Biasing of hyperkinetic behavior rating by diagnostic reports. *Journal of Abnormal Child Psychology*, 1974, 2: 323-329.

New York State Association for Retarded Children, Inc. v. Nelson Rockefeller, No. 72 356, 72 357 (E.D. New York, 1975).

NIEDERMEYER, E., BLUMER, D., HOLSCHER, E., & WALKER, B. Classical hysterical seizures facilitated by anticonvulsant toxicity. *Psychiatrica Clinica*, 1970, 3:71-84.

NISSEN, G. Behavioural disorders in children and the possibilities offered by drugs in their treatment. In: W. Birkmayer (Ed.), *Epileptic Seizures—Behaviour—Pain*. Berne: Hans Huber, 1976.

NISSEN, G., SPILIMBERGO, A., & FLACH, D. *Tegretol bei kindlichen Verhaltensstorunge*. Polycopied manuscript. Basle: Ciba-Geigy. Quoted by Remschmidt (1976).

NUSSBAUM, H., LEFF, W., MATTIA, V., & HILLMAN, E. *Angiology*, 1957, 8:198-200.

OETTINGER, L. & SIMONDS, R. The use of thioridazine in the office management of children's behavior disorders. *Medical Times*, 1962, 90:596-604.

OJEDA, P. Treatment with thioridazine of emotionally disturbed children in a day hospital. *Michigan Medicine*, 1970, 69:215-217.

O'LEARY, K., KENT, R., & KANOWITZ, J.: Shaping data collection congruent with experimental hypotheses. *Journal of Applied Behavior Analysis*, 1975, 8:43-51.

O'LEARY, K., PELHAM, W., ROSENBAUM, A., & PRICE, G. H. Behavioral treatment of hyperkinetic children. An experimental evaluation of its usefulness. *Clinical Pediatrics*, 1976, 15:510-515.

OUNSTED, C. The hyperkinetic syndrome in epileptic children. *Lancet*, 1955, 2:303-311.

OVERALL, J. E. & WOODWARD, J. A. Nonrandom assignment and the analysis of covariance. *Psychological Bulletin*, 1977, 84:588-594

OVERTON, D. State dependent or "dissociated" learning produced with pentobarbitol. *Journal of Comparative and Physiological Psychology*, 1964, 57:3-12.

OVERTON, D. Dissociated learning in drug states (state dependent learning). In: D. Efron (Ed.), *Psychopharmacology: A Review of Progress 1957-1967*. U.S. Government Printing Office, Public Health Service Publication No. 1836, 1968, pp. 918-930.

PAGE, J., BERNSTEIN, J., JANICKI, R., & MICHELLI, F. A multiclinic trial of pemoline in childhood hyperkinesis. In: C. Conners (Ed.), *Clinical Use of Stimulant Drugs in Children*. Amsterdam: Excerpta Medica, 1974, pp. 98-123.

PAINE, R. & OPPE, T. *Neurological Evaluation of Children*. London: Heinemann, 1966.

PALMER, R. (Ed.). *Horizons in Clinical Pharmacology*. New York: Marcel Dekker, 1976.

PARSONAGE, M. Treatment with carbamazepine: Adults. In: J. Penry & D. Daly (Eds.), *Complex Partial Seizures and Their Treatment*. New York: Raven Press. 1975.

PATEL, H. & CRICHTON, J. The neurological hazards of diphenylhydantoin in childhood. *Journal of Pediatrics*, 1968, 73:676-684.

PATTERSON, G. A community mental health program for children. In: L. Hamerlynck, P. Davidson, & L. Acker (Eds.), *Behaviour Modification and Ideal Mental Health Services*. Calgary, Canada: University of Calgary Press, 1969, pp. 130-179.

PATTERSON, G. & COBB, J. A dyadic analysis of "aggressive" behavior. In: J. Hill (Ed.), *Minnesota Symposia on Child Psychology*, 5. Minneapolis: University of Minnesota Press, 1971.

PATTERSON, G. & REID, J. Reciprocity and coercion: Two facets of social systems. In: C. Neuringer and J. Michael (Eds.), *Behavior Modification in Clinical Psychology*. New York: Appleton-Century-Crofts, 1970, pp. 133-177.

PAULSON, G., RIZVI, A., & CRANE, G. Tardive dyskinesia as a possible sequel of long-term therapy with phenothiazines. *Clinical Pediatrics*, 1975, 14:953-955.

PAYNE, D. *The Assessment of Learning: Cognition and Affection*. Lexington, Mass.: D.C. Heath, 1974.

PEKARIK, E., PRINZ, R., LIEBERT, D., WEINTRAUB, S., & NEALE, J. The Pupil Evaluation Inventory: A Sociometric Technique for Assessing Children's Behavior. *Journal of Abnormal Child Psychology*, 1976, 4:83-97.

PENRY, J. Behavioural correlates of generalised spikewave discharge in the electroencephalogram. In: M. Brazier (Ed.), *Epilepsy, Its Phenomena in Man*. New York: Academic Press, 1973.

PENRY, J., PORTER, R., & DREIFUSS, F. Simultaneous recording of absence seizures with videotape and electroencephalography. *Brain*, 1975, 98:427-440.

PETERS, H. Anticonvulsant drug intolerance. *Neurology*, 1962, 12:299.

PETERS, J., DYKMAN, R., ACKERMAN, P., & ROMINE, J. The special neurological examination. In: C. Conners (Ed.), *Clinical Use of Stimulant Drugs in Children*. Amsterdam: Excerpta Medica, 1974, pp. 53-65.

PIERS, E. Parent prediction of children's self-concepts. *Journal of Consulting and Clinical Psychology*, 1972, 38:428-433.

PIERS, E. & HARRIS, D. Age and other correlates of self-concept in children. *Journal of Educational Psychology*, 1964, 55:91-95.

PILLINER, A. & REID, J. The definition and measurement of reading problems. In: J. F. Reid (Ed.), *Reading: Problems and Practices*. London: Ward Lock Educational, 1972, pp. 20-36.

PIND, K. & FAURBYE, A. Concentration of homovanillic acid and 5-hydroxyindoleacetic acid in cerebrospinal fluid after treatment with probenecid in patients with drug induced tardive dyskinesia. *Acta Psychologica Scandinavica*, 1970, 46:323-326.

PINDER, R., BROGDEN, R., SPEIGHT, T., & AVERY, G. Sodium valproate: A review of its pharmacological properties and therapeutic efficiency in epilepsy. *Drugs*, 1977, 13:81-123.

PISCIOTTA, A. Drug induced leukopenia and aplastic anemia. *Clinical Pharmacology and Therapeutics*, 1971, 12:13-43.

PLAA, G. Acute toxicity of antiepileptic drugs. *Epilepsia*, 1975, 16:183-191.

PLATMAN, S. & FIEVE, R. Biochemical aspects of lithium in affective disorders. *Archives of General Psychiatry*, 1968, 19:659-663.

PLATMAN, S. & FIEVE, R. The effect of lithium carbonate on the electroencephalogram of patients with affective disorders. *British Journal of Psychiatry*, 1969, 115:1185-1188.

PLETSCHER, A. Monoamine oxidase inhibitions. *Pharmacological Review*, 1966, 18:121-129.

POLIZOS, P., ENGELHARDT, D., HOFFMAN, S., & WAIZER, J. Neurological consequences of psychotropic drug withdrawal in schizophrenic children. *Journal of Autism and Childhood Schizophrenia*, 1973, 3:247-253.

REFERENCES

POPE, L. Motor activity in brain-injured children. *American Journal of Orthopsychiatry*, 1970, 40:783-794.

PORGES, S., WALTER, G., KORB, R., & SPRAGUE, R. The influences of methylphenidate on heart rate and behavioral measures of attention in hyperactive children. *Child Development*, 1975, 46:727-733.

PORTEUS, S. *The Porteus Maze Test Manual*. London: Harrap, 1967.

POST, R. & GOODWIN, F. Time dependent effects of phenothiazines on dopamine turnover in psychiatric patients. *Science*, 1975, 190:488-489.

POUSSAINT, A. & DITMAN, D. A controlled study of imipramine (Tofranil) in the treatment of childhood enuresis. *Journal of Pediatrics*, 1965, 67:283-290.

POWELL, G., MILLER, J., OLAVESEN, A., & CURTIS, C. Liver as the major organ of phenol detoxification? *Nature*, 1974, 252:234-235.

PREGELJ, S. & BARKAUSKAS, A. Thioridazine in the treatment of mentally retarded children. *Canadian Psychiatric Association Journal*, 1967, 12:213-215.

PRENSKY, A., DE VIVO, D., & PALKES, H. Severe bradykinesia as a manifestation of toxicity to antiepileptic medications. *Journal of Pediatrics*, 1971, 78:700-704.

PRICE, S. & SPENCER, D. A trial of beclamide (Nydrane) in mentally subnormal patients with disorders of behaviour. *Journal of Mental Subnormality*, 1967, 13:75-77.

PRICE-EVANS, D., MANLEY, K., & MCKUSICK, V. Genetic control of isoniazid metabolism in man. *British Medical Journal*, 1960, 2:485-491.

PRICE-EVANS, P., DAVISON, K. & PRATT, R. The influence of acetylator phenotype on the effects of treating depression with phenelzine. *Clinical Pharmacology and Therapeutics*, 1965, 6:430-435.

PRIEN, R., CAFFEY, E., & KLETT, C. The relationship between lithium level and clinical response in acute manics treated with lithium carbonate. *Cooperative Studies in Psychiatry* (Report No. 91). Perry Point, Maryland, VA-NIMH Collaborative Study Group, 1971.

PRIEN, R., CAFFEY, E., & KLETT, C. Relationship between serum lithium levels and clinical response in acute mania treated with lithium. *British Journal of Psychiatry*, 1972, 120:409-414.

PROGER, B., MANN, L., GREEN, P., BAYUK, R., & BURGER, R. Discriminators of clinically defined emotional maladjustment: Predictive validity of the Behavior Problem Checklist and Devereux Scales. *Journal of Abnormal Child Psychology*, 1975, 3:71-82.

PRUITT, A. & DAYTON, P. A comparison of the binding of drugs to adult and cord plasma. *European Journal of Clinical Pharmacology*, 1971, 4:59-62.

PRUITT, A., DAYTON, P., & PATTERSON, J. Disposition of diazoxide in children. *Clinical Pharmacology and Therapeutics*, 1973, 14:73-82.

PRYCE-PHILLIPS, W. & JEAVONS, P. Effect of carbamazepine (Tegretol) on the electroencephalograph and ward behaviour of patients with chronic epilepsy. *Epilepsia*, 1970, 11:263-273.

Psychopharmacology Bulletin, *Special Issue on Pharmacotherapy of Children*, 1973.

PUENTE, R. The use of carbamazepine in the treatment of behavioural disorders in children. In: W. Birkmayer (Ed.), *Epileptic Seizures—Behavior—Pain*. Berne: Hans Huber, 1976.

PUENTE, R., BARRIGA, F., & MORALES, M. T. Estudio doble-ciego con carbamazepina en un grupo de escolares con daño cerebral. Comunicación preliminar. *Medicina (Mexico)*, 1973, 53:97-101. Quoted by Remschmidt (1976).

QUAY, H. Classification. In: H. Quay & J. Werry (Eds.), *Psychopathological Disorders of Childhood* (2nd ed). New York: Wiley—in press.

QUINN, G., HURWIC, M., & PEREL, J. Interspecies differences in drug metabolism. In: E. Usdin and I. Forrest (Eds.), *Psychotherapeutic Drugs, Part I*. New York: Marcel Dekker, 1976.

QUINN, P. & RAPOPORT, J. One-year follow-up of hyperactive boys treated with imipramine or methylphenidate. *American Journal of Psychiatry*, 1975, 132:241-245.

RAAFLAUB, J. On the pharmacokinetics of chlorprothixene in man. *Experientia*, 1975, 15:557-558.

RAITERI, M., ANGELINI, F., & BERTOLLINI, A. Comparative study of the effects of Mianserin, a tetracyclic antidepressant and of imipramine on uptake and release of neurotransmitters in synaptosomes. *Journal of Pharmacy and Pharmacology*, 1976, 28:483-488.

RAJOTTE, P., JILEK, W., PERALES, A., GIARD, W., BORDELEAU, J., & TETREAULT, L. Propriétés antiépileptiques et psychotropes de la carbamazépine (Tégrétol). *Union Medicale du Canada*, 1967, 96:1200-1206.

RANE, A. & SJOQVIST, F. Drug metabolism in the human fetus and newborn infant. *Pediatric Clinics of North America*, 1972, 19:37-49.

RANE, A. & WILSON, J. Clinical pharmacokinetics in infants and children. *Clinical Pharmacokinetics*, 1976, 1:2-24.

RAPOPORT, J. Childhood behavior and learning problems treated with imipramine. *International Journal of Neuropsychiatry*, 1965, 1:635-642.

RAPOPORT, J. Pediatric psychopharmacology and childhood depression. In: D. Klein and R. Gittelman-Klein (Eds.), *Progress in Psychiatric Drug Treatment*, Vol. 2. New York: Brunner/Mazel, 1976.

RAPOPORT, J. Self report, social and emotional functioning measures. In: *Guidelines for Evaluation of Psychoactive Agents in Infants and Children*. Rockville, Md.: Food and Drug Administration—in press.

RAPOPORT, J., ABRAMSON, A., ALEXANDER, D., & LOTT, I. Playroom observations of hyperactive children on medication. *Journal of the American Academy of Child Psychiatry*, 1971, 10:524-534.

RAPOPORT, J. & BENOIT, M. The relation of direct home observations to the clinic evaluation of hyperactive school age boys. *Journal of Child Psychology and Psychiatry*, 1975, 16:141-147.

RAPOPORT, J., PANDONI, C., RENFIELD, M., LAKE, C., & ZIEGLER, M. Newborn dopamine-β-hydroxylase, minor physical anomalies and infant temperament. *American Journal of Psychiatry*, 1977, 134:676-679.

RAPOPORT, J. & QUINN, P. Minor physical anomalies (stigmata) and early developmental deviation: A major biologic subgroup of hyperactive children. *International Journal of Mental Health*, 1975, 4:29-44.

RAPOPORT, J., QUINN, P., BRADBARD, G., RIDDLE, D., & BROOKES, E. Imipramine and methylphenidate treatments of hyperactive boys: A double blind comparison. *Archives of General Psychiatry*, 1974b, 30, 789-793.

RAPOPORT, J., QUINN, P., & LAMPRECHT, F. Minor physical anomalies and plasma-dopamine-beta-hydroxylase activity in hyperactive boys. *American Journal of Psychiatry*, 1974a, 131:386-390.

RASKIN, A., SCHULTENBRANDT, J., REATIG, N., CROUKE, T., & ODLE, D. Depression subtypes and response to phenelzine, diazepam and placebo. *Archives of General Psychiatry*, 1974, 30:66-75.

RAY, O. *Drugs, Society and Human Behavior*. St. Louis: Mosby, 1972.

REACE, A. & MOTOLESE, M. Haemodynamic studies with CIBA, 276 Ba (ludiomil). In: P. Kielholz (Ed.), *Depressive Illness*. Baltimore: Williams & Wilkins, 1972, pp. 161-168.

REICHARDT, C. & ELDER, S. The effects of caffeine on reaction time in hyperkinetic and normal children. *American Journal of Psychiatry*, 1977, 134:144-148.

REILLY, M. J. Pediatric drug dosage. *American Journal of Hospital Pharmacy*, 1972, 29:699-700.

REITAN, R. & DAVISON, L. (Eds.). *Clinical Neuropsychology: Current Status and Applications*. New York: Winston-Wiley, 1974.

REMSCHMIDT, H. The psychotropic effect of carbamazepine in non-epileptic patients, with particular reference to problems posed by clinical studies in children with behavioural disorders. In: W. Birkmayer (Ed.), *Epileptic Seizures—Behaviour—Pain*. Berne: Hans Huber, 1976.

RENARD, P., BANJAC, M., & BARRE, L. Essais cliniques de la thioridazine chez les enfants inadaptes d'age scolaire (Clinical trials with thioridazine in school age children with adaptation difficulties). *Annales Médico-Psychologiques* (Paris), 1962, 120: 578-586.

RENSHAW, D. Thioridazine and urine incontinence. *Journal of the American Medical Association*, 1971, 218:738.

RESNICK, O. The psychoactive properties of diphenylhydantoin: Experiences with prisoners and juvenile delinquents. *International Journal of Neuropsychiatry*, 1967, 3: (Supplement), 30-48.

RETT, A. The so-called psychotropic effect of Tegretol in the treatment of convulsions of cerebral origin in children. In: W. Birkmayer (Ed.), *Epileptic Seizures—Behaviour—Pain*. Berne: Hans Huber, 1976.

RETTIG, J. Chlorpromazine for the control of psychomotor excitement in the mentally deficient: A preliminary study. *Journal of Nervous and Mental Disease*, 1955, 122:190-194.

RETTIG, J., CALDWELL, W., & JOSEPHS, L. A pilot study of trifluoperazine in mentally retarded patients. In: *Trifluoperazine; Clinical and Pharmacological Aspects*. Philadelphia: Lea & Febiger, 1958.

REYNOLDS, E. Chronic antiepileptic toxicity: A review. *Epilepsia*, 1975, 16:319-352.

REYNOLDS, E., CHADWICK, D., & GALBRAITH, A. W. One drug (phenytoin) in the treatment of epilepsy. *Lancet*, 1976, 1:923-926.

REYNOLDS, E. & TRAVERS, R. Serum anticonvulsant concentrations in epileptic patients with mental symptoms. *British Journal of Psychiatry*, 1974, 124:440-445.

RICHENS, A. Drug interactions in epilepsy. *Developmental Medicine and Child Neurology*, 1975, 17:94-95.

RICHENS, A. *Drug Treatment of Epilepsy*. London: Henry Kimpton, 1976.

RIDDLE, K. D. & RAPOPORT, J. A 2-year follow-up of 72 hyperactive boys. *Journal of Nervous and Mental Disease*, 1976, 162:126-134.

RIE, H. Hyperactivity in children. *American Journal of Diseases of Children*, 1975, 130:783-789.

RIE, H., RIE, E., STEWART, S., & AMBUEL, J. Effects of methylphenidate on underachieving children. *Journal of Consulting and Clinical Psychology*, 1976, 44:250-260.

RIESS, W., DUBEY, L., FUNFGELD, E., & IMHOF, P. The pharmacological properties of maprotiline in man. *Journal of International Medical Research*, 1975, 3: (Supplement #2), 16-41.

RIESS, W., RAJOGOPALAN, T., & KEBERLE, H. The metabolism and pharmacokinetics of ludiomil. In: P. Kielholz (Ed.), *Depressive Illness*. Baltimore: Williams & Wilkins, 1972.

RIFKIN, A., QUITKIN, F., CIRILLO, C., BLUMBERG, A., & KLEIN, D. Lithium carbonate in emotionally unstable character disorder. *Archives of General Psychiatry*, 1972, 27:519-523.

RIMLAND, B. Infantile autism: Status and research. In: A Davids (Ed.), *Child Personality and Psychopathology: Current Topics* (Vol. 1). New York: Wiley, 1974, pp. 137-167.

RITSCHEL, W. Dose size and dosing interval determination. *Arzneimittel Forschung*, 1975, 25:1442-1447.

RITVO, E., ORNITZ, E., GOTTLIEB, F., POUSSAINT, A., MARON, B., DITMAN, K., & BLINN,

K. Arousal and non-arousal enuretic events. *American Journal of Psychiatry,* 1969, 126:77-85.

RITVO, E., YUWILER, A., GELLER, E., KALES, A., RASHKIS, S., SCHICOR, A., PLOTKIN, S., AXELROD R., & HOWARD, C. Effects of L-dopa in autism. *Journal of Autism and Childhood Schizophrenia,* 1971, 1:190-205.

RIVERA-CALIMLIM, L., NASRALLAH, H., STRAUSS, J., & LASAGNA, L. Clinical response and plasma levels: Effective dose, dosage schedules, and drug interactions on plasma chlorpromazine levels. *American Journal of Psychiatry,* 1976, 133:646-652.

ROBIN, S. S. & BOSCO, J. J. The social context of stimulant drug treatment for hyperkinetic children. *School Review,* 1976, 85:141-154.

ROBINS, L. Follow up studies. In: H. Quay and J. Werry (Eds.), *Psychopathological Disorders of Childhood* (2nd ed). New York: Wiley—in press (a).

ROBINS, L. Methods of environmental assessment. In *Guidelines for Evaluation of Psychoactive Agents in Infants and Children.* Rockville, Md.: Food and Drug Administration—in press (b).

ROBINSON, D. & BARKER, E. Tricyclic antidepressant cardiotoxicity. *JAMA,* 1976, 236: 2089-2090.

ROBINSON, D., NIES, S., RAVARIS, L., & LAMBORN, K. The monoamine oxidase inhibition phenelzine, in the treatment of depressive—anxiety states. *Archives of General Psychiatry,* 1973, 29:409-413.

RODIN, E., RIM, C., & RENNICK, P. The effects of carbamazepine on patients with psychomotor epilepsy. Results of a double blind study. *Epilepsia,* 1974, 15:547-561.

ROGER, J., GRANGEON, H., GUEY, J., & LOB, H. Psychiatric and psychological effects of ethosuximide treatment in epileptics. *Encéphale,* 1968, 57:407-438.

ROSEN, J. Dilantin dementia. *Transactions of the American Neurological Association,* 1968, 93:273.

ROSENBERG, C. Young drug addicts: Background and personality. *Journal of Nervous and Mental Disease,* 1969, 148:65-73.

ROSVOLD, H., MIRSKY, A., SARASON, I., BRANSOME, E., & BECK, L. A continuous performance test of brain damage. *Journal of Consulting Psychology,* 1956, 20:343-350.

ROUTH, D. & SCHROEDER, C. Standardized playroom measures as indices of hyperactivity. *Journal of Abnormal Child Psychology,* 1976, 4:199-207.

ROUTH, D., SCHROEDER, C., & O'TUAMA, L. Development of activity level in children. *Developmental Psychology,* 1974, 10:163-168.

RUDEL, R. & DENCKLA, M. Relationship of IQ and reading score to visual, spatial, and temporal matching tasks. *Journal of Learning Disabilities,* 1976, 9:42-51.

RUDY, L., HIMWICH, H., COSTA, E., & RINALDI, F. Trifluoperazine in mentally defective patients. In: *Trifluoperazine; Clinical and Pharmacological Aspects.* Philadelphia: Lea & Febiger, 1958.

RUSSO, R., GURURAJ, V., & ALLEN, J. The effectiveness of diphenhydramine HCl in pediatric sleep disorders. *Journal of Clinical Pharmacology,* 1976, 16:284-288.

RUTTER, M. Psychotic disorders in early childhood. In: A. Coppen & A. Walk (Eds.), *Recent Developments in Schizophrenia.* London: Royal Medico-Psychological Association, 1967.

RUTTER, M. Research Report: Institute of Psychiatry, Department of Child and Adolescent Psychiatry. *Psychological Medicine,* 1976, 6:505-516.

RUTTER, M. & GRAHAM, P. The reliability and validity of the psychiatric assessment of the child. I. Interview with the child. *British Journal of Psychiatry,* 1968, 114:563-579.

RUTTER, M., GRAHAM, P., & YULE, W. A neuropsychiatric study in childhood. *Clinics in Developmental Medicine,* Nos. 35/36. London: Heinemann, 1970.

RUTTER, M., SHAFFER, D., & SHEPHERD, M. An evaluation of the proposal for a multiaxial classification of child pyschiatric disorders. *Psychological Medicine,* 1973, 3:244-250.

RUTTER, M., SHAFFER, D., & STURGE, C. *A Guide to a Multi-axial Classification Scheme for Psychiatric Disorders in Childhood and Adolescence.* London: Frowde & Co., 1976.

RUTTER, M., TIZARD, J., YULE, W., GRAHAM, P., & WHITMORE, K. Research report: Isle of Wight studies, 1964-1974. *Psychological Medicine,* 1976, 6:313-332.

RUTTER, M. & YULE, W. Specific reading retardation. In: L. Mann and D. Sabatino (Eds.), *The First Review of Special Education.* Philadelphia, Pennsylvania: J.S.E. Press, 1973, pp. 1-50.

SAFER, D. & ALLEN, R. Single daily dose methylphenidate in hyperactive children. *Diseases of the Nervous System,* 1973, 34:325-328.

SAFER, D. & ALLEN, R. Side effects from long term use of stimulants in children. *International Journal of Mental Health,* 1975, 4:105-118.

SAFER, D. & ALLEN, R. *Hyperactive Children: Diagnosis and Management.* Baltimore: University Park Press, 1976.

SAFER, D., ALLEN, R. & BARR, E. Depression of growth in hyperactive children on stimulant drugs. *New England Journal of Medicine,* 1972, 287:217-220.

SALETU, B., SALETU, M., & ITIL, T. The relationship between psychopathology and evoked responses before, during and after psychotropic drug treatment. *Biological Psychiatry,* 1973, 6:45-74.

SALETU, B., SALETU, M., SIMEON, J., & MARASA, J. Fluphenazine treatment in the psychotic child: Clinical-evoked potential correlations. *Comprehensive Psychiatry,* 1975a, 16:265-278.

SALETU, B., SALETU, M., SIMEON, J., VIAMONTES, G., & ITIL, T. Comparative symptomatological and evoked potential studies with d-amphetamine, thioridazine, and placebo in hyperkinetic children. *Biological Psychiatry,* 1975b, 10:253-275.

SAMUELSSON, B. LSD intoxication in a two year old child. *Acta Pediatrica Scandinavica,* 1974, 63:797-798.

SARAF, K., KLEIN, D., GITTELMAN-KLEIN, R., et al. Imipramine and side effects in children. *Psychopharmacologia,* 1974, 37:265-274.

SARAF, K., KLEIN, D., GITTELMAN-KLEIN, R., GOOTMAN, N., & GREEN, P. EKG effects of imipramine treatment in children. In Press. *Journal of the American Academy of Child Psychiatry,* 1977.

SARAF, K., KLEIN, D., GITTELMAN-KLEIN, G., & GROFF, S. Imipramine side-effects in children *Psychopharmacologia,* 1974, 37:265-274.

SARGANT, W. Treatment of the phobic anxiety state. *British Medical Journal,* 1969, 49.

SATTERFIELD, J. Central and autonomic nervous system function in the hyperactive child syndrome: Treatment and research implications. In: A. Davids (Ed.), *Child Personality and Psychopathology: Current Topics* (Vol. 3), 1976. New York: Wiley, pp. 237-258.

SATTERFIELD, J., ATOIAN, G., BRASHEARS, G., BURLEIGH, A., & DAWSON, M. Electrodermal studies in minimal brain dysfunction children. In: C. Conners (Ed.), *Clinical Use of Stimulant Drugs in Children.* Amsterdam: Excerpta Medica, 1974, pp. 87-95.

SATTERFIELD, J. H. & CANTWELL, D. P. A one year follow up study of treated hyperactive children. Read at the Annual Meeting of the Psychiatric Research Society, Salt Lake City, 1977.

SATTERFIELD, J., CANTWELL, D., LESSER, L., & PODOSIN, R. Physiological studies of the hyperkinetic child: I. *American Journal of Psychiatry,* 1972, 128:1418-1424.

SATTERFIELD, J. & DAWSON, M. Electrodermal correlates of hyperactivity in children. *Psychophysiology,* 1971, 8:191-197.

SATTERLY, D. Cognitive styles, spatial ability, and school achievement. *Journal of Educational Psychology,* 1976, 68:36-42.

SAUNDERS, L. *The Absorption and Distribution of Drugs.* London: Bailliere Tindall, 1974.

SCHAEFER, E. & AARONSON, M. *Classroom Behavior Inventory: Preschool to Primary.* Bethesda, Md.: National Institute of Mental Health, 1966.

SCHAIN, R. *Neurology of Childhood Learning Disorders.* Baltimore: Williams & Wilkins, 1972.

SCHAIN, R. & REYNARD, C. Observations on effects of a central stimulant drug (methylphenidate) in children with hyperactive behavior. *Pediatrics,* 1975, 55: 709-716.

SCHIFINO, et al., unpublished findings, 1969. Quoted by Remschmidt (1976).

SCHILDKRAUT, J. Pharmacology—the effects of lithium on biogenic amines. In: S. Gershon and B. Shopsin (Eds.), *Lithium, Its Role in Psychiatric Research and Treatment.* New York: Plenum, 1973, pp. 51-71.

SCHLEIFER, M., WEISS, G., COHEN, N., ELMAN, M., CVEJIC, H., & KRUGER, E. Hyperactivity in preschoolers and the effect of methylphenidate. *American Journal of Orthopsychiatry,* 1975, 45:38-50.

SCHNACKENBERG, R. Caffeine as a substitute for Schedule II stimulants in hyperkinetic children. *American Journal of Psychiatry,* 1973, 130:796-798.

SCHOU, M. Lithium studies. 3. Distribution between serum and tissues. *Acta Pharmacologica et Toxicologica,* 1958, 15:115-124.

SCHOU, M. Preparations, dosage and control in lithium: Its role in psychiatric treatment and research. In: S. Gershon and B. Shopsin (Eds.), *Lithium ion: Its Role in Psychiatric Research and Treatment.* New York: Plenum, 1973, 51-71.

SCHOU, M. Advances in lithium therapy. *Current Psychiatric Therapies,* 1976, 16: 139-153.

SCHRAG, P. & DIVOKY, D. *The Myth of the Hyperactive Child.* New York: Pantheon, 1975.

SCHULMAN, J. & REISMAN, J. An objective measure of hyperactivity. *American Journal of Mental Deficiency,* 1959, 64:455-456.

SCOTT, K. Recognition memory: A research strategy and a summary of initial findings. *International Review of Research in Mental Retardation,* 1971, 5:83-111.

SEEMAN, P. & LEE, T. Neuroleptic drugs: Direct correlations between clinical potency and presynaptic action and dopamine neurons. In: G. Sedvall, B. Uvnäs, and Y. Zotterman (Eds.), *Antipsychotic Drugs: Pharmacodynamics and Pharmacokinetics.* New York: Pergamon Press, 1976.

SEEMAN, P., STAIMAN, A., LEE, T., & CHAO-WONG, M. The membrane actions of tranquilizers in relation to neuroleptic induced Parkinsonism and tardive dyskinesia. In: I. Forrest, C. Carr, and E. Usdin (Eds.), *Phenothiazines and Structurally Related Drugs.* New York: Raven Press, 1974.

SEGER, E. & HALLUM, G. Methylphenidate in children with minimal brain dysfunction: Effects on attention span, visual-motor skills, and behavior. *Current Therapeutic Research,* 1974, 16:635-641.

SELVINI, A., ROSSI, C., CORALLO, S., & LUCCHELLI, P. Antidepressant treatment with maprotiline in the management of emotional disturbances in patients with acute myocardiac infarction: A controlled study. *Journal of International Medical Research,* 1976, 4:42-49.

SEMMEL, M. Arousal theory and vigilance behavior of educable mentally retarded and average children. *American Journal of Mental Deficiency,* 1965, 70:38-47.

SENN, H., JUNGI, W., KUNZ, H., & POLDINGER, W. Clozapine and agranulocytosis. *Lancet,* 1977, 1:547 (letter).

SERRANO, A. & FORBIS, O. Haloperidol for pyschiatric disorders in children. *Diseases of the Nervous System,* 1973, 34:226-231.

SEWELL, J. & WERRY, J. S. Some studies in an institution for the mentally retarded. *New Zealand Medical Journal,* 1976, 84:317-319.

SHADER, R. *Manual of Psychiatric Therapies: Practical Psychiatry and Psychopharmacology.* Boston: Little Brown, 1975.
SHADER, R. & DIMASCIO, A. *Psychotropic Drug Side Effects.* Baltimore: Williams & Wilkins, 1970.
SHAFFER, D. The association between enuresis and emotional disorder: A review as a literature. In: I. Kolvin, R. MacKeith, & S. Meadow. *Bladder Control in Enuresis* (Clinics in Developmental Medicine, Nos. 48/49) London: Heinemann, 1973, 118-136.
SHAFFER, D. Personal communication, 1977.
SHAFFER, D., MCNAMARA, N., & PINCUS, J. Controlled observations on patterns of activity, attention, and impulsivity in brain-damaged and psychiatrically disturbed boys. *Psychological Medicine,* 1974, 4:4-18.
SHAFFER, D. & STEPHENSON, J. Studies in enuresis I, alpha blockade in local anesthesia in the control of enuresis with the tricyclic antidepressants. Unpublished ms, 1977.
SHAMSIE, S. & BARRIGA, C. The hazards of monoamine oxidase inhibitors in disturbed adolescents. *Canadian Medical Association Journal,* 1971, 104:715.
SHAPIRO, A., SHAPIRO, E., & WAYNE, H. Treatment of Tourette's syndrome. *Archives of General Psychiatry,* 1973, 28:92-97.
SHARPE, D. A controlled trial of trifluoperazine in the treatment of the mentally subnormal patient. *Journal of Mental Science,* 1962, 108:220-224.
SHAW, C., LOCKETT, H., LUCAS, A., LAMONTAGNE, C., & GRIMM, F. Tranquilizer drugs in the treatment of emotionally disturbed children: I. Inpatients in a residential treatment center. *Journal of the American Academy of Child Psychiatry,* 1963, 2:725-742.
SHEARD, M., MARINI, J., BRIDGES, C., & WAGNER, E. The effect of lithium on impulsive aggressive behavior in man. *American Journal of Psychiatry,* 1976, 133:1409-1413.
SHERRILL, R. Six swell exposés that came to practically nothing. *Washington Post,* March 18, 1973.
SHETTY, J. Alpha rhythms in the hyperkinetic child. *Nature,* 1971, 234:476.
SHIELDS, W. & BRAY, P. A danger of haloperidol therapy in children. *The Journal of Pediatrics,* 1976, 88:301-303.
SHINE, L. C. & BOWER, S. M. A one-way analysis of variance for single-subject designs. *Educational and Psychological Measurements,* 1971, 31:105-113.
SHIRKEY, H. Clinical pharmacology in pediatrics. *Clinical Pharmacology and Therapeutics,* 1972, 13:827-830.
SHOPSIN, B. & GERSHON, S. Toxicology of the lithium ion in lithium: Its role in psychiatric research and treatment. In: S. Gershon and B. Shopsin (Eds.), *Lithium ion: Its Role in Psychiatric Treatment and Research.* New York: Plenum Press, 1973, 107-147.
SHOPSIN, B. & KLINE, N. Monamine oxidase inhibitors: Potential for drug abuse. *Biological Psychiatry,* 1976, 11:451-456.
SIBER, G., ECHEVERRIA, R., SMITH, A., PAISLEY, J., & SMITH, D. Pharmacokinetics of gentamicin in children and adults. *Journal of Infectious Diseases,* 1975, 132:637-651.
SIDIROPOULOS, D. & BICKEL, M. Eine tödliche Vergiftung mit Imipramine in Kleiner Dosis bei einem Kleinlind. *Schweizer Medizinische Wochenschrift,* 1971, 101:851-855.
SIEGAL, S. *Nonparametric Statistics for the Behavioral Sciences.* New York: McGraw-Hill, 1956.
SIGG, E. Pharmacological studies with Tofranil. *Canadian Psychiatric Association Journal,* 1959, 4: (Supplement), 75-85.

SILBERSTEIN, R., COOPER, A., MILLER, L., & MANDELL, W. Avoiding institutionalizing psychotic children. *International Journal of Neuropsychiatry*, 1965, 7:144-148.

SILVERMAN, M. & LEE, P. R. *Pills, Profits, and Politics.* Berkeley: University of California Press, 1974.

SIMEON, J., SALETU, B., SALETU, M., ITIL, T., & DASILVA, J. Thiothixene in childhood psychoses. In: I. Forrest, C. Carr, and E. Usdin (Eds.), *Phenothiazines and Structurally Related Drugs.* New York: Raven Press, 1974.

SIMS, V. Review of the wide range achievement test. In *The Third Mental Measurements Yearbook.* New Brunswick, N.J.: Rutgers University Press, 1949, pp. 47-48.

SINGER, I. & ROTENBERG, D. Mechanism of lithium action. *New England Journal of Medicine*, 1973, 289:254-260.

SLEATOR, E., VON NEUMANN, A., & SPRAGUE, R. Hyperactive children: A continuous long-term placebo-controlled follow-up. *Journal of the American Medical Association*, 1974, 229:316-317.

SLOAN, W. The Lincoln Oseretsky motor development scale. *Genetic Psychology monographs*, 1955, 183-252.

SMART, R. & JONES, D. Illicit LSD users—their personality characteristics and psychopathology. *Journal of Abnormal Psychology*, 1970, 75:286-292.

SMITH, W. & LOWREY, J. The effects of diphenylhydantoin on cognitive functions in man. In: W. Smith (Ed.), *Drugs, Development and Cerebral Function.* Springfield, Illinois: Charles C Thomas, 1972.

SMITH, W. & LOWREY, J. The effects of diphenylhydantoin on concentration in the elderly. *Journal of the American Geriatric Society*, 1975, 23:207-211.

SMITH, W., PHILIPPUS, M., & GUARD, H. Psychometric study of children with learning problems and 14-6 positive spike EEG patterns, treated with ethosuximide (Zarontin) and placebo. *Archives of Disease in Childhood*, 1968, 43:616-619.

SMITH, W. & WEYL, T. The effects of ethosuximide (Zarontin*) on intellectual functions of children with learning deficits and cortical brain dysfunction. *Current Therapeutic Research*, 1968, 10:265-269.

SNYDER, S., BANERJEE, S., YAMAMURA, H., & GREENBERG, D. Drugs, neurotransmitters, and schizophrenia. *Science*, 1974, 184:1243-1253.

SNYDER, S., ENNA, E., BIRD, E., BENNETT, J., BYLUND, D., YAMAMURA, H., & IVERSEN, L. Huntington's chorea: Changes in neurotransmitter receptors in the brain. *New England Journal of Medicine*, 1976, 294:1305-1309.

SNYDER, S. & YAMAMURA, H. Antidepressants and the muscarinic acetylcholine receptor. *Archives of General Psychiatry*, 1977, 34:236-239.

SOBLEN, R. & SAUNDERS, S. J. Monoamine oxidase inhibitor therapy in adolescent psychiatry. *Diseases of the Nervous System*, 1961, 22:96-100.

SOLOMONS, G. The hyperactive child. *Journal of the Iowa Medical Society*, 1965, 55:464-469.

SOMMERFELD-ZISKIND, E. & ZISKIND, E. Effect of phenobarbital on the mentality of epileptic patients. *Archives of Neurology and Psychiatry*, 1940, 43:70-79.

SONNEN, A., ZELVELDER, W., & BRUENS, J. A double-blind study of the influence of dipropylacetate on behaviour. *Acta Neurologica Scandanavica*, Supplement 60, 1975, pp. 43-47.

SPITZER, R., ENDICOTT, J., & ROBINS, E. Clinical criteria for psychiatric diagnosis and DSM III. *American Journal of Psychiatry*, 1975, 132:1187-1192.

SPITZER, R. & SHEEHY, M. DSM III: A classification system in development. *Psychiatric Annals*, 1976, 6:448-451.

SPIVACK, G. & SWIFT, M. The classroom behavior of children: A critical review of teacher administered rating scales. *Journal of Special Education*, 1973, 7:55-89.

SPRAGUE, R. L. Psychopharmacology and learning disabilities. *Journal of Operational Psychiatry*, 1972, 3:56-67.

SPRAGUE, R. Recommended performance measures of psychotropic drug investigations. *Psychopharmacology Bulletin,* 1973a, Special Issue, 85-88.
SPRAGUE, R. Minimal brain dysfunction from a behavioral viewpoint. *The Annals of the N.Y. Academy of Sciences,* 1973b, 205:349-361.
SPRAGUE, R. L. Research with preschool children and FDA regulations. In: R. L. Sprague (Chair.), *Hyperactivity: Treatments for Preschool Children.* Symposium presented at the meeting of the Council for Exceptional Children, Atlanta, April 1977 (a).
SPRAGUE, R. L. Psychopharmacotherapy in children. In: M. F. McMillan and S. Henao (Eds.), *Child Psychiatry.* New York: Brunner/Mazel, 1977 (b).
SPRAGUE, R. Performance measures in pediatric psychopharmacology. In *Guidelines for Studies of Psychoactive Drugs in Infants and Children.* Rockville, Md.: U.S. Food & Drug Administration—in press (b).
SPRAGUE, R., BARNES, K., & WERRY, J. Methylphenidate and thioridazine: Learning, reaction time, activity, and classroom behavior in disturbed children. *American Journal of Orthopsychiatry,* 1970, 40:615-628.
SPRAGUE, R. L. & BAXLEY, G. B. Drugs used for the management of behavior in mental retardation. In: N. R. Ellis (Ed.), *Handbook of Mental Deficiency* (2nd ed.). New York: Erlbaum, in press.
SPRAGUE, R., CHRISTENSEN, D., & WERRY, J. Experimental psychology in stimulant drugs. In: C. Conners (Ed.), *Clinical Use of Stimulant Drugs in Children.* Amsterdam: Excerpta Medica, 1974, pp. 141-163.
SPRAGUE, R. L. & GADOW, K. D. The role of the teacher in drug treatment. In: J. J. Bosco and S. S. Robin (Eds.), *The Hyperactive Child and Stimulant Drugs.* Chicago: University of Chicago Press, 1977.
SPRAGUE, R. & SLEATOR, E. Effects of psychopharmacologic agents on learning disorders. *Pediatric Clinics of North America,* 1973, 20:719-735.
SPRAGUE, R., & SLEATOR, E. What is the proper dose of stimulant drugs in children? *International Journal of Mental Health,* 1975, 4:75-118.
SPRAGUE, R. & TOPPE, L. Relationship between activity level and delay of reinforcement in the retarded. *Journal of Experimental Child Psychology,* 1966, 3:390-397.
SPRAGUE, R. L. & WERRY, J. S. Methodology of psychopharmacological studies with the retarded. In: N. R. Ellis (Ed.), *International Review of Research in Mental Retardation,* Vol. 5. New York: Academic Press, 1971.
SPRAGUE, R. & WERRY, J. Psychotropic drugs in handicapped children. In: L. Mann, and D. Sabatino (Eds.), *Second Review of Special Education.* Philadelphia: JSE Press, 1974, pp. 1-50.
SPRING, C., GREENBERG, L., SCOTT, J., & HOPWOOD, J. Electrodermal activity in hyperactive boys who are methylphenidate responders. *Psychophysiology,* 1974, 11: 436-442.
SPRING, C., YELLIN, A., & GREENBERG, L. Effects of imipramine and methylphenidate on perceptual-motor performance of hyperactive children. *Perceptual and Motor Skills,* 1976, 42:459-470.
SPROGIS, G., LEZDINS, V., WHITE, S., MING, C., LANNING, M., DRAKE, M., & WYCKOFF, G. Comparative study on thorazine and serpasil in the mentally defective. *American Journal of Mental Deficiency,* 1957, 61:737-742.
SROUFE, L. Drug treatment of children with behavior problems. In: F. Horowitz (Ed.), *Review of Child Development Research,* Vol. 4. Chicago: University of Chicago Press, 1975, pp. 347-407.
SROUFE, L., SONIES, B., WEST, W., & WRIGHT, F. Anticipatory heart rate deceleration and reaction time in children with and without referral for learning disability. *Child Development,* 1973, 44:267-273.
STACK, J. Chemotherapy in childhood depression. In: A. Annell (Ed.), *Depressive States in Childhood and Adolescence.* New York: Halsted Press, 1972.

STANTON, M. & BARDONI, A. Drug flashbacks: Reported frequency in a military population. *American Journal of Psychiatry*, 1972, 129:751-755.
STEG, J. & RAPOPORT, J. Minor physical anomalies in normal, neurotic, learning disabled and severely disturbed children. *Journal of Autism and Childhood Schizophrenia*, 1975, 5:299-307.
STEPHENS, J. & SHAFFER, J. A controlled study of the effects of diphenylhydantoin on anxiety, irritability and anger in neurotic outpatients. *Psychopharmacologia (Berlin)*, 1970, 17:169-181.
STERN, D., FIEVE, R., NEFF, N., & COSTA, E. The effect of lithium chloride administration on brain and heart norepinephrine turnover rates. *Psychopharmacologia*, 1969, 14:315-322.
STEVENSON, H. Discrimination learning. In: N. Ellis (Ed.), *Handbook of Mental Deficiency*. New York: McGraw-Hill, 1963, pp. 424-438.
STORES, G. Studies of attention and seizure disorders. *Developmental Medicine & Child Neurology*, 1973, 15:376-382.
STORES, G. Behavioural effects of antiepileptic drugs. *Developmental Medicine & Child Neurology*, 1975, 17:647-658.
STORES, G. Behaviour disturbance and type of epilepsy in children attending ordinary school. In: J. Penry (Ed.), *Epilepsy: The Eighth International Symposium*. New York: Raven Press, 1977.
STORES, G. & HART, J. Reading skills of children with generalised or focal epilepsy attending ordinary school. *Developmental Medicine and Child Neurology*, 1976, 18:705-716.
STORES, G., HART, J., & PIRAN, N. Attentiveness and related behaviour in boys and girls with epilepsy attending ordinary school (submitted for publication), 1977.
STORES, G. & PIRAN, N. Dependency in boys and girls with epilepsy. (Submitted for publication), 1977.
STOREY, E. Editorial: The Tetracycline and children's teeth. *Drugs*, 1973, 6:321-323.
SUCKLING, P. Toxic effects of phenothiazine derivatives given for vomiting in children. *South African Medical Journal*, 1966, 40:1073.
SULMAN, F., PFEIFER, Y., & SUPERSTINE, E. Adrenal medullary exhaustion from tropical winds and its management. *Israel Journal of Medical Science*, 1973, 9:1022-1027.
SULZBACHER, S. I. Psychotropic medication with children: An evaluation of procedural biases in results of reported studies. *Pediatrics*, 1973, 51:513-517.
SVENSMARK, O. & BUCHTHAL, F. Diphenylhydantoin and phenobarbital serum levels in children. *American Journal of Diseases of Children*, 1964, 108:82-87.
SWANSON, J. & KINSBOURNE, M. Stimulant-related state-dependent learning in hyperactive children. *Science*, 1976, 192:1354-1357.
SWANSON, J., ROBERTS, W., KINSBOURNE, M., & ZUCKER, K. A time-response-analysis of the effect of stimulant medication on the learning ability of children referred for hyperactivity—submitted for publication 1977.
SWINDLER, G. *Handbook of Drug Interactions*. New York: John Wiley, 1971.
SYKES, D., DOUGLAS, V., & MORGENSTERN, G. The effect of methylphenidate (Ritalin) on sustained attention in hyperactive children. *Psychopharmacologia*, 1972, 25:262-274.
SYKES, D., DOUGLAS, V., WEISS, G., & MINDE, K. Attention in hyperactive children and the effect of methylphenidate (Ritalin). *Journal of Child Psychology and Psychiatry*, 1971, 12:129-139.
TALSO, P. & CLARKE, R. Excretion and distribution of lithium in the dog. *American Journal of Physiology*, 1951, 166:202-208.
TARJAN, G., LOWERY, V., & WRIGHT, S. Use of chlorpromazine in 278 mentally deficient patients. *American Journal of Diseases of Children*, 1957, 94:294-300.
TATSUOKA, M. M. *Multivariate Analysis: Techniques for Educational and Psychological Research*. New York: Wiley, 1971.

TCHICALOFF, M. & GAILLARD, F. Quelques effects indésirables des médicaments antiépileptiques sur les rendements intellectuals. *Revue de Neuropsychiatrie Infantile*, 1970, 18:599-602.
THOMSEN, K. & SCHOU, M. Renal lithium excretion in man. *American Journal of Physiology*, 1968, 215:823-827.
TRAUTNER, E., MORRIS, R., NOACK, C., & GERSHON, S. The excretion and retention of ingested lithium and its effect on the ionic balance of man. *Medical Journal of Australia*, 1955, 42:280-291.
TRICK, K. Double-blind comparison of maprotiline with amitriptyline in the treatment of depressive illness. *International Pharmacopsychiatry*, 1976, 10:193-198.
TRIMBLE, M. & REYNOLDS, E. Anticonvulsant drugs and mental symptoms. *Psychological Medicine*, 1976, 6:169-178.
TUPIN, J., SCHALGENHAUF, G., & CRESON, D. Lithium effects on electrolyte excretion. *American Journal of Psychiatry*, 1968, 125:536-543.
TUPIN, J. & SMITH, D. The use of lithium in aggressive prisoners. *Psychopharmacology Bulletin*, 1973, 9:48.
UCER, E. & KREGER, K. A double-blind study comparing haloperidol with thioridazine in emotionally disturbed, mentally retarded children. *Current Therapeutic Research*, 1969, 11:278-283.
UHLENHUTH, E., STEPHENS, J., DIM, B., & COVI, L. Diphenylhydantoin and phenobarbital in the relief of psychoneurotic symptoms. *Psychopharmacologia*, 1972, 27: 67-84.
VALLARTA, J., BELL, D., & REICHART, A. Progressive encephalopathy due to chronic hydantoin intoxication. *American Journal of Diseases of Children*, 1974, 128: 27-34.
VAN KREVELEN, D. & VAN VOORST, J. Lithium in der Behandlung einer Psychose unklarer Genese bei einem Jugendlichen. *Acta Paedopsychiatrica*, 1959, 26:148-152.
VELIE, L. Is anybody watching? *Reader's Digest*, March 1976, 114-118.
VESSELL, E. & PAGE, J. Genetic control of drug levels in man: Antipyrine. *Science*, 1968, 161:72-73.
VESSELL, E., PASSANANTI, G., & GREENE, F. Impairment of drug metabolism in man by allopurinol and nortriptyline. *New England Journal of Medicine*, 1970, 283: 1484-1488.
VESSELL, E., PASSANANTI, G., GREENE, F., & PAGE, J. Genetic control of drug levels and of the induction of drug metabolising enzymes in man; individual variability in the extent of allopurinol and nortriptyline inhibition of drug metabolism. *Annals of the New York Academy of Sciences*, 1971, 179:752-773.
VOELLER, K. & ROTHENBERG, M. Psychosocial aspects of the management of seizures in children. *Pediatrics*, 1973, 51:1072-1082.
VOGEL, W., BROVERMAN, D., DRAGUNS, J., & KLAIBER, E. The role of glutamic acid in cognitive behavior. *Psychological Bulletin*, 1965, 65:367-382.
VOGEL, H., FEDER, B., HELMCHEN, B., MULLER-OERLINGHAUSER, B., BOHACEK, N., MIHOVICOVIC, M., BRANDL, A., FLEISCHHAUMER, J., & WALCHER, W. Mianserin versus amitriptymine. *International Pharmacopsychiatry*, 1976, 11:25-31.
VON HUNGEN, K. & ROBERTS, S. Neurotransmitter-sensitive adenylate cyclase systems in the brain. In: S. Ehrenpreis and I. Kopin (Eds.), *Reviews of Neuroscience*, Vol. 1. New York: Raven Press, 1974.
WADE, D. Personal communication, 1977.
WADE, M. Effects of methylphenidate on motor skill acquisition of hyperactive children. *Journal of Learning Disabilities*, 1976, 9:48-52.
WAITES, L. & KEELE, D. Fluphenazine in management of disturbed mentally retarded children. *Diseases of the Nervous System*, 1963, 24:113-114.
WAIZER, J., HOFFMAN, S., POLIZOS, P., & ENGELHARDT, D. Outpatient treatment of

hyperactive school children with imipramine. *American Journal of Psychiatry,* 1974, 131:587-591.

WAIZER, J., POLIZOS, P., HOFFMAN, S., ENGELHARDT, D., & MARGOLIS, R. A single blind evaluation of thiothixene with outpatient schizophrenic children. *Journal of Autism and Child Schizophrenia,* 1972, 2:378-386.

WALDMEIER, P., BAUMANN, P., GREENGRASS, P., & MAITRE, L. Effects of chlorimipramine and other tricyclic antidepressants on biogenic amine uptake and turnover. *Postgraduate Medical Journal,* 1976, 52: (Supplement #3), 33-39.

WALDROP, M., PEDERSEN, F., & BELL, R. Minor physical anomalies and behavior in preschool children. *Child Development,* 1968, 38:391-400.

WALKER, D. *Socioemotional Measures for Preschool and Kindergarten Children.* San Francisco: Jossey-Bass, 1973.

WALKER, S., III. Drugging the American child. We're too cavalier about hyperactivity. *Psychology Today,* 1974, 8: No. 7, 43-48.

WALLINGA, J. Use of a phenothiazine derivative, thioridazine, in the treatment of childhood emotional disorders. *Acta Paedopsychiatrica,* 1963, 30:211-225.

WALTER, R. & GROSSMAN, H. Positive spiking—a signal in a search for signficance. *Electroencephalography and Clinical Neurophysiology,* 1963, 15:161-162.

WAPNER, I., THURSTON, D., & HOLOWACH, J. Phenobarbital: Its effect on learning in epileptic children. *Journal of the American Medical Association,* 1962, 182:937.

WARNEKE, L. A case of manic-depressive illness in childhood. *Canadian Psychiatric Association Journal,* 1975, 20:195-200.

WEBER, B. & SULZBACHER, S. Use of CNS stimulant medication in averaged electroencephalic audiometry with children with MBD. *Journal of Learning Disabilities,* 1975, 8:300-303.

WEDKOS, M. Cardiac changes related to phenothiazine therapy with special reference to thioridazine. *Journal of the American Geriatric Society,* 1967, 15:20-28.

WEINBERG, W. & BRUMBACK, R. Mania in childhood. *American Journal of Diseases of Children,* 1976, 130:380-385.

WEINBERG, W., RUTMAN, J., & SULLIVAN, L. et al. Depression in children referred to an educational diagnostic center: Diagnosis and treatment. *Journal of Pediatrics,* 1973, 83:1065-1072.

WEINSTEIN, L. & DALTON, A. Host determinants of response to anti-microbial agents. *New England Medical Journal,* 1968, 279:467-473.

WEISS, B. & LATIES, V. Enhancement of human performance by caffeine and the amphetamines. *Pharmacological Review,* 1962, 14:1-36.

WEISS, C., HEFFELFINGER, J., & BUCHANAN, R. Serial Dilantin levels in mentally retarded children. *American Journal of Mental Deficiency,* 1969, 73:826-830.

WEISS, G. The natural history of hyperactivity in childhood and treatment with stimulant medication at different ages: A summary of research findings. *International Journal of Mental Health,* 1975, 4:213-216.

WEISS, G., KRUGER, E., DANIELSON, U., & ELMAN, M. Effect of long-term treatment of hyperactive children with methylphenidate. *Canadian Medical Association Journal,* 1975, 112:159-165.

WEISS, G., MINDE, K., DOUGLAS, V., WERRY, J., & SYKES, D. Comparison of the effects of chlorpromazine, dextroamphetamine and methylphenidate on the behaviour and intellectual functioning of hyperactive children. *Canadian Medical Association Journal,* 1971a, 104:20-25.

WEISS, G., MINDE, K., WERRY, J., DOUGLAS, V., & NEMETH, E. Studies on the hyperactive child. *Archives of General Psychiatry,* 1971b, 24:409-414.

WEISS, G., WERRY, J., MINDE, K., DOUGLAS, V., & SYKES, D. The effects of dextroamphetamine and chlorpromazine on behavior and intellectual functioning. *Journal of Child Psychology and Psychiatry,* 1968, 9:145-156.

WELSCH V. LITKINS. *Clearinghouse Review,* 1976, 10:(2), 148.

WENDER, P. *Minimal Brain Dysfunction in Children.* New York: John Wiley & Sons, 1971.
WERRY, J. Developmental hyperactivity. *Pediatric Clinics of North America,* 1968a, 15:581-599.
WERRY, J. The diagnosis, etiology, and treatment of hyperactivity in children. *Learning Disorders,* 1968b, 3:173-190.
WERRY, J. Some clinical and laboratory studies of psychotropic drugs in children: An overview. In: W. L. Smith (Ed.), *Drugs and Cortical Function,* (Vol 1). Springfield, Ill: Charles C Thomas, 1970.
WERRY, J. Diagnosis for psychopharmacological studies in children. *Psychopharmacology Bulletin,* 1973, Special Issue (Pharmocotherapy of Children), 89-141.
WERRY, J. Medication for hyperkinetic children. *Drugs,* 1976a, 11:81-89.
WERRY, J. Diet and hyperactivity. *Medical Journal of Australia,* 1976b, 2:281-282.
WERRY, J. The use of psychotropic drugs in children. *Journal of the American Academy of Child Psychiatry,* 1977, 16:446-468.
WERRY, J. Behavior observations and activity measures for use in pediatric psychopharmacology. In *Guidelines for Evaluation of Psychoactive Agents in Infants and Children.* Rockville, Md.: Food and Drug Administration—in press (a).
WERRY, J. Organic factors in childhood psychopathology. In: H. Quay and J. Werry (Eds.), *Psychopathological Disorders of Childhood* (2nd ed.). New York: Wiley—in press (b).
WERRY, J. The childhood psychoses. In: H. Quay and J. Werry (Eds.), *Psychopathological Disorders of Childhood* (2nd Ed.). New York: Wiley—in press (c).
WERRY, J. & AMAN, M. Methylphenidate and haloperidol in children. Effects on attention, memory and activity. *Archives of General Psychiatry,* 1975, 32:790-795.
WERRY, J. & AMAN, M. The reliability and diagnostic validity of the physical and neurological examination for soft signs (PANESS). *Journal of Autism and Childhood Schizophrenia,* 1976, 6:253-262.
WERRY, J., AMAN, M., & LAMPEN, E. Haloperidol and methylphenidate in hyperactive children. *Acta Paedopsychiatrica,* 1976a, 42:26-40.
WERRY, J., AMAN, M., & LAMPEN, E. Imipramine and chlordiazepoxide in enuresis. Paper presented to the Annual NIMH ECDEU Conference, Key Biscayne, Fla. 1976b.
WERRY, J., AMAN, M., & LAMPEN, E. The effect of imipramine and methylphenidate in hyperactive aggressive children. Paper presented to the Annual meeting of the Australia and New Zealand College of Psychiatrists, Brisbane, 1977.
WERRY, J., DOWRICK, P., LAMPEN, E., & VAMOS, M. Imipramine in enuresis—psychological and physiological effects. *Journal of Child Psychology and Psychiatry,* 1975a, 16:289-300.
WERRY, J. & HAWTHORNE, D. Conners teacher questionnaire—norms and validity. *Australian and New Zealand Journal of Psychiatry,* 1976, 10:257-262.
WERRY, J., MINDE, K., GUZMAN, A., WEISS, G., DOGAN, K., & HOY, E. Studies on the hyperactive child. VII: Neurological status compared with neurotic and normal children. *American Journal of Orthopsychiatry,* 1972, 42:441-451.
WERRY, J. & QUAY, H. Observing the classroom behavior of elementary school children. *Exceptional Children,* 1969, 35:461-469.
WERRY, J. & SPRAGUE, R. Hyperactivity. In: C. Costello (Ed.), *Symptoms of Psychopathology.* New York: Wiley, 1970.
WERRY, J. & SPRAGUE, R. Psychopharmacology. In: J. Wortis (Ed.), *Mental Retardation,* (Vol. 4). New York: Grune & Stratton, 1972, pp. 63-79.
WERRY, J. & SPRAGUE, R. Methylphenidate in children—effect of dosage. *Australian and New Zealand Journal of Psychiatry,* 1974, 8:9-19.

WERRY, J., SPRAGUE, R., & COHEN, M. Conners' teacher rating scale for use in drug studies with children. *Journal of Abnormal Child Psychology*, 1975b, 3:217-229.

WERRY, J., WEISS, G., DOUGLAS, V., & MARTIN, J. Studies on the hyperactive child. III. The effect of chlorpromazine upon behavior and learning ability. *Journal of the American Academy of Child Psychiatry*, 1966, 5:292-312.

WERRY, J. & WOLLERSHEIM, J. Behavior therapy with children. *Journal of American Academy of Child Psychiatry*, 1967, 6:346-370.

WHALEN, C. & HENKER, B. Psychostimulants and children: A review and analysis. *Psychological Bulletin*, 1976, 83:1113-1130.

WHALEY-KLAHN, M., LONEY, J., WEISSENBURGER, F., & PRINZ, R. Responses of boys and girls to a behaviorally-focused school attitude questionnaire. *Journal of School Psychology*, 1976, 14:283-290.

WHITEHEAD, P. & CLARK, L. Effect of lithium carbonate, placebo, and thioridazine on hyperactive children. *American Journal of Psychiatry*, 1970, 127:824-825.

WILES, D., KOLAKOWSKA, T., MCNIELLY, A., MANDELBROTE, B., & GELDER, M. Clinical significance of plasma chlorpromazine levels. *Psychological Medicine*, 1976, 6:407-416.

WILK, S., SHOPSIN, B., GERSHON, S., & SUHL, M. Cerebrospinal fluid levels of MHPG in affective disorder. *Nature*, 1972, 235:440-441.

WILLCOX, D., GILLAN, R., & HARE, E. Do psychiatric outpatients take their drugs? *British Medical Journal*, 1965, 2:790-792.

WILSON, J. Compliance with instructions in the evaluation of therapeutic efficacy. *Clinical Pediatrics*, 1973, 12:333-340.

WINSBERG, B. Neuropsychiatric issues in developmental subnormality. In: I. Bialer and M. Sternlicht (Eds.), *The Psychology of Mental Retardation: Issues and Approaches*. New York: Psychological Dimensions Inc., 1977.

WINSBERG, B., BIALER, I., KUPIETZ, S., & TOBIAS, J. Effects of imipramine and dextroamphetamine on behavior of neuropsychiatrically impaired children. *American Journal of Psychiatry*, 1972, 128:1425-1431.

WINSBERG, B., GOLDSTEIN, S., YEPES, L., & PEREL, J. Imipramine and electrocardiographic abnormalities in hyperactive children. *American Journal Psychiatry*, 1975, 132:542-545.

WINSBERG, B., PEREL, J., HURWIC, M., & KLUTCH, A. Imipramine protein binding and pharmacokinetics in children. In: I. Lomest & E. Usdin (Eds.), *The Phenothiazines and Structurally Related Drugs*. New York: Raven Press, 1974a.

WINSBERG, B., PEREL, J., YEPES, L., & BOTTI, E. Imipramine plasma levels and behavioral response in hyperkinetic/aggressive children. Submitted for publication, 1977.

WINSBERG, B., PRESS, M., BIALER, I., & KUPIETZ, S. L. Dextroamphetamine and methylphenidate in the treatment of hyperactive/aggressive children. *Pediatrics*, 1974b, 53:236-241.

WINSBERG, B., YEPES, L., & BIALER, I. Pharmacological management of children with hyperactive/aggressive/inattentive behavior disorders. *Clinical Pediatrics*, 1976, 15:471-477.

WINSCHEL, J. & LAWRENCE, E. Short-term memory: Curricular implications for the mentally retarded. *Journal of Special Education*, 1975, 9:395-408.

WOLFSON, I. Clinical experience with serpasil and thorazine in treatment of disturbed behavior of mentally retarded. *American Journal of Mental Deficiency*, 1957, 62:276-283.

WOLPERT, A. & FARR, D. Psychotropics and their effect on the EKG in children. *Diseases of the Nervous System*, 1975, 36:435-436.

WOLPERT, A., HAGAMEN, M., & MERLIS, S. A comparative study of thiothixene and trifluoperazine in childhood schizophrenia. *Current Therapeutic Research*, 1967, 9:482-485.

WOLRAICH, M., DRUMMOND, T., SALOMON, M., O'BRIEN, M., & SIVAGE, C. Effects of methylphenidate alone and in combination with behavior modification procedures on the behavior and academic performance of hyperactive children. *Journal of Abnormal Child Psychology*—in press.

WONG, G. & COCK, R. Long-term effects of haloperidol on severely emotionlly disturbed children. *Australian and New Zealand Journal of Psychiatry*, 1971, 5:296-300.

WOODBURY, D., PENRY, J., & SCHMIDT, R. (Eds.). *Antiepileptic Drugs*. New York: Raven Press, 1972.

WORDARSKI, J., FELDMAN, R., & PEDI, S. The comparison of antisocial and prosocial children on multicriterion measures at summer camp. *Journal of Abnormal Child Psychology*, 1975, 3:255-274.

Wyatt v. Aderholt, 508 F.2d 1305 (1974).

Wyatt v. Stickney, 344 F. Supp. 387 (1972).

YEPES, L., BALKA, E., WINSBERG, B., & BIALER, I. Amitriptyline and methylphenidate treatment of behaviorally disordered children. *Journal of Child Psychology and Psychiatry*, 1977, 18:39-52.

YEPES, L. & WINSBERG, B. Vomiting during neuroleptic withdrawal in children. *The American Journal of Psychiatry*, in press.

YOLLES, S. Recent research on LSD, marijuana and other dangerous drugs. In: R. Horman and A. Fox (Eds.), *Drug Awareness*. New York: Avon, 1970, pp. 67-82.

YOSS, R. & MOYER, N. The pupillogram of the hyperkinetic child and the underachiever. *Abstracts of the 7th Colloquium on the Pupil*. Rochester, Minn.: Mayo Clinic, 1971.

YOSS, R. 1975—cited in Barkley 1977 (see above).

YOUNG, G. & TURNER, R. CNS stimulant drugs and conditioning treatment of nocturnal enuresis. *Behaviour Research Therapy*, 1965, 3:93-101.

ZAHN, T., ABATE, F., LITTLE, B., & WENDER, P. Minimal brain dysfunction, stimulant drugs and autonomic nervous system activity. *Archives of General Psychiatry*, 1975, 32:381-387.

ZEAMAN, D. & HOUSE, B. The role of attention in retardate discrimination learning. In: N. R. Ellis (Ed.), *Handbook of Mental Deficiency*. New York: McGraw-Hill, 1963, pp. 159-223.

ZERAHN, K. Studies on the active transport of lithium in the isolated frog skin. *Acta Physiologica Scandinavica*, 1955, 33:347-358.

ZIMMERMAN, F. Explosive behavior anomalies in children on an epileptic basis. *New York State Journal of Medicine*, 1956, 56:2537-2543.

ZRULL, J., WESTMAN, J., ARTHUR, B., & RICE, D. An evaluation of methodology used in the study of psychoactive drugs in children. *Journal of the American Academy of Child Psychiatry*, 1966, 5:284-291.

INDEX

Abnormal Involuntary Movement Scale (AIMS), 69
Absorption, 5
 children in, 15
Academic achievemnt
 drug effects and, 99-101
 drugs in combination with remedial education, 100
 lithium and, 322
 stimulants and, 185-186
 tricyclic antidepressants and, 217
Academic Underachievemnt Disorder, 165
Acetazolamide, 307
Acetophenazine, 250, 251, 261
Acetylation, 11
Acetylcholine, 22
 antipsychotic drugs and, 240
Achievement tests, 95
Action
 of drugs, 19, 21
 potential, 21
Activan
 see lorazepam
Activity (Motor)
 antidepressants and, 216, 229
 antipsychotics and, 244
 benzodiazepines and, 339
 lithium and, 322
 measures of, 58-63
Actometer, 62
Adjustment reactions, 161, 163
Adolescent disorders, 146
Adverse drug effects, 23 (see also individual drugs)
 classification, 24
 death from, 24
Aggressive Conduct Disorder, 162
Aggressiveness, lithium in, 325
Agranulocytosis, 252
 antidepressants and, 219

Akathisia, 250
Albutoin, 281, 288
Alcohol (see also depressants, general), 333-335, 340, 350, 352
Amitryptiline, 163, 209, 213, 217, 224
Amphetamines (see also stimulants), 171-207
 history of, xiii
Amylobarbitone
 cognitive function and, 291, 313
Anafranil (see clomipramine)
Analysis of covariance, 128
Analysis of variance, 128
Anatensol (see fluphenazine)
Anesthesia, stages of, 330
Anesthetic agents, 334
Anorexia Nervosa, 162
Antianxiety drugs, 164, 329-346
 antimuscarinic sedatives, 341-342
 anxiety in, 345
 cellular action of, 332
 classification, 334
 clinical indications, 342-346
 dependence, 335
 disinhibition, 333
 enzyme induction, 335
 general depressants, 334
 pharmacology, 331
 selective depressants, 334
 sleep, 335
 sleep disorders in, 342-344
 withdrawal symptoms, 335
Anticholinergic agents (see also antiparkinson drugs), 259
Anticholinergic effects
 of antipsychotic drugs, 248, 249
 tricyclic antidepressants and, 210, 212, 214, 215
Anticonvulsants (see antiepileptic drugs)

401

Antidepressants (see also MAOI, tricyclics, quadricyclics), 208-233
  activity and, 216, 229
  agranulocytosis and, 219
  anxiety in, 218, 222, 223, 232, 233
  antisocial behavior in, 221
  arrhythmias, 220
  attention and, 88
  blood brain barrier, 210, 212
  blood pressure, 215, 219
  blurred vision, 214
  cardiotoxicity, 212, 216, 219, 220, 223
  chlordiazepoxide and, 230
  cholinergic rebound symptoms, 224
  classes, 209
  clinical indications, 220-225, 231, 232-233
  cognitive style and, 89
  constipation, 214
  depression, in, 218, 222, 232, 233
  dryness of mouth, 214
  effects, 214-219, 228-230
  enuresis, in, 209, 214-215, 216-224, 232-233
  ethics and, 232
  flushing, 220
  hyperactivity in, 216, 217, 221, 223
  impulsivity in, 217
  insomnia, 214, 218
  intelligence and, 91
  interactions, 220, 231
  learning disorder and, 217, 223
  methylphenidate, comparative efficacy, 217, 222
  methylphenidate, interaction with, 220
  obsessional disorder in, 229, 233
  platelet MAO and, 228
  pharmacology, 210, 226
  phenobarbital and, 230
  phenothiazines, interaction with, 220
  phenothiazines, similarity to, 208, 209
  phobias in, 229, 231, 233
  Porteus Maze test and, 96, 217
  psychiatric disorders in, 214, 216, 218, 221, 229, 232
  psychosis and, 229
  REM sleep, 214, 228
  school phobia in, 209, 214, 217, 222, 225
  sedation, 220
  seizures, 219
  separation anxiety in, 218, 222, 231
  serotonin and, 212, 233
  short term memory and, 90
  side effects, 219, 220
  stimulants and, 216, 221, 223
  structure, 209
  tachycardia, 215, 220
  transmitter reuptake, 212
  urinary retention, 214
  weight loss, 220
  withdrawal symptoms, 215
Antiepileptics (see also individual drugs)
  adequate trial, 310
  administration, 280
  adverse behavioral effects, 274, 277, 279, 290, 312-315
  adverse physical effects, 279, 314
  antipsychotics and, 259
  change of treatment, 310
  choice of, 276, 309
  classification, 280
  cognitive function and, 290-292
  common structure, 279, 280
  contraindications, 280
  controlled studies, 278-279
  dosages, 280
  EEG and, 310
  half lives, 279
  idiosyncracy to, 279
  indications, 280
  intelligence and, 91
  interaction with non-drug treatment, 280
  interaction with other drugs, 280
  international glossary of, 280
  intoxication, 279
  limitations, 311
  mechanisms of action, 278
  metabolism related to age, 282
  misuse, 315
  pharmacology, 278
  placebo response, 315
  precautions, 280
  psychotropic effects, 274, 315
  serum levels, 279, 310-311
  side effects, 279, 312-314
  single daily dose, 309
  single drug treatment, 310
  treatment emergent effects, 279, 312-314
Antihelminthics, antipsychotics and, 259
Antihistamines (see antimuscarinic sedatives)
Antimedication movement, xv-xvi
Antimuscarinic sedatives
  antianxiety drugs as, 341-342
  clinical effects, 341
  hallucinogens and, 347
  pharmacology, 341
Antiparkinson drugs, 249

INDEX 403

Antipsychotics, 139, 145, 157, 158, 159, 234-273
  actions, 239-243
  activity level and, 244
  akathisia, 250
  anticonvulsants and, 259
  antihelminthics and, 259
  Anxiety Disorders in, 271-272
  attention and, 88
  blood pressure, 254
  chemical structure, 234-236
  clinical indications, 260-272
  cognitive function and, 245-247
  diuretics and, 259
  doses, 272-273
  drowsiness, 247
  drug interactions, 258-260
  dry mouth, 248
  dystonic reactions, 249
  EEG and, 243-244
  evoked potentials, 244
  extent of use, 109
  extrapyramidal symptoms, 249-251, 256, 258
  5-hydroxyindoleacetic acid (5-HIAA) and, 240
  gamma-amino butyric acid and, 240
  Gilles de la Tourette syndrome in, 271
  glaucoma, 259
  homovanillic acid (HVA) and, 240
  intelligence and, 91
  interactions, 258-260
  jaundice, 253-254
  learning, 241-247
  metabolism, 237-238
  paired associate learning and, 88
  parkinsonism and, 250, 251
  petition on, 131
  Porteus Mazes and, 95
  psychosis in, 260-264
  serum levels, 237-239
  short term memory and, 90
  side effects and toxicity, 247-258
  tardive dyskinesia, 256
Antisocial behavior
  antidepressants in, 221
Anxiety
  antianxiety drugs in, 345
  antidepressants in, 218, 222, 223, 232, 233
  measures of, 65
Anxiety Disorders, 163-164
  antipsychotic drugs in, 271-272
Anxiolytic (see antianxiety drugs)
Apparent volume of distribution (V_d), 11
Arithmetic skills, 165

Arrhythmias antidepressants with, 220
Articulation Disorder, 166
Assent to treatment, and research, 114, 115, 118
Atarax (see hydroxyzine)
Atropine, 341
Attention
  antidepressants and, 88
  antipsychotics and, 88
  hyperactivity in, 80-81
  mental retardation in, 84-85
  specific learning disorders in, 83
  stimulant drugs and, 87
Attention Deficit Disorders (see also hyperactivity), 155
  diagnosis and pharmacotherapy, 159-160, 162, 167, 198
  lithium in, 325
Atypical childhood psychosis, 158
Aura, 277
Autism (see psychosis)
  hallucinogens in, 352
  levodopa in, 352
  megavitamin therapy in, 354
  thyroid and, 353
Automatisms, 277

Barbiturates (see also individual drugs and depressants, general), 280, 288-293, 334
  disturbed behavior and, 278, 279
  sleep disorders and, 343
Beclamide, 308
Bed-wetting (see enuresis)
Behavior
  definition of, 46
  measures of, 46-58
  lithium and, 322
  observations, 56
  rating scales, 47-56
  stimulants, 186-188
Behavior Disorders (see psychiatric disorders)
Behavior Modification
  drugs and, 102-104
  stimulants and, 193-194
Behavior observations and learning, 98
Behavior Problem Checklist (BPC), 49
Behavior therapy (see behavior modification)
Behavior toxicity
  antipsychotic drugs and, 251
Benadryl (see diphenhydramine)
Bender Visual Motor Gestalt test

antipsychotic drugs and, 92
stimulant drugs and, 92
Benuride (see pheneturide)
Benzedrine (see amphetamine)
Benzodiazepines, 164, 336-341
　activity, 339
　clinical effects, 302, 339
　dependence, 340
　diphenyldantoin and, 287, 302
　drug interactions and, 340
　EEG, 302, 339
　enzyme induction, 339
　epilepsy and, 281, 301-302
　indications, 303
　interactions, 302
　muscle relaxation, 339
　pharmacology, 301, 337
　phenytoin and, 287, 302
　psychomotor function and, 339
　psychotropic effects, 301-302
　REM sleep, 339
　side effects, 302, 340
　sites of action, 338
　sleep disorders and, 343
　sodium valproate and, 302
　treatment emergent effects, 302, 340
　withdrawal symptoms, 340
Benztropine mesylate, 249
Bioavailability, 6
　effect on metabolism, 10
Biotransformation, 8, 9
Blood-brain barrier, 7
　antidepressants and, 210, 212
Blood dyscrasias
　antipsychotics and, 252
　propanediols and, 340
Blood pressure
　antidepressants and, 215, 219
　antipsychotics and, 254
　monoaxine oxidase inhibitors and, 229
Body surface area, 17
Brain, entry of drugs, 7
Brandy, 334
Bromides, 288
Bufotenin, 347
Butyrophenones (see also antipsychotics), 234, 236, 263

Caffeine (see also stimulants), 171-207
California Personality Inventory, 46
Cannabis (see Hallucinogens)
Cannaboids, 347
Carbamazepine, 276, 281, 294
　antiepileptic effects, 295

clinical effects, 295-297
diphenylhydantoin and, 287
effect on EEG, 295
indications in psychiatric disorders, 298
indications in seizure disorders, 298
metabolite, 294
pharmacology, 294
phenytoin and, 287
psychiatric disorders in, 296-297
psychotropic effects, 295-297
side effects, 297
structure, 294
therapeutic range, 295
treatment emergent effects, 297
tricyclic antidepressants, 294
Cardiotoxicity of antidepressants, 212, 216, 219, 220, 223
Cardiovascular reactions of antipsychotics, 254
CAT, 46
Catecholamines, 22
　stimulants and, 174
Cell membrane, 4, 21
Celontin (see methsuximide)
CGI (see Clinical Global Impressions)
Chelating substances, 354
Chemical structure, 21
Child, definition of, vii
Child psychiatric (see psychiatric)
Childhood psychoses (see psychosis, pervasive developmental disorders)
Children's Behavior Inventory (CBI), 50, 52, 54
Children's Diagnostic Classification (CDS), 44
Children's Manifest Anxiety Scale, 65
Children's Personal Data Inventory (CPDI), 42
Children's Psychiatric Rating Scale (CPRS), 45, 53
Children's Symptom History, 42
Chloral hydrate (see also depressants, general), 334, 343
Chlordiazepoxide (see also benzodiazepines), 301, 337, 339
　antidepressants and, 230
Chlorpromazine (see also antipsychotics), 163, 248, 249, 250, 251, 252, 253, 254, 255, 258, 262
　antimuscarinic sedative as, 342
　hyperactivity in, 267
　mental retardation in, 264
　psychosis in, 260-262
　seizures and, 251-252
　sleep disorders and, 343

Chlorprothixene (see thioxanthenes, antipsychotics)
Chromosomal abnormalities, hallucinogens and, 350
Classroom Behavior Inventory, 50
Clearance, 12
Clinical Global Impressions (CGI), 52, 53, 64
Clinical trials (see drug studies)
Clomipramine, 212, 233
Clonazepam (see also Benzodiazepines), 276, 301, 302
   diphenylhydantoin and, 302
   phenytoin and, 302
   sodium valproate and, 305
Clozapine, 241, 249, 252
Cogentin (see benztropine)
Cognitive deficits
   hyperactivity in, 80-82
   mental retardation, 84-85
   specific learning disorders, 83-84
Cognitive function
   antianxiety drugs and, 334, 339
   antiepileptics and, 290-291
   antipsychotics and, 245-247
   drugs and, 87-94
   lithium and, 322
   measures of, 87-101
   psychomotor function, 339
   stimulants and, 181-185
   tricyclic antidepressants and, 216-217
Cognitive style
   antidepressants and, 89
   hyperactivity in, 81-82
   specific learning disorders in, 83
   stimulant drugs and, 89
Commission (see National Commission)
Compartments, 6, 11
Compazine (see prochlorperazine)
Compliance, 26
Conduct disorders, 155, 209, 218, 231
   diagnoses and pharmacotherapy, 159, 161-162
   socialized, 161, 162
   stimulants in, 198
   undersocialized, 161
Conjugation, 10
Conners' Parent Questionnaire (PQ), 51
Conners' Teacher Questionnaire (TQ), 48, 49
Consent, informed, 114, 115, 118
Convulsive equivalent syndrome, 284, 314
Correlation coefficients, 127-128
Council on Exceptional Children, 111
CPZ (see chlorpromazine)

Cyclic AMP
   antipsychotic drugs and, 240
   lithium and, 319
   stimulants and, 174
Cylert (see pemoline)
Cyproheptadine, 163

Dalmane (see flurazepam)
Davids Hyperkinetic Scale, 50
Deaner (see deanol)
Deanol (see also stimulants), 171-207
Delinquency, 162
Depakine (see sodium valproate)
Dependence
   antianxiety drugs, 335
   hallucinogens, 351
Depolarization, 21
Depot preparation, 6
Depressants (see antianxiety drugs)
Depressants, general, 334-337
   psychomotor function and, 334
   REM sleep, 335
Depressants, selective (see also benzodiazepines), 336-341
Depression
   antidepressants in, 218, 222, 232, 233
   children in, 208, 219, 222, 223, 231
   measures, 65
   somatic symptoms and, 223
Dermatologic toxicity
   antipsychotic drugs and, 255, 258
Design of drug studies, 121-126, 128
Desipramine, 210, 212, 233
Desmethyl-imipramine, 209
Devereux Elementary School Behavior Rating Scale, 49
Dexedrine (see dextroamphetamine)
Dextroamphetamine (see also stimulants), 171-207
Diabetes and monoamine oxidase inhibitors (MAOI), 229
Diabetes insipidus and lithium, 324
Diagnosis, measures of, 44
Diagnosis in child psychiatry
   American (DSM III), 141-154
   classification systems of, 136-167
   criteria for, 149-151
   DSM III, 141-154
   ICD-9, 141-146, 151-166
   indications for pharmacotherapy, 155-167
   International (ICD-9), 141-146, 151-166
   pharmacotherapy and, 155-167
   principles of, 137-140
Diamox (see Acetazolamide)

Diazepam, 337-341
  chemical structure, 335
  clinical effect in epilepsy, 301, 302
  cognitive function and, 291, 313
  epilepsy and (see also benzodiazepines), 301-303, 313
  indications in epilepsy, 303
  pharmacology, 302
  psychotropic effects, 302
  release and aggression, 333
Dibenzoxazepines (see dibenzoxapines)
Dibenzoxapines, 234, 238
Dihydroindolones, 234
Dilantin (see diphenylhydantoin)
Diphenhydramine, 249, 341, 346
  extrapyramidal symptoms in, 249
  sleep disorders and, 343
Diphenylhydantoin (phenytoin), 276, 281-287
  abnormal EEGs and, 284, 287
  benzodiazepines and, 287
  carbamazepine and, 287
  chemical structure, 276, 281
  clinical effects in epilepsy, 283
  cognitive function and, 283, 285, 286, 287, 312-314
  cosmetic effects, 284, 314
  degenerative disorders and, 285
  encephalopathy, 285
  epileptic equivalent and, 284
  half life, 282
  increased seizure frequency and, 310
  indications, 287
  interactions, 281, 287, 306, 310
  methylphenidate and, 286
  neurological impairment and, 284-286, 314
  pharmacology, 281-283
  preparations, 281
  psychiatric disorder, 283-286, 287, 312, 314
  psychotropic effects, 283-284
  side effects, 284-286, 312, 314
  sulthiame and, 286, 306, 310
  therapeutic range, 282
  treatment emergent effects, 284-286, 312, 314
Disintegrative Psychosis, 158
Disinhibition
  antianxiety drugs and, 333
  hallucinogens and, 349
Dissociation constant (pKa), 4
Dissociative Disorders, 146
Dissociation of learning, 105-106
Distribution, 6, 7

children in, 15, 17
efficacy and, 7
interactions and, 25
toxicity and, 7
Diuretics and antipsychotics, 259
DMT, 347
Dopamine and antipsychotic drugs, 239-241
Dosage
  body surface area and, 19
  learning and, 107
  modifications for children, 19
Dose-response relationship, 20
Dosage and Treatment Emergent Systems Scale (DOTES), 72
Double blind, 118, 120, 121
Doxepin, 220
DPH (see Diphenylhydantoin)
Drug Action, 19, 21
Drug interactions (see also interactions of various drugs), 25
Drug overdose, 25
Drug-receptor interaction, 20
Drug studies
  checklist for, 123-124
  design of, 121-126, 128
  ethics of, 113-115
  guidelines for, 119-121
  regulation of, 12-113, 115-119, 129-131
  statistics in, 126-128
Drug usage patterns, 109-110
Drugs
  classification of, xiii-xiv
  name chemical, xii-xiv
  name generic, xii-xiv
  name trade, xii, xiv
  psychotherapy and, 101-104
  terminology of, xiii
DSM III, 141-154
  field trials, 150
  ICD-9 and, 144-146, 151-154
Dyskinesia (see tardive dyskinesia), 158, 160
Dysphoria, 218, 219
Dystonic reactions and antipsychotics, 249

Eating disorders, 162
ECDEU assessment manual, 40
ECG (see EKG)
EEG
  abnormalities of, 284, 287, 314-315
  antipsychotics and, 243-244
  benzodiazepines and, 339
  classification of seizures, 277

INDEX 407

epilepsy in, 277, 284, 287, 314-315
evoked potentials, 7
lithium and, 320
monoamine oxidase inhibitors and, 228
quadracyclics and, 214
reliability, 315
stimulants and, 180
tricyclic antidepressants and, 214
Elavil (see amitryptilene)
Elective mutism, 161
Electroencephalogram (see EEG)
Electronic measurs, 62
Electropupillography, stimulants and, 181
Elimination of drugs, 8
  rate constant (Ke), 12
  screening, 72
  thioridazine and, 255
  tricyclic antidepressants and, 216, 219, 225
Encopresis, 155
  diagnosis and treatment, 166
Enuresis, 155
  antidepressants in, 214-215, 216-224, 232-233
  antipsychotic drugs and, 254
  diagnosis and treatment, 166
  stimulants in, 195-196
Enuresis diurnal
  antidepressants in, 221
Enzyme induction
  antianxiety drugs, 335
  benzodiazepines and, 339
Epanutin (see Diphenylhydantoin)
Epilepsy (see also Seizures)
  causes, 275
  classification, 275-277
  clinical types, 275-277
  definition, 275
  diagnostic features, 277
  equivalents, 284, 315
  generalisations about, 312
  International Bureau for, 280
  international classification, 275
  misdiagnosis, 277, 314-315
  psychosocial complications, 275, 277, 315
  subgrouping by EEG type, 312
  subgrouping by sex, 312
Epileptic equivalents, 284, 315
Epilim (see Sodium Valproate)
Equanil (see Meprobamate), 355
Ethics
  antidepressants and, 232
  children and, 113-115, 125
  drug studies and, 113-115

stimulants and, 205-207
Ethosuximide, 276, 298, 299-301
  chemical structure, 298, 299
  clinical effects in epilepsy, 299, 300-301
  cognitive function and, 300, 312
  diphenylhydantoin and, 286
  fourteen and six per second positive spike and, 299
  interactions, 300
  pharmacology, 299
  psychiatric disorder and, 299-301
  psychotropic effects, 300
  sodium valproate and, 305
  therapeutic levels, 299
  treatment emergent effects, 300
Ethotoin, 281, 288
Evoked potentials (see EEG)
Extrapyramidal system antipsychotics and, 249-251, 256, 258
Eye toxicity antipsychotics and, 258

Factitious Disorders, 145
Family Environment, measures of, 43
Fast acetylation, 11
FDA (U.S. Food and Drug Administration), 112, 116, 117, 119, 122, 130, 131
  efficacy requirements, 113, 115, 116, 118, 121
  guidelines for children, 40, 119, 122, 134
  measures, 40
  monitoring of drugs, 119, 120, 130, 132, 133
  safety of drugs and, 113, 115, 116, 118, 119, 121
Feingold diet, 354
  Federal committee on, 35
First order kinetics, 11
First pass metabolism, 10
5-hydroxyindoleacetic acid (5-HIAA), antipsychotics and, 240
Flashback, 350
Fluphenazine (see also antipsychotics), 250, 251, 252, 254, 255, 257, 262
  mental retardation in, 266
  psychosis in, 261, 262, 263
Flurazepam, 337, 338, 343
Food additives
  Federal committee on, 135
Food and Drug Administration (see FDA)
Fourteen and six per second positive spike, 299, 315
  ethosuximide and, 299
Frostig Test of Visual Perception, 92

Gamma-amino butyric acid (GABA), 22, 304
　antipsychotics and, 240
　inhibition by sodium valproate, 304
Galvanic skin response, 71
Gemonil (see metharbital)
Gilles de la Tourette syndrome
　antipsychotics in, 271
　diagnosis and pharmacotherapy, 160
　haloperidol in, 271
　thioridazine in, 271
Glaucoma
　antipsychotics and, 259
　tricyclic antidepressants and, 224
Glue sniffing, 335
Glutamic acid, 354
Goitre, lithium and, 321
Growth, stimulants and, 191
Growth Hormone, stimulants and, 191

Haldol (see Haloperidol)
Half-life (T½), 12
Haloperidol (see also antipsychotics), 250, 251, 253, 254, 257
　extrapyramidal reactions and, 248
　Gilles de la Tourette Syndrome in, 271
　hyperactivity in, 268, 269
　mental retardation, 265, 266
　psychosis in, 261, 262, 263
Hallucinogens, 346-353
　clinical effects, 349
　dependence, 351
　indications, 351
　patterns of use, 348
　pharmacology, 348
　side effects, 350
　types of, 347
Hepatic toxicity (see liver toxicity)
History
　developmental, 42
　measures of, 42
　medical, 42
　perinatal, 42
Homovanillic acid (HVA), antipsychotics and, 240
Hydantoins, 281-287 (see also individual drugs)
Hydroxyzine, 341
Hydroxyzine, sleep disorders and, 343
HVA (see homovanillic acid)
Hyoscine (see scopolamine)
Hyperactivity (see also activity, attention deficit disorders)
　antianxiety drugs in, 346

antidepressants in, 216, 217, 220, 221, 223
antipsychotics in, 271
chelating substances in, 354
chlorpromazine in, 267
cognitive deficits in, 80-82
cognitive styles in, 81-82
diagnosis of, 139, 146-149, 159
diet and, 354
haloperidol in, 268, 269
inattention in, 80-81
lead and, 354
lithium in, 325
perceptual function in, 81
phenobarbital and, 290
stimulants in, 196-198
thioridazine in, 268, 269, 270
Hyperkinetic Conduct Disorder, 159
Hyperkinetic Reaction of Childhood (see also hyperactivity), 139, 159
Hypersensitivity to drugs, 24
Hypertensive crises, monoamine oxidase inhibitors with, 230
Hysteria, 145

ICD-9, 141-146, 151-154
Idiographic, 32
Idiosyncracy to drugs, 24
Illinois Test of Psycholinguistic Abilities (ITPA), 93
　stimulant drugs and, 93
Imipramine (see also antidepressants, tricyclics), 209, 210, 213, 214-220, 221-223, 224, 225, 233, 294, 343
IND (Investigational Exemption for New Drug), 118, 119
Indolealkylamines, 347
Infantile Autism, 157, 158 (see also psychosis)
Insomnia, 342
　antidepressants and, 214, 218
Intelligence, 90-91
　antidepressants and, 91
　antiepileptic drugs and, 91
　antipsychotics and, 91
　stimulant drugs and, 90-91
Interactions (see drug interactions)
International Bureau for Epilepsy, 280
International Classification of Diseases (see ICD-9)
International Classification of Seizures, 275
International Glossary of Anticonvulsants, 280
Interviews

activity estimates and, 59
  reliability of, 44-45
Intoxication, alcoholic, 335
Intramuscular route, 6
Intravenous route, 5
Introverted Disorder, 164
Ionisation, 4
IQ, 156
IRB (Institutional Review Board), 114, 129
Isle of Wight measures
  child, 44-45
  parent, 44-45
  teacher, 49-50
Isocarboxazide, 229, 226

Jaundice
  antipsychotics and, 253, 254
  monoamine oxidase inhibitors and, 229

Kinetics
  first order, 11
  zero order, 12
Kraepelin, 154

Labelling of drugs, 116, 131
Laboratory tests
  antipsychotics and, 252-254
  routine, 72
Largactil (see chlorpromazine)
Laroxyl (see amitriptyline)
Laudanum, 334
Lawsuit, 111, 112
  Benskin v. Taft City Schools, 134
  Gary W. v. Louisiana, 133
  New York ARC v. Rockefeller, 133, 134
  Welch v. Likins, 112
  Wyatt v. Stickney, 111, 132
Lead, hyperactivity and, 354
Learning
  antianxiety drugs and, 334, 339
  antidepressants and, 87-107, 216-217
  antiepileptics and, 87-107, 290-291
  antipsychotics and, 87-107, 245-247
  dose titration and, 245-247
  drug effects on, 87-107
  measures of, 87-101
  phenobarbital and, 291
  stimulants and, 87-107, 181-185
  tricyclics antidepressants and, 216-217
Learning disorders
  antidepressants in, 217, 223
  stimulants in, 198
Leukopenia antipsychotics and, 252

Levodopa, 352
Librium (see chlordiazepoxide)
Lidone (see molindone)
Limbic system, benzodiazepines and, 338
Lipid Solubility, 4
Lithium, 316-329
  academic achievement and, 322
  activity and, 322
  aggressiveness in, 325
  attention deficit disorder with hyperactivity in, 325
  blurred vision and, 323
  cardiovascular system and, 321
  clinical indications, 324, 326, 329
  cognitive function and, 322
  contraindications, 326
  diabetes insipidus and, 324
  dosages, 326
  EEG and, 320
  EKG and, 321
  endocrine system and, 321
  gastrointestinal tract and, 321, 323
  goitre and, 321
  hyperactivity in, 325
  hypothyroidism and, 321
  interactions, 324
  manic-depressive illness in, 324
  mechanism of action, 318-319
  mood and, 323
  neuromuscular system and, 321, 323
  periodic behavior disorder in, 328
  pharmacology, 317-319
  poisoning, 323
  polydipsia and, 323
  polyuria and, 323
  psychosis in, 326
  serum levels, 317
  side effects, 320, 323-324
  sleep and, 320
  sodium and, 318
  thyroid and, 321
  tremor and, 323
  withdrawal effects and, 328
Liver Toxicity
  antipsychotics and, 253, 254
  monoamine oxidase inhibitors and, 229
Lorazepam, 339
Louisville Behavior Checklist, 52
Loxapine (see dibenzoxapines)
Loxitane (see loxapine)
LSD, 347
Ludiomil (see maprotiline)
Luminal (see phenobarbital)

Mania, 223

Manic-depressive illness, lithium in, 324
MAO, platelet, antidepressants and, 228
MAOI (see Monoamine oxidase inhibitors)
Maprotiline, 208-210, 212, 214, 219, 220, 223, 225
Marijuana, 347
Marplan (see isocarboxazide)
Massachusetts law on drugs and children, 129, 134
Measures, 29-78
  activity, 58-63
  anxiety, 65
  background, 41
  behavior, 46-58
  biochemical, 67
  chaos in, 39
  Children's Personal Data Inventory (CPDI), 42
  Children's Symptom History (CSH), 42
  correct, 38
  current, 39-78
  depression, 65
  descriptive, 32
  diagnosis, 44
  electroencephalographic, 70
  electronic, 62
  family environment, 43
  FDA and, 40
  general aspects, 29-39
  good characteristics of, 29
  history, 42
  idiographic, 32
  interview, 44-45
  Isle of Wight, 45, 49
  laboratory, 67
  mechanical, 35, 62
  minor congenital anomalies, 67
  mood, 63
  motor function, 69
  neurological, 68
  NIMH and, 40
  nomothetic, 32
  observations, 33, 56
  parent, 50
  parenting, 43
  peer, 55
  personality, 46
  physical, 66-73
  physician, 53
  plasma drug concentration, 14
  predictive, 32
  preschool children for, 50
  psychophysiological, 70
  psychosocial, 41-66
  purposes, 31
  ratings, 34, 47-56
  reference sources, 41
  relevance, 31
  scope of, 35
  sensitivity, 30
  self image, 63
  self reports, 35
  side effects, 71
  teacher, 48
  techniques, 33
  tests, 34
Medical model, 136
Medication error, 26
Megavitamin therapy, 353
Mellaril (see thioridazine)
Memory (see short term memory)
Mental Retardation, 152, 156-157
  antipsychotics in, 264-267
  attention in, 84-85
  cognitive deficits in, 84-86
  diagnosis, 156-157
  glutamic acid in, 354
  haloperidol in, 265, 266
  performance of auditory-visual integration in, 85
  psychopharmacological treatment, 157
  stimulants in, 199
  stimulus selection in, 85
  thioridazine in, 265
  thyroid in, 353
  trifluoperazine in, 265, 266
Meprobamate (see antianxiety drugs)
  chemical structure, 336
Mesantoin (see methoin)
Mescaline, 347
Metabolism, 8, 9
  bioavailability and, 10
  children in, 17-18
  first pass, 10
  genetic control, 10
  incompetent systems, 25
  interactions involved, 26
  liver diseases and, 10
Methylphenidate (see also stimulants), 171-207
  antidepressants and, 220
  antidepressants, comparative efficacy and, 217, 222
  antiepileptics and, 286
  diphenylhydantoin and, 286
Methobarbital, 288
Methoin, 281, 287
Methsuximide, 298, 301

Methysergide, 351
Mianserin, 210, 212
Michigan, regulations on drug use, 130
Milontin (see phensuximide)
Miltown (see meprobamate), 335
Minimal brain dysfunction (see also hyperactivity, learning disorders), 159
Minor congenital anomalies, 67
MMPI, 46, 65
Modicate (see fluphenazine)
Mogadon (see nitrazepam)
Molindone, 250, 251, 263
Monoamine oxidase inhibitors (MAOI) (see also antidepressants), 208, 221, 224, 225, 227, 228, 232
  blood pressure and, 229
  cardiovascular system and, 229
  chemical structure, 209, 225, 226
  chlordiazepoxide and, 230
  classes, 225, 226
  clinical indications, 231-232, 232-233
  diabetes and, 229
  dose-response characteristics, 228
  drug interactions, 231
  EEG, 228
  hypertensive crises with, 230
  hypoglycemic action, 229
  hypotension and, 229, 230
  jaundice, 229
  phenobarbital and, 230
  pharmacology, 226-227
  poisoning with, 230
  side effects, 229, 230
  tyramine-containing foods and, 230
Monoamines, lithium and, 318
Mood
  lithium and, 323
  measures, 63
  stimulants and, 189
Motor activity (see activity, hyperactivity)
Motor function, measures, 69
Motor Tic Disorder, 160
Motor-Verbal Tic Disorder (see Gilles de la Tourette)
Multiaxial diagnostic system, 150-153
Muscle relaxation
  benzodiazepines and, 339
Mysoline (see primidone)

Names of drugs, xviii
Narcotics (see opiates)
Nardil (see phenelzine)
National Commission for Protection of Subjects, 113, 114, 115, 134

National Institute of Mental Health (see NIMH)
Navane (see thiothixene)
NCDEU, 40 (see also ECDEU)
NDA (New Drug Application), 117, 119
Nerve impulse, 21
Neuroleptics (see antipsychotics)
Neurological, measures, 68
Neuropsychological Battery, 70
Neurosis, 164, 165
Neurotransmitter, 22
Nightmares, 343
Night terrors, 343
NIMH (National Institute of Mental Health), 40, 113, 129
Nitrazepam, 276, 301, 303, 337, 339
Nomothetic, 32
Non-compliance, 26
Nondrug treatment and drug interactions, 101-104
Norepinephrine, antipsychotics and, 259
Norpramin (see desipramine)
Nydrane (see beclamide)

Observations
  activity, 61
  behavioral, 56-58
  definition, 33
Obsessional disorder, antidepressants in, 229, 233
Octopamine, 349
  antipsychotics and, 239-241
Opiates (see also depressants, general), 334, 335, 350
  antidepressants and, 259
Oppositional disorder, 165
Oral route of administration, 5
Oseretsky test, 70
Ospolot (see sulthiame)
Overanxious Disorder, 163
Oxazepam, 337, 343
Oxidation of drugs, 10

Paired associate learning
  antipsychotics and, 88
  stimulant drugs and, 88
Papez circuit, 22
Parent measures, 50
Parenting, measures of, 43
Pargyline, 226
Parkinsonism, antipsychotics and, 250-251
Parnate (see tranylcypromine)
Pediatric psychopharmacology
  definition of, vii
  history of, xiii

social aspects of, xv
Peer measures, 55
Peganone (see ethotoin)
Pellagra, 353
PEMA (see phenylethylmalonamide)
Pemoline, 171-207
Pentothal (see thiopentone)
Perceptual function, 91
Periactin (see cyproheptadine)
Periodic behaviour disorder, lithium and, 328
Permatil (see fluphenazine)
Perphenazine, 249, 250, 251, 255, 261, 268
Personality
  measures of, 46
  stimulants and, 188
Pertofrane (see desipramine)
Pervasive Developmental Disorders (see also psychosis), 157-158
Pharmacokinetics, 3, 7, 11
  pediatric variations in, 15
Phenacemide, 307
Phenelzine, 226, 229
Phenergan (see promethazine)
Phenethylamines, 347
Pheneturide, 286, 292, 307
  clinical effects in seizure disorders, 307
  diphenylhydantoin and, 286, 308
  phenobarbital and, 292
  treatment emergent effects, 308
Phenobarbital, 276, 288-292, 306
  antidepressants and, 230
  antiepileptic drugs and, 287, 292
  chemical structure, 288
  clinical effect in seizure disorders, 289
  cognitive function and, 290-292
  contraindications, 292
  developmental delay and, 291
  hyperkinetic behavior and, 290
  indications, 292
  intellectual deterioration and, 290-292
  interactions, 287, 292
  pharmacology, 288-289
  psychiatric disorders and, 290-292
  psychotropic effects, 289, 292
  side effects, 290-292
  therapeutic range, 289
  treatment emergent effects, 290-292
Phenomenology, 138, 154
Phenothiazines (see also antipsychotics), 234, 235, 236
  antidepressants, interaction with, 220
  antidepressants similarity to, 208, 209
  petition on, 131
Phensuximide, 298, 301

Phenylethylmalonamide, 293
Phenytoin (see diphenylhydantoin)
Phobic Disorders, 154, 164
  antidepressants in, 229, 231, 233
Physical and Neurological Examination for Soft Signs (PANESS), 69
Physical Examination, 66
Piers Harris Self-Image Scale, 64
pKa, 4
Placebo, drug trials in, 120, 121, 125
Placental transfer, 7, 16
Plasma drug concentration, 14
Plasma protein binding, 7, 8
Plateau levels, 12
Poisoning
  lithium, 323
  tricyclic antidepressants, 215, 220, 230
Polypharmacy, 130
Porteus Maze Test, 93
  antidepressants and, 95, 217
  antipsychotics and, 95
  stimulant drugs and, 93
  tricyclic antidepressants and, 217
PQ (see Conners' Parent Questionnaire)
Primidone, 276, 288, 292-294, 306, 310
  chemical structure, 288, 292
  clinical effects, 293
  contraindications, 294
  idiosyncratic response, 293-294, 310
  indications, 294
  interactions, 294, 306
  pharmacology, 292-293
  treatment emergent effects, 293-294
Prochlorperazine, 245, 261
Prochlorpromazine (see prochlorperazine)
Prognosis, 138
Prolixin (see fluphenazine)
Promethazine, 341
Prominal (see methobarbital)
Propanediols (see also depressants, selective), 336-341
Prostaglandins, antipsychotic drugs and, 240
Protein binding, 7, 8
  changes, 8
  children in, 15
  interactions, 25
Psilocybin, 347
Psychedelics (see hallucinogens)
Psychiatric, definition of, xix
Psychiatric disorders
  classification, 136-167
  epilepsy and, 275, 277, 284, 315
  etiology, 138, 145

pharmacotherapy of, 136-167
Psychogenic attacks, 277
Psychomotor function (see cognitive function)
Psychophysiological measures, 70
Psychoses
 antianxiety drugs in, 346
 antidepressants in, 229
 antipsychotics in, 260-264
 chlorpromazine in, 260-262
 diagnosis and pharmacotherapy of, 144, 158
 haloperidol in, 261, 262, 263
 lithium in, 326
 thioridazine in, 261
 trifluoperazine in, 261, 262, 264
Psychotherapy, 101-104
 drug treatment and, 102
Psychotomimetics (see hallucinogens)
PTQ (see Conners' Parent Teacher Questionnaire), 49
Pupillography, 71

Quadracyclics
 chemical structure, 208, 209
 clinical indications, 222, 225, 233
 EEG and, 214
 effects, 214, 216, 218
 toxicity, 220

Ratings
 activity of, 59
 behavior of, 47-56
 definition, 34
Rawolfia alkaloids (see reserpine)
Reading skills, 165
Receptors, 19
 affinity, 20
 efficacy, 20
Regulation of drugs, 112, 115, 117, 130, 133
Relationship problems, 165
Reliability, 29
REM Sleep
 antidepressants and, 214, 228
 benzodiazepines and, 339
 depressants general and, 335
Renal excretion, 8, 9
 children in, 17, 18
 drug effects and, 9
 interactions in, 26
Research (see drug studies)
Reserpine, 264
Retardation, mental law and drug use in, 109, 112, 117, 131

Right
 Constitutional, 112, 131, 132
 least restrictive, 132
 to education, 131
 to treatment, 131
Risk, research in, 114
Ritalin (see methylphenidate)
Rivotril (see clonazepam)
Rocky Mountain Educational Laboratory Scale, 49
Rorschach, 46
Running record, 56
Rutter Scales (see Isle of Wight Scales)

Salivary Drug concentration, 14
Schizophrenia (see also psychoses), 144, 145, 158
 antianxiety drugs in, 346
 antidepressants in, 229
 antipsychotic drugs and, 260-264
 hallucinogens and, 352
 megavitamin therapy in, 353
 thyroid and, 353
School Phobia (Separation Anxiety Disorder), 163, 167
 antidepressants in, 209, 214, 217, 222, 225
 diagnosis, 163
 pharmacotherapy, 164, 167
Scopolamine, 341
Sedation
 antidepressants and, 220
 antiepileptics and, 285, 290, 297, 305
 antihistamines and, 342
 antimuscarinics and, 342
 antipsychotics and, 247, 273
 benzodiazepines and, 338
 indications for, 344-345
 nature of, 329
 physiological basis of, 331
 v. tranquilization, 332
Sedatives (see antianxiety drugs)
Seizures (see also epilepsy)
 absence, 276-277
 akinetic, 276
 antidepressants in, 219
 antipsychotic drugs and, 251-252
 atonic, 276
 classification, 275-277
 clonic, 276
 co-existence with psychogenic attacks, 277
 complex partial, 276-277
 complex symptomatology with, 276
 elementary symptomatology with, 276
 focal, 276, 277

generalised, 276
grand mal, 275, 276
major, 275
minor, 275
myoclonic, 276
petit mal, 275, 276
psychological precipitants, 312
psychomotor, 276
secondary generalised, 277
television induced, 314
temporal lobe, 276
tonic, 276
tonic-clonic convulsion, 276, 277
Selectivity of drug effects, 23
Self image measures, 63
Self ratings, 63
Self reports, definition, 35
Separation Anxiety Disorders (see also school phobia), 163, 167, 218, 222, 231
Serenace (see haloperidol)
Serepax, Serax (see oxazepam)
Serotonin, 22
　antidepressants and, 212, 233
　antipsychotic drugs and, 239
　hallucinogens and, 347, 348
　lithium and, 319
Serpasil (see reserpine)
Serum drug concentration, 14
Short term memory, 89-90
　antidepressants and, 90
　antipsychotics and, 90
　stimulant drugs and, 89
Shyness Disorder, 163
Side effects
　classification of, 23
　measures, 71
　regulations on, 118-121
Sinequon (see doxepin)
Single compartments model, 11
Skin conductance, stimulants and, 180-181
Skin reactions (see dermatological toxicity)
Sleep, 329
Sleep disorders
　antianxiety drugs in, 342-344
　treatment of, 342-345
　types, 342-345
Slow acetylators, 11
Sodium valproate, 276, 281, 303-306
　antianxiety drugs and, 305, 310
　antidepressant drugs and, 305
　chemical structure, 303-304
　clinical effects in seizure disorders, 304
　clonazepam and, 305
　cognitive function and, 304

ethosuximide and, 305
hypnotic effect of, 305
interactions, 305
pharmacology, 303
phenobarbital and, 305
psychiatric disorders and, 304-305
psychotropic effects, 304-305
sedative drugs and, 305, 310
tardive dyskinesia and, 305
therapeutic range, 304
treatment emergent effects, 305
Solacen, (see tybamate)
Somatoform Disorders, 146
Somnambulism, 343
Special education
　drug usage in, 110, 134
Special Symptoms, 160
Specific Developmental Disorders (see also learning disorders and enuresis), 198
　diagnosis and pharmacotherapy, 152, 165-166
　stimulants in, 198
Specific Learning Disorders, 82-84
　auditory-visual integration in, 83
　cognitive deficits in, 83-84
　cognitive style in, 83
　definition, 82
　inattention in, 83
Speech Disorders, 160, 165, 166
State dependent learning, 105-106
State-Trait Anxiety Scale, 65
Statistics
　analysis of covariance, 128
　analysis of variance, 128
　correlation, 127, 128
　drugs studies and, 126-128
　non-parametric, 127
　time-series analysis, 128
Steady state, drug concentration at, 12
Stelazine (see trifluoperazine)
Stemetil (see prochlorperazine)
Stereotyped Movement Disorders, 160
Stimulants
　absorption, 173
　academic achievement and, 99-101, 185-186
　activity and, 179-180
　appetite suppression and, 177
　attention and, 87
　Attention Deficit Disorders in, 159, 198
　behavior and, 186-188
　behavior modification and, 103-104, 193-194
　cardiovascular system and, 177

catecholamines and, 174
chemical structures of, 172
classes of, 171-172
clinical administration of, 200-205
clinical indications, 195-198
cognitive function and, 87-101, 181-188
cognitive style and, 89
conduct disorders and, 162, 198
contraindications, 199
criticism of use, 110-111
cyclic AMP and, 174
diagnosis and, 138
dosage, 202-204
dose response, 174-175
EEG and, 180
electropupillography and, 181
enuresis in, 195-196
ethics and, 205-207
extent of use, 109-110
growth and, 191
growth hormone and, 191
half life, excretion, 173-174
history of, xiii
hyperactivity in, 196-198
intelligence and, 90-91
interactions with, 192-193
learning disorders and, 87-101, 198
litigation, 134
mental retardation in, 157
metabolic system and, 179
mood and, 189
musculoskeletal system and, 178
Paired Associate Learning and, 88
personality and, 188
physiological effects, 176-178
Porteus Mazes and, 93
prediction of effect, 190
psychophysiological effects, 181
public concern and, 110-111
renal system and, 178
respiratory system and, 176
short term memory and, 89
side effects, 190-192
site and mode of action, 174
skin conductance and, 180-181
specific developmental disorders and, 198
state dependent learning, 105-106
stomach and, 178
time action relationship, 174-175
treatment emergent effects, 190-192
treatment—non drug and, 193-195
tutoring and, 194-195
weight and, 190-191
Studies (see drug studies)

Stuttering, 161
Subcutaneous route, 6
Succinimides, 281, 298
Sulthiame, 306-307
cognitive function and, 306-307
diphenylhydantoin and, 286, 307, 310
pharmacology, 306
phenobarbital serum levels and, 292
primidone and, 306
psychiatric disorders in, 307
seizure disorders in, 306
treatment emergent effects, 306-307
Synapse, 22

Taractan (see chlorprothixene)
Tardive dyskinesia, 256
Taxonomy, 136, 139
Teacher measures, 48
Team prescription, 112, 132
Tegretol (see carbamazepine)
Tests
definition, 34
projective, 46
psychological, 55
T½, 12
Thalidomide, 116, 118
Thiopentone, 331, 334
Thioridazine (see also antipsychotics), 247, 249, 251, 253, 255, 257, 258, 262
anticholinergic effects, 248-249
antimuscarinic sedative as, 342
enuresis and, 254
extrapyramidal reactions and, 248-249
Gilles de la Tourette's syndrome in, 271
hyperactivity in, 268, 269, 270
mental retardation in, 265
psychosis in, 261
seizures and, 252
sleep disorders and, 343
Thiothixene, 250, 251, 253, 255, 257, 261, 263
Thioxanthenes (see also thiothixine), 234, 236
Thorazine (see chlorpromazine)
Thyroid substances, 353
Time sampling, 57
Time series analysis, 128
Tindal (see acetophenazine)
Titration
relationship to learning, 107
Tofranil (see imipramine)
Tourette's Disease (see Gilles de la Tourette)
Toxic effects, 71

TQ (see Conners' Teacher Questionnaire), 48
Trade Names of drugs, xii, xiv
Tranquilization
  compared to sedation, 332
  definition, 332
Tranquilizers
  major, 333
  minor, 333
Transmitter substance, 22
Tranylcypromine, 229
Treatment-emergent effects (see Side Effects)
Treatment—non drug with drug, 101-105, 193-195
Trials (see drug studies)
Tricyclic antidepressants, 208-225
  absorption, 210
  academic achievement and, 217
  activity and, 216
  alpha adrenergic activity, 213
  anticholinergic effects, 210, 212, 214, 215
  chemical structure, 209
  conduct disorders in, 221-222
  cognitive function and, 87-97, 216, 217
  dose-response relationships, 213, 214
  EEG, 214
  effects, 215-219
  EKG and, 216, 219, 225
  excretion, 211, 212
  glaucoma and, 224
  indications, 221-224
  interactions, 221
  long term treatment with, 222, 233
  pharmacology, 210-214, 219
  poisoning and, 215, 220, 230
  Porteus Maze test and, 217
  serum levels, 210, 213
  side effects, 208, 211, 212, 214, 217, 219, 220, 222, 224
Tridione (see troxidone)
Trifluoperazine, 249, 250, 251, 252, 257, 261, 262
Trifluopromazine, 271
Trilafon (see perphenazine)
Triodothyronine (T^3), 353
Troxidone, 308-309
Tryptanol (see amitryptiline)
Tutoring, stimulants and, 194-195
Tybamate, 337
Tybatran (see tybamate)

Tyramine, monoamine oxidase inhibitors (MAOI) and, 230

Underachievers, 165
Urinary toxicity, antipsychotics and, 254-255

Validity, 30
Valium (see diazepam)
Variable
  dependent, 33
  independent, 32
  interval, 38
  nominal, 37
  ordinal, 37
  ratio, 38
Vd, 11
Vesprin (see trifluopromazine)
Vastaril (see hydroxyzine)
Vitamins, 353
Volume of distribution, 11

Water
  extra-cellular, 16
  soluble compounds, excretion of, 9
  total body, 16
Wechsler Intelligence Scale for Children (see WISC)
Weight
  antidepressants and, 220
  antipsychotic drugs and, 255
  stimulants and, 190, 191
Wepman test of auditory discrimination, 93
Werry-Weiss-Peters Activity Scale, 60
Wetting (see enuresis)
Wide Range Achievement Test (WRAT), 95
WISC (Wechsler Intelligence Scale for Children), 29, 34, 90-91
  drug effects on, 94-97, 182, 300
Withdrawal symptoms
  antianxiety drugs, 335
  antidepressants, 215
  antipsychotic drugs, 257, 273
  benzodiazepines, 340
  lithium and, 328
Work output and effectiveness, 99

Zorontin (see ethosuximide)
Zero order kinetics, 12

Date Due

	MAY 05 1992		